Nutrition and Diet Research Progress

nova
Medicine & Health
New York

Nutrition and Diet Research Progress

Chlorella and Its Health Benefits
Mubarak Marutholi, PhD (Editor)
2022. ISBN: 978-1-68507-887-4 (Softcover)
2022. ISBN: 978-1-68507-911-6 (eBook)

A Biochemical View of Vitamins
Dorota Bartusik-Aebisher, PhD, DSc (Editor)
David Aebisher, PhD, DSc (Editor)
2022. ISBN: 978-1-68507-494-4 (Hardcover)
2022. ISBN: 978-1-68507-573-6 (eBook)

Grape Pomace in Health and Disease Prevention
Veronica Sanda Chedea, PhD (Editor)
2022. ISBN: 978-1-68507-425-8 (eBook)
2021. ISBN: 978-1-68507-409-8 (Hardcover)

Spirulina and Its Health Benefits
Jaylee Cochran (Editor)
2021. ISBN: 978-1-68507-018-2 (Softcover)
2021. ISBN: 978-1-68507-084-7 (eBook)

What to Know about Carotenoids
Robert M. Albert (Editor)
2021. ISBN: 978-1-68507-105-9 (Softcover)
2021. ISBN: 978-1-68507-164-6 (eBook)

More information about this series can be found at
https://novapublishers.com/product-category/series/nutrition-and-diet-research-progress/

Kathryn Woltjer
Editor

Curcumin and Its Role in Health and Disease

nova
Medicine & Health
New York

Library of Congress Cataloging-in-Publication Data

ISBN: 979-8-88697-491-1

Published by Nova Science Publishers, Inc. † New York

Contents

Preface

This book contains eight chapters discussing curcumin and its role in health and disease. Chapter One evaluates curcumin's role in cancer prevention. Chapter two reviews curcumin's function as a natural systemic disease modulator. Chapter three looks at the effects of curcumin supplantation and exercise training on Alzheimer's disease and age-associated cognitive decline. Chapter Four Focuses on the antiviral effects of curcumin, with a special emphasis on the COVID-19 virus. Chapter Five examines green extraction techniques for curcumin, synthetic approaches, as well as its anti-inflammatory, antioxidant, and anti-neoplastic effects. Chapter Six reviews the possible effects of immune responses to the preventive combined effects of exercise training and curcumin supplementation in chronic disease. Chapter Seven is a mini review of the essential therapeutic effects of curcumin. The Eighth and final chapter examines the promises and challenges of Curcumin in medical research.

Chapter 1 - Cancer is a leading cause of death worldwide. Modern scientific and medical research faces significant challenges in developing new anticancer therapeutics with increased efficacy and fewer side effects. Most of the anticancer drugs that are available on the market are associated with limited efficacy, severe side effects, and are also very expensive. Therefore, finding anticarcinogenic agents that come with the minimum number of drawbacks is of utmost importance. In this context, the use of phytochemicals as chemotherapeutic agents in cancer treatment is receiving attention as they possess minimal side effects. Among them, curcumin, derived from *Curcuma longa* L. (Zingiberaceae), has been reported to have significant chemo-preventive activity. Recent scientific research has identified the mode of action, pathways involved and molecules targeted by curcumin in order to stand against cancer. Curcumin has antioxidant, anti-inflammatory, and regenerative properties, so it has been shown to protect against neuronal disorders, heart disease, liver injury, various skin diseases, gastric disorders, and kidney malfunctions in addition to cancer. With the expanding implications of curcumin in treating multiple pathophysiological conditions and a better understanding of its functional biology, it is not surprising that there is an increasing focus on its therapeutic exploitation for sake of cancer treatment. Many clinical trials have already been completed for its use in cancer treatment. This chapter focuses on the diverse molecular targets modulated by curcumin that contribute to its efficacy against various human cancers. Cancer cells cope with microenvironmental stress to adapt to the constantly changing cellular nutrient supply, energy, oxidative and immune conditions posed by the invariably increasing number of cancer cells and also by the host cells. Curcumin is capable of targeting most of these vulnerable points, making it an attractive therapeutic agent. It fulfils the characteristics of an ideal chemopreventive agent with its low toxicity, affordability, and easy accessibility. Here the authors focus on the potential of curcumin in cancer prevention, its molecular targets, and its action mechanisms. Further information from different pharmacodynamics as well as more clinical trials is necessary to conclude the chemopreventive evaluation of curcumin has been discussed as well.

Chapter 2 - In the prevention and treatment of various diseases, a variety of preparations based on medicinal plants are now generally acknowledged and well-documented. The main advantages of traditional medicine in underdeveloped nations are safety and affordability. As diferuloylmethane, curcumin is a naturally occurring polyphenol that is mostly produced in the rhizomes of plant roots. Curcumin has a long history of usage in conventional medicine, although its therapeutic effects and health advantages are still little understood. The therapeutic benefits of curcumin include the treatment of malignancies, neurodegenerative, ocular, and COVID diseases as well as inflammatory and digestive disorders, rheumatic and skin issues, and tumors. Apoptosis-related genes, cytokines, enzymes, and other targets have all been found in certain studies to be modulated by curcumin. Furthermore, little is known about the biological mechanisms that underlie these activities. The authors will examine some of the known molecular targets and biological processes of curcumin in this chapter. The processes through which curcumin functions in neuroprotection and/or mental health disorders will be covered in this chapter. The authors will also talk about curcumin's protective role in how bone may impact neurological function.

Chapter 3 - Aging is associated with cognitive impairment and is a major risk factor for neurological disorders, including dementia and Alzheimer's disease (AD). AD is a progressive neurodegenerative disease characterised by gradual loss of memory and motor activity. Although the exact pathogenesis of AD is not fully understood, there is ample evidence that oxidative stress and inflammation may play a critical role in the underlying mechanisms of cognitive impairment and AD. Curcumin is a chemical component of turmeric (*Curcuma longa*), a natural compound with antioxidant and anti-inflammatory properties proposed to combat neurological dysfunction, reduce neuro-degenerative diseases such as AD, protect the hippocampus, and treat cognitive dysfunction. Epidemiological evidence links regular physical exercise to improved age-related cognitive function, lower risk for dementia, reduced pathological changes in the central nervous system, and reduced atrophy of brain executive function. Regular physical exercise reduces inflammatory cytokines and increases the production of brain-derived neurotrophic factors, especially in the hippocampus, which is the main center of learning and memory formation. Exercise can also enhance the antioxidant protection of the hippocampus and induce positive effects of brain-derived neurotrophic factor (BDNF) on neurons. Therefore, the synergic effects of regular exercise training and curcumin supplementation may be considered an effective strategy for dealing with neurological and cognitive disorders. In this chapter, the authors assess the combined effects of physical exercise and curcumin supplementation on the reduction in cognitive function due to aging and AD.

Chapter 4 - Plant derived biomolecules are said to possess various pharmacological actions. Curcumin obtained from rhizomes of *Curcuma longa*, is the primary bioactive molecule which exhibits antiviral, antinociceptive, anti-inflammatory, antipyretic and anti-fatigue effects. Recent studies reveal that curcumin also shows antiviral activity against many viruses such as dengue, hepatitis, zika, chikungunya, etc. Few research studies revealed that curcumin has binding potential to target a variety of SARS-Cov-2 proteins. This chapter covers antiviral activity of curcumin with special focus on its role in inhibiting COVID-19 virus. These findings will be utilized to develop therapeutic lead using curcumin against COVID-19.

Chapter 5 - Curcumin is a useful natural product applied in Medicine including treatment and diagnosis. In this regard, it has been used for treatment of neurodegenerative diseases and as anti-inflammatory and anticancer agents. This natural product can be obtained by extraction from a natural source (turmeric powder) or via synthetic approaches (batch and/or flow chemistry). Herein, the authors describe general green extraction methods using alternative media and synthetic procedures for curcumin through continuous flow chemistry as well as its production in up-scale, high purity, and low cost for medical use. Moreover, some recent advances on pharmacological effects of curcumin as anti-inflammatory, antioxidant and anti-neoplastic agents are reported and discussed. In this chapter, the authors did not produce a systematic review; instead, they highlighted selected green extraction methods (using alternative solvents) and synthetic procedure (combining batch and flow chemistry) for curcumin and its possibilities and limitations as a medicine.

Chapter 6 - Numerous studies have confirmed curcumin's anti-inflammatory and antioxidant effects due to its biological activities. Also, the positive effects of curcumin on various immune system indices have been established in multiple studies. Acute and chronic responses to physical exercise can be effective in physiological responses and, at the same time, innate and adaptive immune responses. It has been suggested that regular physical exercise can effectively prevent several diseases, including cancer, cardiovascular disease, neuromuscular disorders, and diabetes. Adipose tissue is considered the leading risk factor for chronic diseases. The possible effects of curcumin on adipose tissue and the proven positive effects of exercise training on weight control can be effective in modulating immune system responses in adipose tissue and preventing weight gain. In addition, according to new studies, higher intensities of physical exercise are effective in preventing some chronic diseases. However, this exercise is associated with further muscle damage and inflammation. It has been suggested that curcumin can modulate the inflammatory responses created following intensive physical exercise. The synergistic effects of exercise training and curcumin supplementation modulate immune responses effectively. The physiological and metabolic effects of exercise training combined with curcumin supplementation can probably be effective in preventing chronic disease by improving immune responses.

Chapter 7 - Curcumin is the essential bioactive constituent of *Curcuma longa* that has diverse disease healing effects that majorly includes antibacterial, anticancer, antidiabetic and anti-inflammatory. Curcumin has the potential to exhibit broad-spectrum antibacterial efficacy by a mechanism that includes ROS generation, membrane damage and cell death. The anticancer effectiveness of curcumin has been rigorously investigated, and it is chiefly mediated by inhibition of cyclin D1, preventing NF-ƙB activation and increasing reduced glutathione levels (GSH) in cancerous cells. Curcumin can show good antidiabetic activity using principles that involve enhancing uptake of glucose by increasing GLUT2, GLUT3 and GLUT4 gene expressions, decreasing glucose levels in hepatic cells, increasing release of insulin from pancreatic cells, decreasing resistance to insulin. The anti-inflammatory role of curcumin is largely due to the downregulation of key pathways that include lipooxygenase and cyclooxygenase pathways, thereby inhibiting the generation of important inflammation regulators, such as pro-inflammatory leukotrienes and prostaglandins. However, the aforesaid healing potency of curcumin is limited up to a definite scale due to its large size of particle, retarded aqueous dissolution, limited stability that results in decreased bioavailability and cellular uptake. All these shortcomings linked to curcumin can be addressed by synthesizing nanocurcumin as well as conjugating/loading nanocurcumin to another therapeutically bioactive nanoparticle to develop nanoconjugates/nanocomposites of curcumin having reduced size of particle, improved dissolution in water, enhanced stability and bioavailability thereby resulting in increased level of therapeutic efficacy. Moreover, such curcumin based nanoconjugates/nanocomposites, due to improved properties, can also exhibit multi-targeting therapeutic efficacy.

Chapter 8 - Turmeric (*Curcuma longa* L. (Zingiberaceae)) is a popular spice with medicinal properties that has been extensively used in Ayurveda and Chinese traditional medicine for centuries. Curcumin or [(E,E)-1,7-bis (4-hydroxy-3-methoxy-phenyl)-1,6-heptadiene-3,5-ione] is the active component of turmeric and is widely used in the pharmaceutical industry. It is a highly versatile pigment with medicinal properties viz., anticancer, anti-inflammatory, anti-microbial and so on. Curcumin absorbs strongly near 425 nm and, due to its ligand binding properties, it has found extensive use in textile industry as well. It also exhibits strong emission near 570 nm which makes it an excellent choice for cellular imaging and spectroscopic study. However, despite such multifold applications, one of the greatest challenges posed in the application of curcumin is its poor bioavailability. Being a phenolic moiety, curcumin is predominantly hydrophobic which limits its availability in aqueous or biological media. Research is now being focused upon developing media such as microemulsions, mixed micelle systems etc., to increase the solubility of curcumin. This review gives an overview of the application of curcumin in health, the existing challenges in relation to bioavailability of curcumin and current research being done to overcome the same.

Chapter 1

Curcumin and Its Role in Cancer Prevention

Sayanta Sarkar[1]
and Parames C. Sil[2,*]
[1]Department of Life Science and Bio-Technology, Jadavpur University, Jadavpur, Kolkata, India
[2]Division of Molecular Medicine, Bose Institute, Kolkata, India

Abstract

Cancer is a leading cause of death worldwide. Modern scientific and medical research faces significant challenges in developing new anticancer therapeutics with increased efficacy and fewer side effects. Most of the anticancer drugs that are available on the market are associated with limited efficacy, severe side effects, and are also very expensive. Therefore, finding anticarcinogenic agents that come with the minimum number of drawbacks is of utmost importance. In this context, the use of phytochemicals as chemotherapeutic agents in cancer treatment is receiving *attention* as they possess minimal side effects. Among them, curcumin, derived from *Curcuma longa* L. (Zingiberaceae), has been reported to have significant chemopreventive activity. Recent scientific research has identified the mode of action, pathways involved and molecules targeted by curcumin in order to stand against cancer. Curcumin has antioxidant, anti-inflammatory, and regenerative properties, so it has been shown to protect against neuronal disorders, heart disease, liver injury, various skin diseases, gastric disorders, and kidney malfunctions in addition to cancer. With the expanding implications of curcumin in treating multiple patho-physiological conditions and a better understanding of its functional biology, it is not surprising that there is an increasing focus on its

* Corresponding Author's Email: parames@jcbose.ac.in.

In: Curcumin and Its Role in Health and Disease
Editor: Kathryn Woltjer
ISBN: 979-8-88697-491-1

therapeutic exploitation for sake of cancer treatment. Many clinical trials have already been completed for its use in cancer treatment. This chapter focuses on the diverse molecular targets modulated by curcumin that contribute to its efficacy against various human cancers. Cancer cells cope with microenvironmental stress to adapt to the constantly changing cellular nutrient supply, energy, oxidative and immune conditions posed by the invariably increasing number of cancer cells and also by the host cells. Curcumin is capable of targeting most of these vulnerable points, making it an attractive therapeutic agent. It fulfils the characteristics of an ideal chemopreventive agent with its low toxicity, affordability, and easy accessibility. Here we focus on the potential of curcumin in cancer prevention, its molecular targets, and its action mechanisms. Further information from different pharmacodynamics as well as more clinical trials is necessary to conclude the chemopreventive evaluation of curcumin has been discussed as well.

Keywords: curcumin, cancer, chemopreventive potential, molecular signalling

Abbreviations

5-FU	Fluoropyrimidine
β-FGF	Basic fibroblast growth factor
Akt	Ak strain transforming
ALK	Anaplastic lymphoma kinase
ALT	Alanine aminotransferase
AP-1	Activator protein 1
AR	Androgen receptor gene
AST	Aspartate aminotransferase
BAX	Bcl-2-associated X protein
Bcl-2	B-cell lymphoma 2
CAP	Capecitabine
CAT	Catalase
CBP	CREB-binding protein
CDK	Cyclin-Dependent Kinases
Chk	Checkpoint Kinase
c-myc	Cellular myelocytomatosis viral oncogene homolog
DEN	Diethylnitrosamine
EGFR	Epidermal growth factor receptor
EMT	Epithelial to mesenchymal transition

ERK	Extracellular signal-regulated kinase
EZH2	Enhancer of zeste homolog 2
EZRI	Ezrin
Fen1	Flap endonuclease
FOXO	Forkhead box transcription factors
GST	Glutathione S transferase
HBV	Hepatitis B
HCV	Hepatitis C
HER	Human epidermal growth factor receptor
HES1	Hairy and enhancer of split-1
HIF-1α	Hypoxia-inducible factor-1
IRI	irinotecan
IκB-alpha	Nuclear factor of kappa light polypeptide gene enhancer in B-cells inhibitor, alpha
JNK	c-Jun N-terminal kinase
LC3	Microtubule-associated protein 1A/1B-light chain 3
LOX	Lysyl oxidase
MAP kinase	Mitogen-activated protein kinase
MMP	Matrix metalloproteinase
mTOR	Mammalian target of rapamycin
NF-κB	Nuclear factor kappa B
Nrf2	Nuclear factor erythroid 2–related factor 2
NSCLC	Non-small-cell lung cancer
OX	Cxaliplatin
p70S6K	Ribosomal protein S6 kinasebeta-1
PARP	Poly (ADP-ribose) polymerases
PGC-1α	Peroxisome proliferator-activated receptor-gamma coactivator
PHOX2B	Paired-like homeobox 2b
PI3K	Phosphoinositide 3-kinase
PSA	Prostate-specific antigens
ROS	Reactive oxygen species
SCLC	Small cell lung cancer
SOD	Superoxide dismutase
SREBP1	Sterol regulatory element-binding transcription factor 1
STAT	Signal transducer and activator of transcription
TFF1/pS2	Trefoil factor 1
TGF-β	Transforming growth factor beta
TIMP-1	TIMP metallopeptidase inhibitor 1

TNBC	Triple-negative breast cancer
TNF-α	Tumour Necrosis Factor alpha
TRIM	Tripartite motif
VCAM	Vascular cell adhesion protein
VEGF	Vascular endothelial growth factor
Wnt	Wingless-related integration site

Introduction

Over the past few decades, phytochemicals have become the focus of attention for their medicinal values by several scientists. Several serious side effects and many other disadvantages of modern synthetic medicines developed by pharmaceutical companies make natural compounds with less or no toxic effects suitable choices for the disease of anticipation and prevention. In Asia, especially in India and China, medical practitioners apply turmeric to treat various illnesses. Since ancient times, traditional medicines in Ayurveda, Unani, Siddha, and Chinese medicine describe the importance of curcumin in the prevention of various diseases (Hatcher et al. 2008). Curcumin has been isolated from the rhizome of the turmeric plant, which has been a part of the Indian household for its colour, taste, and antimicrobial properties for generations (Kanai 2014). Curcumin, a natural polyphenol that belongs to the Zingiberaceae (ginger) family, specifically, *Curcuma longa*, originated in southeast Asia (Sharma et al. 2010, Prasad et al. 2014). Other than curcumin, turmeric also contains two curcuminoids, but in a lesser amount, which are demethoxycurcumin and bisdemethoxycurcumin. In traditional Ayurvedic treatment, turmeric paste was recommended to be applied topically over wounds, burns, and other skin infections due to its beneficial antimicrobial properties. Because of its anti-inflammatory effects, people with coughs and other respiratory disorders often take turmeric as an ayurvedic medicine. Turmeric also gives relief to patients suffering from indigestion or other mild gastrointestinal diseases. In this regard, western civilization was introduced to turmeric as a spice after the 14th century, when European travellers first discovered Asia and came to know about Asian culture. In 1280 A.D., Venetian merchant and explorer Marco Polo mentioned turmeric in his writings when he visited the Asian continent (Tiwari et al. 2012). It was mentioned in his book that native Indian and Chinese people often used a spice having all the beneficial roles of saffron. Searching for spices, the Portuguese sailor Vasco de Gama came to India long before Marco Polo, about 500 years before 1280 AD, when he introduced turmeric into the European culture for the first time (Aggarwal et al. 2007, Aggarwal and Shishodia 2004). After advances in science and technology, Vogel was able to isolate curcumin in 1842. In 1910, its overall chemical structure was characterised by Lampe and Milobedeska.

Although it is unknown how cancer originated, it is known that at least 300 to 500 genes are altered in the case of cancer. Therefore, cancer is a result of a disorder in cellular function at multiple steps. Most of the anticancer drugs, available on the market are found to modulate a single target and many times fail to show satisfactory results. Many pharmaceutical companies have increased their interest and investment in developing multi-targeted therapies using natural phytochemicals due to the lack of efficacy, harmful side effects, and high cost of mono-targeted therapies. Many plant-based natural compounds show multi-targeted actions, and besides, they are very safe to use and inexpensive to manufacture; thus, they become a suitable choice for pharmaceutical companies. Regardless of what the cause of cancer is, whether it is a genetic factor or lifestyle, the uncontrolled growth of cells in cancer can put human life at risk, if not treated properly. Over 1.9 million new cancer cases are estimated to be diagnosed in the United States in 2022. In the United States, approximately 609360 deaths from cancer are anticipated in 2022 (Siegel et al. 2022). These mortality rates raise serious concern about the development of effective anticancer drugs and the search for new compounds to overcome the hurdles in cancer therapy. The development of cancer is a gradual process, that takes an incubation time of 20-30 years. Before the final development of metastatic cancer, at the very beginning, there is hyperplasia due to initial carcinogen exposure, followed by dysplasia with mild, moderate, and severe symptoms, and then advanced to carcinoma (Haddad and Shin 2008). Scientists are working on finding various effective strategies, from chemoprevention to surgical operations, to prevent or slow down the process of the development of cancer (Lippman and Hawk 2009, Pollack et al. 1984, Brennan et al. 1995, Calle et al. 2003, Thaker et al. 2006, Kenfield et al. 2011). For cancer prevention, many approaches like chemotherapy, radiotherapy, and synthetic drugs are available, but they are very costly and sometimes beyond the reach of normal people to obtain. On the other hand, they sometimes alter the actions of normal genes, causing serious health problems. The term "chemoprevention" was first mentioned by M. B. Sporn in the year 1976. By chemoprevention, he meant the manner of prevention of cancer development by synthetic or natural compounds. One particular milestone in breast cancer research was the approval of tamoxifen, a selective oestrogen receptor modulator (SERM), by the Food and Drug Administration (FDA) after positive large-scale clinical trials in 1998 (Cuzick et al. 2002). The field of cervical cancer chemoprevention research gained noticeable momentum when the FDA approved the vaccine for HPV cervical cancer in the year of 2009 after positive randomised controlled clinical trials. On the other hand, sulindac, celecoxib, and aspirin failed to give desirable data against colorectal cancer after several clinical trials (Giardiello et al. 1993, Steinbach et al. 2000, Baron et al. 2003). The selenium and vitamin E cancer prevention trial (SELECT) also gave no hope for lung and prostate cancer prevention (Lippman and Hawk 2009). After so many disappointing negative results of chemotherapeutic agents, researchers have now shifted their focus to finding compatible multi-targeted natural compounds. During chemotherapy, patients receive a certain dose of a chemotherapeutic agent for a long period of time. The toxicity or side effects could hamper the patient's health.

Unlike synthetic compounds, natural compounds are usually consumed by people in their normal lives, making natural compounds a much safer choice for cancer treatment. Among so many natural compounds, curcumin has received special attention for its multitargeted cancer prevention strategy, ease of use, and low cost of production. The amount of data describing the protective effects of curcumin in combating different types of cancer is increasing. This book chapter represents the recent work on curcumin in the prevention and treatment of different types of cancers.

Breast Cancer

Breast cancer is the second most common cancer in women (Siegel et al. 2021). Approximately 2.3 million cases of breast cancer were reported worldwide in the year 2020 (Siegel et al. 2021). Treatments for breast cancer include surgical resection, radiation, and chemotherapy (Loibl et al. 2021). Immunotherapy and hormone therapy have recently developed into more effective therapies (Loibl et al. 2021). Despite the effectiveness of current therapies, challenges to their side effects and resistance development need to be resolved (Loibl et al. 2021). In this regard, the trials of anticancer compounds from medicinal plants provide solutions to these challenges. Curcumin and its analogues exhibit multiple beneficial effects against breast cancer. In this section, we will discuss some in vitro and in vivo anticancer properties of curcumin and its analogues in breast cancer.

The oestrogen receptor (ER) regulates transcription upon ligand binding and its interaction with the ER-responsive element (ERE) is crucial for the regulation of gene expression. ER-mediated changes in gene expression for growth induction are majorly regulated by pS2 and TGF-β in ER-positive cells. Curcumin inhibits the proliferation, reduces the expression of oestrogen receptor responsive genes (pS2, TGF-β), and suppresses ERE-CAT activity of ER-positive cells (MCF-7) in the presence of oestrogen (Mo et al. 2012, Paramita et al. 2018, Shao et al. 2002). Moreover, it downregulates MMP-2, VEGF, β-FGF, and TIMP-1 to inhibit invasive properties in ER-negative MDA-MB-231 cells (Shao et al. 2002). In the same cells, curcumin shows synergistic effects with epigallocatechin (EGCG) in inducing G2/M cell cycle arrest (Chung and Vadgama 2015). The combination of both also reduces tumour volume along with a significant decrease in the levels of VEGFR-1 in athymic nude mice (Somers-Edgar et al. 2008). In these mice, curcumin alone reduces Akt and EGFR levels (Somers-Edgar et al. 2008). This study identified a method to reduce the amount of effective curcumin dose that could be beneficial in chemotherapy treatment for patients that were otherwise taking a high amount of the same. Moreover, the mechanism of curcumin-mediated Akt suppression involves its degradation by the autophagy pathway (Akkoc et al. 2015, Guan et al. 2016).

Curcumin also affects the nuclear factor kappa-light-chain-enhancer of activated B cells (NF-κB) signalling to exert its anti-tumor activity. NF-κB signalling regulates transcription and cytokine signalling to regulate cell survival. In MDA-MB-231 and BT-483, it downregulates the expression of NF-κB regulated genes (Liu et al. 2009). It also reduces the expression of cyclin D1 in MDA-MB-231 cells and the expression of CDK4 in BT-483 cells to block the proliferation of these breast cancer cells (Liu et al. 2009). Moreover, the administration of curcumin downregulates the expression of MMP-1 in both these cells to reduce the invasiveness of breast tumors (Table 1).

The growth of triple-negative breast cancer (TNBC) MDA-MB-231 cells is dependent on EGFR signaling. Curcumin decreases the levels of EGFR and, thereby, the proliferation of the same, providing an efficient treatment option for TNBC patients.

Table 1. The effects of curcumin therapy in breast cancer

In vitro/In vivo	Dosage	Duration	Major outcomes	Reference
MCF-7 cell line	10,20, 30 µg/mL	24, 48, 72 h	Inhibition of cell proliferation	(Calaf, Ponce-Cusi, and Carrion 2018)
			Reduction in cell viability	
MDA-MB-231 cell line	15-19 µM	24, 48, 72 h	Inhibition of cell proliferation	(Abuelba et al. 2015)
			Reduction in cell viability	
MDA-MB-231 cell line	10, 50 µM	48 h	Inhibition of cell proliferation	(Bimonte et al. 2015)
			Decrement in cell migration	
			Induction of apoptosis	
MCF-7, MDA-MB-231 cell line	30 µM	48 h	Induction of apoptosis	(Calaf, Ponce-Cusi, and Carrion 2018)
MDA-MB-231 cell line	10, 20, 30 µM	48 h	Decreased cell proliferation	
			Induction of apoptosis	(Chiu and Su 2009)
MCF-7 cell line	10, 25 µM	24 h	Attenuated cell growth	(Choudhuri et al. 2002)
			Induction of apoptosis	
T47D cell line	30 µM	24, 48 h	Decreased cell viability	(Coker-Gurkan et al. 2019)
			Induction of apoptosis	
MCF-7 cell line	30 µM	24, 48 h	Decreased cell viability	(Coker-Gurkan et al. 2018)
			Induction of apoptosis	
MDA-MB-231 cell line	50 µg/mL	24 h	Decreased cell viability	(Fan et al. 2016)
			Induction of apoptosis	
MDA-MB-231 cell line	50 µg/mL	48 h	Inhibition of cell proliferation	(Ghosh et al. 2021)
			Induction of apoptosis	
			Cell cycle arrest	
MCF-7 cell line	1 mM	24 h	Decreased invasion	(Hashemzehi et al. 2018)
			Decreased cell growth	
4T1 cell line	50 µg/mL	48 h	Decreased cell viability	(He et al. 2019)
T47D, MCF-7 cell line	10, 30 µM	72 h	Decreased cell proliferation	(Hu et al. 2018)
			Induction of apoptosis	

In vitro/In vivo	Dosage	Duration	Major outcomes	Reference
MDA-MB-435 cell line	10, 25, 50, 75 μM	12, 24, 48 h	Decreased cell proliferation	(Hua et al. 2010)
			Cell cycle arrest	
MDA-MB-231 cell line	50 μg/mL	24 h	Induction of apoptosis	(Ji et al. 2020, Jiang et al. 2013)
MCF-7, LCC2, LCC9 cell line	10, 30 μM	24, 48, 72, 96 h	Decreased colony formation	
			Induction of apoptosis	
MCF-7 cell line	10 μg/mL	24 h	Induction of apoptosis	(Jin et al. 2017)
BT-474 cell line	10 μg/mL	72 h	Decreased cell proliferation	(Lai et al. 2012)
Balb/c mice	5mg/kg; IV, IP		Decreased tumor volume	(Fathy Abd-Ellatef et al. 2020)
Female ACI mice	1000 ppm; implant	-	Decreased tumor volume	(Bansal et al. 2014)
Foxn1nu/nu female mice	0.6%; Diet		Decreased tumor volume	(Bimonte et al. 2015)
Swiss albino mice	10 mg/kg; IV	-	Decreased tumor volume	(Ghosh et al. 2021)
Balb-neuT mice	58.2 mg	-	Decreased tumor volume	(Grill et al. 2018)
Kunming mice	10 mg/kg; IV	-	Decreased tumor volume	(Lv et al. 2015)
Transgenic BALB-neuT mice	6-50 μM		No tumor	(Masuelli et al. 2013)
Sprague-Dawley rat	2.5 mg; IV	-	Decreased tumor volume	(Vakilinezhad et al. 2019)

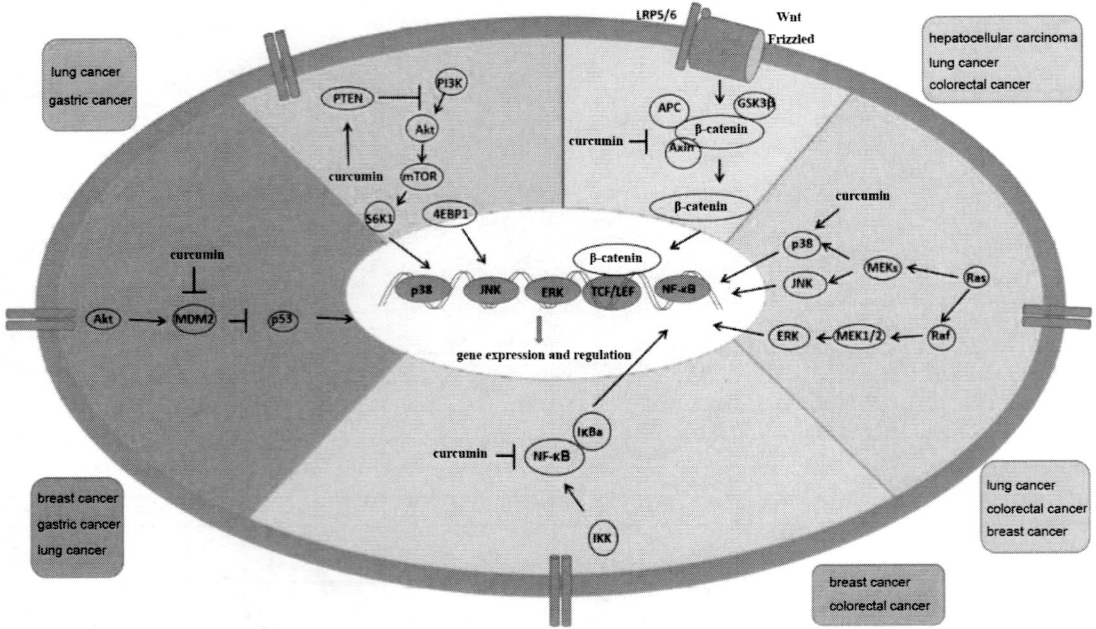

Abbreviation: AKT, v-akt murine thymoma viral oncogene; PI3K, phosphatidylinositol 3-kinase; mTOR, mammalian target of rapamycin; PTEN, phosphatase and tensin homolog; MAPK, mitogen-activated protein kinase; MMP, matrix metalloproteinase; ERKs, extracellular regulated protein kinases; JNK, c-Jun N-terminal kinase; APC, adenomatous polyposis coli; Dvl, Disheveled; GSK3β, glycogen synthase kinase 3β; LRP5/6, low-density lipoprotein receptor-related protein 5/6; TCF/LEF, T-cell factor/lymphoid enhancer-binding factor; JAK/STAT, Janus kinase/signal transducers and activators of transcription; MDM2, murine double minute 2; NF-κB, nuclear factor kappa B; IKK, Inhibitory-κB kinase.

Figure 1. (Continued).

Figure 1. Molecular pathways targeted by curcumin in different cancers: In breast, gastric, and lung cancer, curcumin inhibits the cell proliferation pathways by enhancing the PTEN activity. PTEN inhibits the Akt activation by inhibiting PI3K levels. Akt Activates mTOR, phosphorylation of p70S6K1 (S6K1) and 4E-BP1which activates various cell proliferation pathways. Various growth factors lead to activation of the MEK, which further leads to activation of the ERK1/2, p38, and JNK signaling molecules to initiate the gene expression. Curcumin regulates the activation of p38 and thereby p38-induced gene expression in lung, colorectal, and breast cancer. The phosphorylation and translocation of β-catenin by various inducers into the nucleus leads to its binding with TCF/LEF co-transcription factors that ultimately induces the Wnt-mediated gene transcription. Curcumin inhibits the Wnt/β-catenin pathway in hepatocellular, lung, and colorectal cancer. Curcumin enhances the anti-tumor activity of p53 and thereby inhibits the Akt-induced activation of MDM2 in breast, gastric, and lung cancer. Curcumin enhances the anti-tumor activity by inhibiting the NF-κB signaling pathway in breast, and colorectal cancer.

Matrix metalloprotease-9 (MMP-9) plays a crucial function in cancer cell invasion. Curcumin suppresses MMP-9 expression in a mechanism that involves inhibition of NF-κB and AP-1 signalling (Tong et al. 2016). Curcumin-mediated reduced activation of MAP kinases (p38 and JNK) also has an inhibitory effect on MMP-9 expression (Yao, Lin, et al. 2015). This study signifies the role of curcumin in reducing the invasiveness of breast cancer cells and the molecular mechanism underlying this function.

JIMT1 cells are HER2 positive and show resistance to trastuzumab. Immunoliposome-mediated delivery of curcumin in JIMT1 cells lowers the IC_{50} and increases the HER2 overexpressed cell selectivity in comparison to free or liposome-mediated curcumin delivery (Hosseini et al. 2019). This delivery system provides a better option to treat breast cancers that are otherwise resistant to conventional therapies (Mock, Jordan, and Selvam 2015).

Curcumin also targets the DNA repair process to selectively kill breast cancer cells. Flap endonuclease (Fen1) overexpression is one of the risk factors in the development of breast cancer. Curcumin regulates Nrf2-dependent Fen1 expression (Chen et al. 2014). Curcumin treatment in MCF-7 cells reduces Nrf2 translocation into the nucleus, which then becomes unavailable to bind at the Fen1 promotor, leading to reduced Fen1 expression (Chen et al. 2014). Breast cancer cell proliferation is adversely affected in the absence of Fen1 (Chen et al. 2014).

Cancer cells depend on a higher rate of protein synthesis for their growth, which is fulfilled by high activation of mTOR signalling (Figure 1). Effects of curcumin on the mTOR pathway are also reported to exhibit its anti-tumor activity (Beevers, Zhou, and Huang 2013). Curcumin inhibits mTOR activation, as well as mTOR-dependent activation of its downstream effectors p70S6K and 4E-BP1 (Beevers, Zhou, and Huang 2013).

Liver Cancer

Liver cancer is the sixth most frequently occurring cancer in the world. Liver cancer patients have only a 5-year life expectancy after treatment. Such a low survival rate makes it challenging for researchers to find more efficient cures for liver cancer. Cirrhosis, hepatitis virus infection, and steatosis are the risk factors for hepatocellular carcinoma (HCC), which accounts for more than 90% of cases of liver cancer (Llovet et al. 2021). Its progression includes certain biochemical reactions such as inflammation and increased reactive oxygen species (Llovet et al. 2021).

Hepatitis B virus (HBV), which is one of the risk factors for HCC, is treated by interferons and nucleoside analogues (Llovet et al. 2021). Another better therapy is the use of peroxisome proliferator-activated receptor-alpha (PGC-1α) inhibitors (Llovet et al. 2021; Shlomai, Paran, and Shaul 2006). Curcumin significantly suppresses PGC-1α and inhibits HBV infection (Rechtman et al. 2010). Notably, curcumin administration along with nucleoside analogues synergistically inhibits HBV replication (Rechtman et al. 2010). Curcumin also suppresses hepatitis C virus (HCV) infection by inhibiting its replication via PI3K/Akt/SREBP1 signaling (Kim et al. 2010).

Curcumin has protective effects against liver toxicity. Curcumin induces liver apoptosis in liver cancer cells. Administration of the curcumin analogue, EF24, in mouse liver cancer cells, induces apoptosis with an increase in the levels of BAX, cleaved PARP, and a decrease in Bcl-2 levels (Cianciulli et al. 2016). Curcumin also downregulates BCL-2 expression in SMMC-7721 human liver cancer cells (Yu et al. 2011). Additionally, curcumin upregulates P53 expression in liver cancer cells. However, BCL-2 expression changes are not P53 dependent, indicating a different function of curcumin-induced P53 in liver cancer inhibition. In mouse liver cancer cells, it induces Chk1 activation and arrests the cells in the G2/M phase of the cell cycle, inhibiting the proliferation of liver cancer cells (Figure 1). Curcumin regulates cell proliferation and apoptosis in liver cancer cells by inhibiting the Wnt/β-catenin pathway (Ahn et al. 2010). Besides inducing cancer cell death, curcumin also prevents tumour progression by reducing the invasiveness of hepatocytes. It does so by downregulating the activation of TNF-α which plays a prominent role in tumour cell malignancy (Aggarwal, Gupta, and Sung, 2013).

In liver toxicity, glutathione S transferase (GST) activity is reduced; however, in vivo curcumin supplementation increases GST activity (El-Ashmawy et al. 2006, Garcia-Nino et al. 2013, Soliman, Baiomy, and Yassin 2015).It also balances the activity of alanine aminotransferase (ALT) and aspartate aminotransferase (AST), which are otherwise higher in conditions of hepatotoxicity (Garcia-Nino et al. 2013, Reyes-Gordillo et al. 2008, Zhao et al. 2014). Cancer cells proliferate in conditions of high reactive oxygen species by inducing the levels of hypoxia-inducible factor-1 (HIF-1α). One of the modes of action of curcumin to reduce tumorigenesis is by inhibiting HIF-1α so that cancer cells become unable to cope with high levels of ROS (Zhao et al. 2014). In addition, curcumin decreases the levels of MMP-9, VCAM-1, and integrins, which are necessary for metastasis and invasion (Ohashi et al.

2003, Aggarwal, Kumar, and Bharti 2003). Curcumin protects the liver against DEN-induced HCC in mice by controlling TGF-β and p38 signalling pathways (Reyes-Gordillo et al. 2008, Yao et al. 2012, Zhang, Rui, and Yan 2014). It also reduces angiogenesis factors like VEGF in HepG2 cells to suppress tumorigenesis (Aggarwal, Kumar, and Bharti 2003, Gao et al. 2015). When administered with paclitaxel, curcumin shows synergistic effects in Hep3B cells by downregulating the activity of NF-κB (Fan et al. 2014; Aggarwal, Kumar, and Bharti 2003). Similarly, curcumin with pterostilbene reduces ethanol-induced metastasis by suppressing lysyl oxidase (LOX) expression in liver cancer patients (Huang et al. 2013, Aggarwal, Kumar, and Bharti 2003). Moreover, in vivo treatment of curcumin with piperine synergistically lowers DEN-induced HCC features in rats (Patial et al. 2015). Most notably, nanoparticle-coated curcumin shows synergy with sorafenib treatment by inhibiting tumour volume and metastasis in HCC cells (Hu et al. 2015). Multiple nano-formulations have been tested to enhance the bioavailability and solubility of curcumin to treat HCC (Table 2).

Lung Cancer

Lung cancer is the leading cause of death due to cancer, and approximately 2 million people die each year due to lung cancer. It is of two types, including small cell lung cancer (SCLC) and non-small-cell lung cancer (NSCLC), of which NSCLC is the predominant one, accounting for more than 80% of cases of lung cancer (Thai et al. 2021). Current treatments for lung cancer include chemotherapeutic drugs such as paclitaxel, docetaxel, cisplatin, gemcitabine (Thai et al. 2021), etc. Curcumin-affected proliferation, apoptosis, metastasis, and signalling pathways in lung cancer are discussed in this section.

Tumor suppressor genes set a crucial line of defence against tumorigenesis and their altered activity leads to uncontrolled cell proliferation. A key tumour suppressor is p53, which regulates cell proliferation, apoptosis, tumorigenic transformation, and many important cellular functions through its downstream genes such as p21, B-cell lymphoma (BCL), BCl-2 associated protein (Bax), cellular myelocytomatosis viral oncogene homolog (c-myc), etc. (Figure 1). Curcumin upregulates the expression of p53, which results in the stimulation of apoptosis in lung cancer cells (Ye et al. 2015).

One of the crucial functions of autophagy is to suppress cancer cells. Curcumin analogues have been investigated to modulate autophagy proteins

Table 2. The effects of curcumin therapy in liver cancer

In vitro/In vivo	Dosage	Duration	Major outcomes	References
Human hepatocyte L02 cells	2.5 or 5 mM/0.1% DMSO	2 h pre-treatment then incubated for4 or 24 h with QCT	Prevents oxidative stress and inhibit the rises of SOD activity and GSH level	(Patial et al. 2015)
Rat HSCs-6	0.15 μM	3 h pre-treatment then incubated with GO for 2 h	Nuclear expression levels of Nrf2 and the levels of GSH were increased expression of smooth muscle α-actin (α-SMA) was suppressed	(Hu et al. 2015)
Male Wistar rats	100 mg/kg (I.P.)	Pre-treatment for 1 h	Down-regulation of nitric oxide synthase 2 (NOS-2), nitric oxide (NO) levels and lipid peroxidation	(Galaly, Ahmed, and Mahmoud 2014)
Male Wistar albino rats (*Rattus novegiccus*)	50 mg/kg/day in corn oil (oral)	14 days	Reduction of tumor necrosis factor-α (TNF-α) levels, increase of catalase, SOD and GST activities in liver	(Lee et al. 2016)
Male Wistar rats	100 mg/kg/day in Carboxymethyl cellulose (CMC) (oral)	28 days	Down-regulation of Rac1, NADPH oxidase-1 (NOX1)	(Park et al. 2000)
Female Wistar Albino rat	100 mg/kg (I.P.)	30 min pre-treatment before I/R	Reduction of NO, TNF-α	(Cao et al. 2015)
Male Albino Wistar rats	200 mg/kg in corn oil (oral)	1st = 24 h before APA 2nd = 2 h after APAP 3rd = 12 h after APAP	Down-regulation of pro-apoptotic protein Bax and CD68	(Shapiro et al. 2006)
Male albino rats	20 mg/kg/every other day in 1% CMC (oral)	21 days	Alteration in proapoptotic protein caspase-3, Bax and antiapoptotic protein B-cell lymphoma-2 (Bcl-2) protein expressions	(Kaur et al. 2006)

in lung cancer cells. ZYX01, a curcumin analogue, upregulates autophagy to inhibit the proliferation of NSCLC cells (Zhou, Wang, et al. 2019). MOMI-1, which is also an analogue of curcumin, increases the levels of Beclin and LC3-I/II with a decrease in p62 (Zhou, Shi, et al. 2019). This results in upregulation of autophagy and reduced proliferation of A549 lung cancer cells due to cell cycle arrest in the G0/G1 phase. One of the regulatory mechanisms of autophagy by curcumin is through the Akt signalling axis, which is a potent modulator of autophagy (Zhang et al. 2019). Additionally, mTOR is a negative regulator of autophagy and plays a prominent role in tumour growth. Curcumin inhibits Akt/mTOR signalling in A549 lung cancer cells, increasing autophagy proteins Beclin-1 and the LC3-II/I ratio (Zhang et al. 2019). It is noteworthy that curcumin supplementation induces apoptosis in NSCLC by autophagy induction. Phosphoinositide 3-kinase (PI3K) activation is the hallmark of tumorigenesis and its signalling suppression is prominently used in cancer cure. Inhibitors of TRIM26 have been used to target PI3K signalling, which suppressed lung cancer growth. Curcumin can inhibit PI3K signalling and thereby suppress the invasiveness of tumour cells (Table 3).

The epidermal growth factor receptor (EGFR) produces growth and differentiation signals in response to ligand binding. Mutation in EGFR that results in its constitutive activation or overexpression is responsible for uncontrolled cellular proliferation, leading to epithelial to mesenchymal transition (EMT) and promoting lung cancer progression (Bethune et al. 2010). Curcumin inhibits EMT by suppressing EGFR signalling, thus suppressing invasiveness in NSCLC cells (Shaik et al. 2019).

Chemotherapy is effective in reducing the tumour cells and tumour volume. However, resistance to chemotherapy is becoming a challenging task nowadays. Doxorubicin is extensively used in lung cancer chemotherapy. Co-supplementation of curcumin with doxorubicin enhances its efficacy towards lung cancer cells and reduces cancer cell migration by inhibiting MMP-2 and HIF-1α signalling (Jyoti et al. 2017).

Cancer stem cells have a major influence on the process of tumorigenesis and its relapse post-treatment. Curcumin adversely affects tumor sphere formation to inhibit tumorigenesis in A549 and H1299 lung cancer cells. Curcumin administration induces apoptosis and inhibits proliferation in these cells (Zhu et al. 2017). It also inhibits the Wnt/β-catenin pathway, which is crucial to maintaining cancer stem cells. Curcumin suppresses Sonic Hedgehog pathway proteins to downregulate the activity of lung cancer stem cells (Zhu et al. 2017).

Table 3. The effects of curcumin therapy in lung cancer

In vitro/In vivo	Dosage	Duration	Major outcomes	References
A549 and H1299 cells	0.78–100 μM	48 h	Induced apoptotic with palladium, activation of caspase-3 and -7	(Tunc et al. 2017)
A549 cells	4 μM	12 and 24 h	Curcumin derivative, MHMD activated caspase-3, 8, 9, and PARP to induce apoptosis	(Zhou, Cao, and Du 2015)
A549 cell line	100 μM	24 h	Decreased proliferation & metastasis, GSK-3β	(Eren and Betul 2016)
A549 cells	5, 10, 15, 20, 30, 40, and 50 μM		Induced ROS, apoptosis, ATP	(Hossein-zadehdehkordi, Adelinik, and Tashakor 2015)
A549 and H460 cells	5, 10, and 20 μM	12 h	Increased sensitivity towards chemotherapy, decreased proliferation	(Kim, Baek, and Lee 2015)
H1299 cells	10 μM	8, 16, and 24 h	Induced necrosis via the mitochondrial pathway	(Li et al. 2015)
A549 cells	5, 10, and 20 μM	24 hr	Induced apoptosis, upregulated mir-192-5p, downregulated PI3K/Akt signaling	(Jin et al. 2015)
NCI-H460 human lung cancer cells	2 μM		Induced DNA damage, and inhibited cell metastasis	(Jiang et al. 2015)
A549 cells	5, 10, 20, 30, 40, 50, and 60 μM	24 h	Reduced cell proliferation, invasion, MMP-9	(Fan et al. 2015)
A549 and H460 cells	1 and 5 μM	24 h	Reduced DNA methylation of a tumor suppressor to induce its expression	(Jiang et al. 2015)
Drug-sensitive (A549, SPC-A-1, LTEP-G-2) and drug-resistant (A549/DDP) lung cancer cells	0.6, 1.2, 2.1, and 4.2 μM	24 h	Inhibited AKT, ERK, p-GP; increased ROS, apoptosis	(Ai et al. 2016)

Table 3. (Continued)

In vitro/In vivo	Dosage	Duration	Major outcomes	References
A549 and H1299 cells	10, 20, 30, 40, 50, 60, 70, and 80 μM	24 h	Induced apoptosis, calcium signaling	(Xu et al. 2015)
A549 lung cancer cells	20, 40, and 80 μM	24 h	Induced apoptosis, autophagy	(Zhou, Cao, and Du 2015)
A549 cells	0, 1.25, 2.5, 5, 10, and 20 μM	24 h	Increased sensitization to chemotherapy via BRCA signaling	(Xu et al. 2015)
H460 and A427 cells	0, 5, and 15 μM	48 h	Upregulated miR-192–5p/215 via p53, induced apoptosis	(Ye et al. 2015)
Human NSCLC cell lines 95D and A549 cells	0, 15, and 30 μM	24 h	Reduced proliferation, and invasiveness via the Wnt/β-catenin pathway	(Lu, Wei, and Xi 2014)
A549 cells	0, 12.5, 25, 50, and 100 μM	24 h	Suppressed metastasis and invasion via adiponectin/MMP downregulation	(Tsai et al. 2015)
A549 cells	0, 15, 30, 45, and 60 μM		Inhibited metastasis via GLUT1/MT1-MMP2 downregulation	(Liao et al. 2015)
H460 cell line	0.5, 1, 2, 4, and 8 μM	72 h	A curcumin analog, JZ534 stimulated cell cycle arrest, apoptosis via activation of p53, caspase-3, and Bax	(Wu et al. 2015)

EZH2 (enhancer of zeste homolog 2) is a polycomb group of epigenetic modulator proteins and supports tumour progression via regulating cell growth and invasion. Its overexpression is reported in several cancers, such as hepatic, pancreatic, etc. EZH2 inhibitors are used in cancer treatment. Curcumin downregulates EZH2 at both the mRNA and protein level (Wu et al. 2016). It also suppresses EZH2-dependent NOTCH1 expression, which arrests cells in the G1 phase of the cell cycle and attenuates cell growth and migration of lung cancer cells (Wu et al. 2016).

Gastric Cancer

Gastric cancer is the fifth most common cancer worldwide. More than 1 million new cases of gastric cancer were diagnosed worldwide. Gastric cancer is mostly diagnosed at the later stages, and therefore, patients have less than 1 year of survival. Chemotherapy, surgery, phototherapy, and radiotherapy are conventional treatment methods for gastric cancer (Van Cutsem et al. 2016). All of these show the cure but have side effects, and cancer cells become resistant to these therapies. 5-fluorouracil (5-FU) along with adriamycin and mitomycin C, cisplatin along with 5-FU, doxorubicin and methotrexate, and oxaliplatin along with 5-FU and leucovorin are the chemotherapeutic combinations to cure gastric cancer (Van Cutsem et al. 2016). Gastric cancer patients may benefit from curcumin administration alone or in combination with ongoing chemotherapeutic molecules. In this section, we will elaborate on the usage of curcumin alone or in combination to reduce gastric cancer.

Signal transducer and activator of transcription 3 (STAT3) is a transcription factor that regulates growth and cytokine response in cells. Its signalling is crucial in making gastric cells resistant to chemotherapy. Yoshida et al. (2018) show that co-treatment of curcumin with 5-FU shows synergistic effects in promoting gastric cancer cell death via STAT3 suppression. Curcumin administration also enhances the anti-tumoral response of doxorubicin and etoposide in SGC-7901 cells by suppressing NF-κB activation and its downstream signalling (Notarbartolo et al. 2005).

Curcumin's anti-tumor effects are not only reported in vitro, but there are several studies available for its in vivo tumour suppression (Table 4). Curcumin shows its protective effects against the N-methyl-Nitrosourea-induced gastric cancer rat model. It does so by reducing IκB-alpha levels (Sintara et al. 2012). In another mouse model of gastric cancer, curcumin suppresses lymphatic vessel density, which reduces gastric cancer metastasis

(Da et al. 2015). Moreover, curcumin and 5-FU have additive effects in reducing xenograft tumour growth (Koo et al. 2004). In the tobacco smoke-induced gastric cancer mouse model, curcumin reduces the activity of all three MAP kinases (ERK, JNK, and p38 kinase) to suppress tumour growth and elevate E-cadherin to reverse epithelial to mesenchymal features (Liang et al. 2015).

It suppresses metastasis by inhibiting TGF-β signalling in gastric cancer cells (Davoodvandi et al. 2021). Expression of Notch1 and Hes1 is also downregulated in this process (Yao, Zheng, et al. 2015). In AGS cells, it inhibits MMP-2 and MMP-9 to suppress metastasis (Silva et al. 2018). In GC cells, curcumin reduces metastasis by inhibiting Ezrin (EZRI), which is upregulated in the metastasizing process in several cancers (Cai et al. 2013). When administered with 5-fluorouracil and oxaliplatin, curcumin synergistically impedes BGC-823 cell proliferation and promotes cell death by activation of caspases, PARP (Guan et al. 2016).

Curcumin destabilises the mitochondrial membrane potential and, thereby, induces cell death in MGC-803 cells (Zhang et al. 2015). In SGC-7901 and BGC-823 cells, it reduces the cancer cell number by decreasing cell proliferation and inducing apoptosis (Cai et al. 2009). Some microRNAs (mir-33b) are regulated by curcumin, which has adverse effects on cancer cell growth (Sun et al. 2016). Curcumin affects certain cellular pathways to regulate cancer cell proliferation and cell death. The JNK pathway is one such pathway that is activated by stress stimuli and activated by curcumin to induce apoptosis of cancer cells (Figure 1). In KATO-III cells, curcumin elevates levels of cyclin D and B to arrest the cell cycle and promotes PARP activation to induce apoptosis (Moragoda, Jaszewski, and Majumdar, 2001).

There are several drug-delivery systems to enhance the efficacy of curcumin in gastric cancer. Curcumin supplementation through the microsponge system increases its retention and availability in the gastric region of rabbits (Arya and Pathak 2014). Additionally, curcumin-loaded nanostructured lipid carriers (NLCs) also enhance their bioavailability. Curcumin, along with etoposide loaded into these lipid carriers, has been tested for better-sustained release, cell adhesion, uptake, and availability in the mouse xenograft model (Jiang et al. 2016).

Table 4. The effects of curcumin therapy in gastric cancer

In vitro/In vivo	Dosage	Duration	Major outcomes	References
SGC-7901 cell lines	50 μM	12,24,48,72 h	Reduced c-Myc, lncRNA H19 expression, Increased p53 expression	(Liu et al. 2016)
MGC-803 cells	15 μM	24,48,72 h	Reduction of cell viability, colony formation, and migration-induced apoptosis by caspase-3/8, Bcl-2, and Bax pathways	(He et al. 2017)
BGC-823, SGC-7901, MNK-28 cell line	0-200 μM	24,48,72 h	Formation of AVOs, induced apoptosis, increased autophagy	(Li et al. 2017)
BGC-823 cell line	3.125, 6.25, 12.5, 25.0 μM	48,72 h	Decreased Bcl-2 protein and mRNA levels, increased Bax and caspase-3, 8, and 9 expressions	(Yang et al. 2017)
SGC-7901 cells	50 μM	24,48,72,96 h	Increased miR-34a, G0/G1 cell cycle arrest, reduced Bcl-2, CDK4, cyclin D1	(Sun et al. 2019)
MGC-803 cells	0, 10, 15, and 20 μM	24,48,72 h	Inhibited lymphangiogenesis, blocked HMGB1/VEGF-D, increased cell death	(Zhou et al. 2017)
AGS cell line	0.0001- 1 μM	24 h	Reduced cell proliferation, increased autophagy and apoptosis, high p53 activation	(Fu et al. 2018)
AGS cell line	30 μM	24,48,72 h	Increased PTEN activity, low miRNA-21 expression, blocked PI3K signaling	(Li et al. 2017)

Colorectal Cancer

Colorectal cancer (CRC) is the second-most mortality-causing cancer worldwide. Surgery, neoadjuvant radiotherapy, chemotherapy, and immunotherapy are the currently used therapies to treat CRC. Current chemotherapy drugs for CRC include fluoropyrimidine (5-FU), oxaliplatin (OX), irinotecan (IRI), and capecitabine (CAP) (Xie, Chen, and Fang 2020). Despite the development of effective therapies, cases are rapidly increasing with increasing resistance to chemotherapy, including side effects. As a result, medications with low side effects and the ability to selectively kill resistant cells are desperately needed. Curcumin shows both effects on colorectal cancer and prevention.

With its well-known cell cycle arrest property in cancer cells, curcumin halts HCT-116 cells in the G2/M phase of the cell cycle (Mosieniak et al. 2012). It can also prevent exit from the G1 phase by inhibiting the CDK2 activity in the HCT116 colon cancer cell line (Lim et al. 2014). miR-27a and miR34a are tumour suppressors in CRC and curcumin administration upregulates the levels of both in CRC cells (Mosieniak et al. 2012). Curcumin inhibits miR-21 to suppress metastasis and miR-20a, and also miR-17-5p to inhibit specificity protein-mediated cancer cell growth (Gandhy et al. 2012, Mudduluru et al. 2011).

Curcumin induces cell death in CRC cells via a variety of mechanisms. One such pathway is tumour necrosis factor ligand-mediated cell death. Another is NF-κB mediated, which increases reactive oxygen species (ROS) production and superoxide dismutase (SOD) and induces cell death via the extrinsic apoptotic pathway (Ismail et al. 2019). In Caco2 and HT29 cells, curcumin abrogates EGFR signalling, which is usually needed for cancer cells' growth and metastasis as well (Zhen et al. 2014). In colon cancer cells, curcumin upregulates levels of p53 to induce G2 cell cycle arrest and apoptosis (DiMarco-Crook et al. 2020).

Curcumin's effect on cancer stem cells is useful in treating chemoresistant colorectal cancer cells (Wang et al. 2012). Usually, cancer stem cells are the ones that develop resistance to regular treatment (Cai et al. 2018). Curcumin and its analogues chemo-sensitize these cells efficiently.

Since its low bioavailability, nano-formulations of curcumin have been developed to target colorectal cancer (Wong et al. 2019). Curcumin-loaded exosomes such as NCT01294072; NCT01294072; NCT01294072; NCT01294072; NCT01294072 induce immunological response against CRC.

Table 5. The effects of curcumin therapy in colorectal cancer

In vitro/In vivo	Dosage	Duration	Major outcomes	References
5-FU resistant HCT8 cells	10 μM	24 h	Increase sensitivity to 5-FU by increasing Nrf2	(Zhang et al. 2018)
HCT116, SW620 cells	0,2,4,8,16 μM	24,48,72 h	Decrease proliferation and increase autophagy by decreasing YAP	(Zhu et al. 2018)
Irinotecan resistant LoVo cells	0-40 μM	24 h	Increase apoptosis of cancer stem cells	(Su et al. 2018)
HCT116, DLD1, HCT15 cells and HCT116-xenograft	0-10 μM	0-12 h	Decrease xenograft tumor growth by decreasing SIRT1	(Lee et al. 2018)
LoVo, HT29 cells	0-20 μM	24 h	Increase ROS generation, ER stress	(Huang et al. 2017)
SW480, LoVo cells	0-50 μM	24 h	Decrease adhesion and proliferation by increasing AMPK and decreasing NF-κB, uPA and MMP9	(Adeyeni et al. 2016)
DLD1 cells	6.25, 12.5, 25 μM	48 h	Increase apoptosis by decreasing BMI1	(Zhang et al. 2016)
HT29, LoVo, DLD1 and their corresponding oxaliplatin resistant cells	1.25-30 μM, 5-40 μM	24,48 h	Increase sensitivity to oxaliplatin by decreasing NF-κB	(James et al. 2015)
SW620 cells			Decrease EMT progression by decreasing NKD2, Wnt, CXCR4	(Shakibaei et al. 2015)
Patient-derived colorectal liver metastases xenografts	5 μM	2 weeks	Decrease cancer stem cell phenotypes and increase anti-proliferative and pro-apoptotic effects	(Toden et al. 2015)

Human trials for CRC with curcumin are in progress. Nano-lipid curcumin supplementation in food was tested in Phase II clinical trials (Wong et al. 2019).This formulation enhances curcumin absorption and increases the survival rate of CRC patients. Oxaliplatin is the standard chemotherapeutic drug for CRC treatment. However, curcumin delivery through liposomes provides a better cure for CRC in Lovo cells (Table 5). In Colo25 cells, liposomal curcumin shows anticancer effects similar to oxaliplatin. In some cases, curcumin is given in combination with oxaliplatin, and this combination shows synergy in reducing CRC (Li et al. 2007). Liposomal encapsulation of curcumin along with doxorubicin also enhances the effects of doxorubicin in C26 cell growth inhibition (Sesarman et al. 2018). It does so by inhibiting the activation of NF-κB and reducing protein levels required for tumorigenesis (Sesarman et al. 2018). Calcium carbonate encapsulated liposome-mediated delivery of curcumin shows significantly higher anticancer effects in HCT116 cells in comparison to free curcumin (Chen et al. 2019). Another nano-formulation for better bioavailability of curcumin is the use of β-CD-curcumin which shows greater toxicity at low doses in SW-620 cells (Rahman et al. 2012). Curcumin delivery through micelles increases its solubility in water, therefore, making it easily deliverable in the form of injections. In colon cancer C-26 cells, this formulation decreases the cytotoxicity of curcumin (Wong et al. 2019). There are several tested formulations of curcumin with a variety of nanoparticles that enhance its anticancer effects against colorectal cancer. Nanoparticle-coated curcumin enhances the anti-tumoral effects of camptothecin (CPT) in C-26 cells, arrests the cell cycle in HT29 cells, and reduces toxicity in non-cancerous NCM460 cells (Xie et al. 2017). There are many other curcumin delivery systems that have been tested that are summarised in the table.

Prostate Cancer

Prostate cancer is a cancer of the reproductive organ in men. It is the second-most common cancer worldwide and the fifth-leading cause of cancer-related deaths in men. Its treatment includes prostatectomy, radiation therapy, cryosurgery, hormone therapy, and chemotherapy. Chemotherapeutic drugs for prostate cancer treatment are docetaxel, cabazitaxel, bevacizumab, thalidomide, prednisone (Sandhu et al. 2021), etc. Various risk factors target androgen signalling to induce prostate cancer initiation and progression, though androgen-independent prostate cancer relies on overexpression of the androgen receptor gene (AR) or hyperactive AR (Sandhu et al. 2021). Additionally, androgen metabolism plays a crucial role in prostate growth while the oestrogen receptor β negatively regulates it (Sandhu et al. 2021).

Curcumin is used as a phytochemical chemopreventive compound for prostate cancer. It modulates both androgen and oestrogen signalling to regulate the growth and proliferation of prostate cancer cells. Curcumin blocks androgen synthesis by reducing the expression of steroidogenic proteins (CYP450, CYP11A1, and HSD3B2) in LNCaP and 22Rv1 prostate cancer cells, thereby leading to apoptosis and reduced growth of these cells (Ide et al. 2018). Another study reveals the inhibitory role of curcumin on androgen receptor expression via the Wnt/β-catenin pathway in LNCaP cells (Choi, Lim, and Hong 2010). Curcumin suppresses the colony-forming capacity in LNCaP and PC3 cells with a reduced level of androgen receptors, activator protein-1 (AP-1), NF-κB, and CREB-binding protein (CBP) (Nakamura et al. 2002). This study reveals the in vitro suppressive function of curcumin in the cancer cell transformation process. Curcumin also downregulates prostate-specific antigens (PSA), which are stimulated by androgen in LNCaP cells (Tsui et al. 2008). It is known to arrest prostate cancer cells at the G2/M phase of the cell cycle and induce cell death by reducing the expression of androgen receptors in LNCaP and PC3 cells (Guo et al. 2013). This study deconstructs a technique that could be used in patients with androgen-independent prostate cancer (Table 6). Curcumin increases the anticancer effects of existing chemotherapeutic drugs; therefore, could be used in combinatorial chemotherapy for treating prostate cancer patients. When co-administered with docetaxel, curcumin synergistically induces anti-proliferative and apoptotic effects in PC3 and DU145 cells (Banerjee et al. 2017). Anticancer properties of curcumin have also been validated in prostate cancer in vivo models. Curcumin significantly reduces testosterone levels in the prostate tissue of transgenic mice with prostate adenocarcinoma (TRAMP) (Ide et al. 2018). Moreover, curcumin slows the growth of prostate tumours in the LNCaP xenograft model (Hong, Lee, and Choi 2015). Curcumin administration has improved the conditions of human prostate cancer patients. In a phase II trial of 30 castration-resistant prostate cancer (CRPC) patients, curcumin in combination with docetaxel improved their response to anti-androgen therapy (Mahammedi et al. 2016). This combination reduced the serum PSA levels, but it did not improve the survival response. Therefore, the prostate cancer curative effects of curcumin are yet to be established in clinical trials.

Table 6. The effects of curcumin therapy in prostate cancer

In vitro/In vivo	Dosage	Duration	Major outcomes	References
LNCaP and 22Rv1 cells	0-50 μM	0, 24, 48 and 72h	Decreased the expression of steroidogenic	(Ide et al. 2018)
Transgenic adenocarcinoma of the mouse prostate (TRAMP) model	200 mg/kg/d	1 month	Acute regulatory proteins, CYP11A1 and HSD3B2	(Choi, Lim, and Hong 2010)
LNCaP cells	10-100 μM	24 h	Cyclin D1 and c-myc, the target gene of the β-catenin were decreased	(Nakamura et al. 2002)
LNCaP and PC-3 cells	50 μM	24 h	Downregulation of transactivation and expression of androgen receptor (AR), activator protein-1 (AP-1), nuclear factor-kB (NF-kB), and CREB (cAMP response element-binding protein)-binding protein (CBP)	(Tsui et al. 2008)
LNCaP cells	0-80 μM	24, 48 and 72h	Inhibition of methyltrienolone (R1881) and interleukin-6 (IL-6) mediated prostate-specific antigen (PSA) gene expression	(Guo et al. 2013)
LNCaP and PC-3 cells	20,40 μM	24 h	Upregulation of the protein level of NF-κB inhibitor IκBα and downregulation of protein levels of c-Jun and AR.	(Banerjee et al. 2017)
PCa cells	0-50 μM	24 h	Modulates the expression of RTKs, PI3K, phospho-AKT, NF-kappa B, p53, and COX-2	(Hong, Lee, and Choi 2015)
Balb/c nude mice	500 mg/kg/bw	4 weeks	Decreased AR expression	(Mahammedi et al. 2016)
Patients with chemotherapy-naïve metastatic castration-resistant prostate cancer (CRPC)	6,000 mg/day	1 week	Positive prostate-specific antigen (PSA)	(Ohtsu et al. 2002)
PC-3 and DU-145 cells	1 μM	24 h	Inhibition of androgen receptor-mediated prostate cancer growth	(Ohtsu et al. 2002)

Due to the effective *in vitro* and *in vivo* therapeutic results of curcumin in prostate cancer samples, various analogues of curcumin have also been characterised and evaluated in the field of prostate carcinoma treatment in the hope of improved efficacy over curcumin itself (Ohtsu et al. 2002). Dimethylcurcumin (ASC-J9), a curcumin analog, acts as an androgen antagonist. ASC-J9 blocks prostate tumour growth in the CWR-22Rv1 xenograft mouse model. It perturbs the ligation between androgen receptors and their coregulators in LNCaP cells to suppress androgen receptor activation (Ohtsu et al. 2002). Likewise, other curcumin analogues also show toxic effects on prostate cancer (Ohtsu et al. 2002). Numerous studies point out the beneficial role of curcumin in combating prostate cancer by various mechanisms. However, the potential effects of curcumin and its analogues in prostate cancer treatment need further validation through extensive clinical trials.

Neuroblastoma

A neuroblastoma is a tumour of the nervous system found in several areas of the body. Since it originates from immature nerve cells, neuroblastoma is the third most common cancer in children (Park, Eggert, and Caron 2008). Neuroblastoma is caused by mutations in the anaplastic lymphoma kinase (ALK) gene, the PHOX2B gene, amplification of the MYCN oncogene, duplication of the LMO1 gene, copy number variation in the NBPF10 gene, and other factors (Park, Eggert, and Caron 2008).Risk factors for these changes include chemical exposure during the gestational period, smoking, alcohol consumption, and birth factors. Treatments include surgery, chemotherapy, radiation, stem cell transplantation, monoclonal antibody therapy, and the use of isotretinoin. Commonly used chemotherapeutic drugs for neuroblastoma are cisplatin, carboplatin, cyclophosphamide, etoposide, doxorubicin, and vincristine (Park, Eggert, and Caron 2008). Naxitamab is a newly US-approved chemotherapeutic drug used in combination with granulocyte-macrophage colony-stimulating factor (GM-CSF) (Markham 2021).

The anticancer properties of curcumin have been explored to overcome the shortcomings of conventional chemotherapy in neuroblastoma. The growth and survival of cancer cells are fulfilled by high Akt and NF-κB activity (Fresno Vara et al. 2004, Taniguchi and Karin 2018). Curcumin inhibits the growth and induces apoptosis in neuroblastoma cells by decreasing the activation of Akt and NF-κB; increasing the activity of p53, and caspases (Jee et al. 1998). Moreover, PTEN, a tumour suppressor and Akt regulator, is downregulated in most cancer cells to induce tumorigenesis (Cantley and Neel 1999). Curcumin blocks tumour growth by increasing the levels of PTEN in neuroblastoma cells (Picone et al. 2014). The resultant increase and nuclear translocation of FOXO3a activate pro-apoptotic proteins Bim, FAS-L, and caspase-8 and induce cell death (Picone et al. 2014, Sukumari-Ramesh et al. 2011). Curcumin also modulates other pathways for inducing cancer cell death. It destabilises mitochondrial membrane potential (MMP) with a decrease in the anti-apoptotic form of BCl-2 associated with an increase in Bax levels and thereby results in the death of neuroblastoma cells (Kalashnikova et al. 2017). Another regulation of cancer cell death by curcumin is ERK1/2 and HIF-1α mediated upregulation of p53 in SK-N-MC and N2a neuroblastoma cells (Parandavar and Yazdanparast 2017, Sidhar and Giri 2017). Both proteins negatively regulate p53 and their levels are significantly reduced by curcumin to upregulate p53 levels. Inducing cell cycle arrest by upregulation of p27 and p21 is another mechanism to inhibit the proliferation of neuroblastoma cells by curcumin (Picone et al. 2014, Namkaew et al. 2018). Curcumin inhibits GSK-3β regulated degradation of α-synuclein via autophagy that reduces amyloidogenesis in the SH-SY5Y neuroblastoma cells (Song et al. 2020).

Despite inducing cell death and growth arrest of neuroblastoma cells, curcumin also inhibits their migration and metabolism. It downregulates matrix metalloprotease MMP-2 by increasing its inhibitor TIMP-1 levels to reduce the metastasis of SH-SY5Y neuroblastoma cells (Namkaew et al. 2018). Cancer cells depend on the high rate of metabolism for their survival and growth, which is maintained by the high activity of metabolising enzymes. Curcumin perturbs the conversion of pyruvate into lactate, reducing the rate of glycolysis and gluconeogenesis essential for cancer cell growth by decreasing the activity of lactate dehydrogenase, aldolase, enolase, and glyceraldehyde-3-phosphate dehydrogenase (D'Aguanno et al. 2012).

Curcumin in combination with other beneficial alkaloids shows promising toxicity against neuroblastoma. When administered with berberine, it synergises the cytotoxic effects on neuroblastoma cells. This reduces the working concentration of berberine and the side effects caused by it at a high dosage (Maiti, Plemmons, and Dunbar 2019). Likewise, the curcumin and piperine combination enhances cytotoxicity in SH-SY5Y neuroblastoma cells

Table 7. The effects of curcumin therapy in neuroblastoma

In vitro/In vivo	Dosage	Duration	Major outcomes	References
LAN5 NB cells	15 μM	3,5,24 h	Inhibition of AKT and Foxo3a nuclear translocation	(Picone et al. 2014)
SK-N-AS and SK-N-BE cells	0-100 μM	24 h	Reduction in NF-κB, Bcl-2 and Bcl-xL expression	(Sukumari-Ramesh et al. 2011)
SK-N-AS and IMR-32 cells	50, 100,250 μM	72 h	Induction of Cellular Hypoxia and ROS-mediated Apoptosis	(Kalashnikova et al. 2017)
N2a cells	0-50 μM	24 h	Induce expression of group of pro-apoptotic Bex genes	(Parandavar and Yazdanparast 2017)
SH-SY5Y cells	0-50 μM	24 h	Suppression of growth and 3D tumor migration	(Sidhar and Giri 2017)
SH-SY5Y cells	2.5-20 μM	12,24 h	Regulation of autophagy by controlling transcription factor EB (TFEB) through the inhibition of GSK-3β	(Namkaew et al. 2018)
SH-SY5Y cells	40 μM	24 h	Inhibition of the ubiquitin–proteasome system	(Song et al. 2020)
U-87MG and U-251MG cells	50-200 μM	24 h	Inhibition of PI3K/Akt/mTOR pathway	(D'Aguanno et al. 2012)
SH-SY5Y cells	5-100 μM	24 h	Significant cytotoxic effects	(Maiti, Plemmons, and Dunbar 2019)

(Baspinar et al. 2018). Moreover, curcumin aids in the anticancer effects of conventional chemotherapeutic compounds used for the treatment of neuroblastoma. Co-administration of curcumin with cisplatin or doxorubicin induces the rate of cell death in SH-SY5Y, SH-EP-1, SK-N-AS, and LAN5 neuroblastoma cells (Namkaew et al. 2018, Sukumari-Ramesh et al. 2011, Rajkumar et al. 2016). Finally, the clinical trials could support the prominent anticancer agent in neuroblastoma treatment.

Conclusion

Over the past few years, curcumin has gone through various experimental studies and clinical trials to prove its potential as a natural anticancer compound. The establishment of curcumin as an anticancer agent helped to open a gateway for many other natural compounds for study for future drug development. Over the past few decades, researchers around the world have been trying to find some therapeutic approaches with strong potential to fight against cancer. For many years before scientific advancement, mother nature provided us with food, fire, and shelters to build up strength and immunity. Now in the current scenario, cancer is one of the biggest problems for our life sustainability, which is also caused by environmental factors. When nature creates a poison like cancer, it must also have a cure for the same, which we need to find out. Among many bioactive natural compounds, the most promising molecule, curcumin shows multi-targeted activity by modulating genes involved in various cell signalling pathways. The inadequate intake, fast cellular degradation, and rapid removal from the system put curcumin in a quarry of whether it is the right representative of choice or we should wait for some other compounds. Even after so many trials, there are still some doubts and disputes about the significance of the action of curcumin as a cancer-curing agent. For instance, it is not exactly known whether higher anticancer effects are attributed to the original compound or its derivatives. These findings also help scientists to understand the drug and ways to improve drug delivery to improve the bioavailability of curcumin. Many trials are involved in increasing the solubility and bioavailability of curcumin and targeting drug delivery exactly to the site of action. With these promising shreds of evidence, the application of curcumin for cancer treatment could be possible shortly.

References

Abuelba, H., C. E. Cotrutz, B. A. Stoica, L. Stoica, D. Olinici, and T. Petreus. 2015. "In vitro evaluation of curcumin effects on breast adenocarcinoma 2D and 3D cell cultures."*Rom J Morphol Embryol* 56 (1):71-6.

Adeyeni, T. A., N. Khatwani, K. San, and U. R. Ezekiel. 2016. "BMI1 is downregulated by the natural compound curcumin, but not by bisdemethoxycurcumin and dimethoxycurcumin." *Physiol Rep* 4 (16). doi: 10.14814/phy2.12906.

Aggarwal, B. B., S. C. Gupta, and B. Sung. 2013. "Curcumin: an orally bioavailable blocker of TNF and other pro-inflammatory biomarkers."*Br J Pharmacol* 169 (8):1672-92. doi: 10.1111/bph.12131.

Aggarwal, B. B., A. Kumar, and A. C. Bharti. 2003. "Anticancer potential of curcumin: preclinical and clinical studies." *Anticancer Res* 23 (1A):363-98.

Aggarwal, B. B., and S. Shishodia. 2004. "Suppression of the nuclear factor-kappaB activation pathway by spice-derived phytochemicals: reasoning for seasoning." *Ann N Y Acad Sci* 1030:434-41. doi: 10.1196/annals.1329.054.

Aggarwal, B. B., C. Sundaram, N. Malani, and H. Ichikawa. 2007. "Curcumin: the Indian solid gold." *Adv Exp Med Biol* 595:1-75. doi: 10.1007/978-0-387-46401-5_1.

Ahn, J., H. Lee, S. Kim, and T. Ha. 2010. "Curcumin-induced suppression of adipogenic differentiation is accompanied by activation of Wnt/beta-catenin signaling." *Am J Physiol Cell Physiol* 298 (6):C1510-6. doi: 10.1152/ajpcell.00369.2009.

Ai, Y., B. Zhu, C. Ren, F. Kang, J. Li, Z. Huang, Y. Lai, S. Peng, K. Ding, J. Tian, and Y. Zhang. 2016. "Discovery of New Monocarbonyl Ligustrazine-Curcumin Hybrids for Intervention of Drug-Sensitive and Drug-Resistant Lung Cancer." *J Med Chem* 59 (5):1747-60. doi: 10.1021/acs.jmedchem.5b01203.

Akkoc, Y., O. Berrak, E. D. Arisan, P. Obakan, A. Coker-Gurkan, and N. Palavan-Unsal. 2015. "Inhibition of PI3K signaling triggered apoptotic potential of curcumin which is hindered by Bcl-2 through activation of autophagy in MCF-7 cells." *Biomed Pharmacother* 71:161-71. doi: 10.1016/j.biopha.2015.02.029.

Arya, P., and K. Pathak. 2014. "Assessing the viability of microsponges as gastro retentive drug delivery system of curcumin: optimization and pharmacokinetics." *Int J Pharm* 460 (1-2):1-12. doi: 10.1016/j.ijpharm.2013.10.045.

Banerjee, S., S. K. Singh, I. Chowdhury, J. W. Lillard, Jr., and R. Singh. 2017. "Combinatorial effect of curcumin with docetaxel modulates apoptotic and cell survival molecules in prostate cancer." *Front Biosci (Elite Ed)* 9 (2):235-245. doi: 10.2741/e798.

Bansal, S. S., H. Kausar, M. V. Vadhanam, S. Ravoori, J. Pan, S. N. Rai, and R. C. Gupta. 2014. "Curcumin implants, not curcumin diet, inhibit estrogen-induced mammary carcinogenesis in ACI rats." *Cancer Prev Res (Phila)* 7 (4):456-65. doi: 10.1158/1940-6207.CAPR-13-0248.

Baron, J. A., B. F. Cole, R. S. Sandler, R. W. Haile, D. Ahnen, R. Bresalier, G. McKeown-Eyssen, R. W. Summers, R. Rothstein, C. A. Burke, D. C. Snover, T. R. Church, J. I. Allen, M. Beach, G. J. Beck, J. H. Bond, T. Byers, E. R. Greenberg, J. S. Mandel, N. Marcon, L. A. Mott, L. Pearson, F. Saibil, and R. U. van Stolk. 2003. "A randomized trial of aspirin to prevent colorectal adenomas." *N Engl J Med* 348 (10):891-9. doi: 10.1056/NEJMoa021735.

Baspinar, Y., M. Ustundas, O. Bayraktar, and C. Sezgin. 2018. "Curcumin and piperine loaded zein-chitosan nanoparticles: Development and in-vitro characterisation." *Saudi Pharm J* 26 (3):323-334. doi: 10.1016/j.jsps.2018.01.010.

Beevers, C. S., H. Zhou, and S. Huang. 2013. "Hitting the golden TORget: curcumin's effects on mTOR signaling." *Anticancer Agents Med Chem* 13 (7):988-94. doi: 10.2174/1871520611313070004.

Bethune, G., D. Bethune, N. Ridgway, and Z. Xu. 2010. "Epidermal growth factor receptor (EGFR) in lung cancer: an overview and update." *J Thorac Dis* 2 (1):48-51.

Bimonte, S., A. Barbieri, G. Palma, D. Rea, A. Luciano, M. D'Aiuto, C. Arra, and F. Izzo. 2015. "Dissecting the role of curcumin in tumour growth and angiogenesis in mouse model of human breast cancer." *Biomed Res Int* 2015:878134. doi: 10.1155/2015/878134.

Brennan, J. A., J. O. Boyle, W. M. Koch, S. N. Goodman, R. H. Hruban, Y. J. Eby, M. J. Couch, A. A. Forastiere, and D. Sidransky. 1995. "Association between cigarette smoking and mutation of the p53 gene in squamous-cell carcinoma of the head and neck." *N Engl J Med* 332 (11):712-7. doi: 10.1056/NEJM199503163321104.

Cai, X. Z., W. Y. Huang, Y. Qiao, S. Y. Du, Y. Chen, D. Chen, S. Yu, R. C. Che, N. Liu, and Y. Jiang. 2013. "Inhibitory effects of curcumin on gastric cancer cells: A proteomic study of molecular targets." *Phytomedicine* 20 (6):495-505. doi: https://doi.org/10.1016/j.phymed.2012.12.007.

Cai, X. Z., J. Wang, X. D. Li, G. L. Wang, F. N. Liu, M. S. Cheng, and F. Li. 2009. "Curcumin suppresses proliferation and invasion in human gastric cancer cells by downregulation of PAK1 activity and cyclin D1 expression." *Cancer Biol Ther* 8 (14):1360-8. doi: 10.4161/cbt.8.14.8720.

Cai, Z., Y. Cao, Y. Luo, H. Hu, and H. Ling. 2018. "Signalling mechanism(s) of epithelial-mesenchymal transition and cancer stem cells in tumour therapeutic resistance." *Clin Chim Acta* 483:156-163. doi: 10.1016/j.cca.2018.04.033.

Calaf, G. M., R. Ponce-Cusi, and F. Carrion. 2018. "Curcumin and paclitaxel induce cell death in breast cancer cell lines." *Oncol Rep* 40 (4):2381-2388. doi: 10.3892/or.2018.6603.

Calle, E. E., C. Rodriguez, K. Walker-Thurmond, and M. J. Thun. 2003. "Overweight, obesity, and mortality from cancer in a prospectively studied cohort of U.S. adults." *N Engl J Med* 348 (17):1625-38. doi: 10.1056/NEJMoa021423.

Cantley, L. C., and B. G. Neel. 1999. "New insights into tumor suppression: PTEN suppresses tumor formation by restraining the phosphoinositide 3-kinase/AKT pathway." *Proc Natl Acad Sci U S A* 96 (8):4240-5. doi: 10.1073/pnas.96.8.4240.

Cao, L., W. Ding, J. Du, R. Jia, Y. Liu, C. Zhao, Y. Shen, and G. Yin. 2015. "Effects of curcumin on antioxidative activities and cytokine production in Jian carp (Cyprinus carpio var. Jian) with CCl4-induced liver damage." *Fish Shellfish Immunol* 43 (1):150-7. doi: 10.1016/j.fsi.2014.12.025.

Chen, B., Y. Zhang, Y. Wang, J. Rao, X. Jiang, and Z. Xu. 2014. "Curcumin inhibits proliferation of breast cancer cells through Nrf2-mediated down-regulation of Fen1 expression." *J Steroid Biochem Mol Biol* 143:11-8. doi: 10.1016/j.jsbmb.2014.01.009.

Chen, Y., Q. Du, Q. Guo, J. Huang, L. Liu, X. Shen, and J. Peng. 2019. "A W/O emulsion mediated film dispersion method for curcumin encapsulated pH-sensitive liposomes in the colon tumor treatment." *Drug Dev Ind Pharm* 45 (2):282-291. doi: 10.1080/03639045.2018.1539099.

Chiu, T. L., and C. C. Su. 2009. "Curcumin inhibits proliferation and migration by increasing the Bax to Bcl-2 ratio and decreasing NF-kappaBp65 expression in breast cancer MDA-MB-231 cells." *Int J Mol Med* 23 (4):469-75. doi: 10.3892/ijmm_000 00153.

Choi, H. Y., J. E. Lim, and J. H. Hong. 2010. "Curcumin interrupts the interaction between the androgen receptor and Wnt/beta-catenin signaling pathway in LNCaP prostate cancer cells." *Prostate Cancer Prostatic Dis* 13 (4):343-9. doi: 10.1038/pcan.2010.26.

Choudhuri, T., S. Pal, M. L. Agwarwal, T. Das, and G. Sa. 2002. "Curcumin induces apoptosis in human breast cancer cells through p53-dependent Bax induction." *FEBS Lett* 512 (1-3):334-40. doi: 10.1016/s0014-5793(02)02292-5.

Chung, S. S., and J. V. Vadgama. 2015. "Curcumin and epigallocatechin gallate inhibit the cancer stem cell phenotype via down-regulation of STAT3-NFkappaB signaling." *Anticancer Res* 35 (1):39-46.

Cianciulli, Antonia, Rosa Calvello, Chiara Porro, Teresa Trotta, Rosaria Salvatore, and Maria Antonietta Panaro. 2016. "PI3k/Akt signalling pathway plays a crucial role in the anti-inflammatory effects of curcumin in LPS-activated microglia." *International Immunopharmacology* 36:282-290. doi: https://doi.org/10.1016/j.intimp.2016.05.007.

Coker-Gurkan, A., D. Bulut, R. Genc, E. D. Arisan, P. Obakan-Yerlikaya, and N. Palavan-Unsal. 2019. "Curcumin prevented human autocrine growth hormone (GH) signaling mediated NF-kappaB activation and miR-183-96-182 cluster stimulated epithelial mesenchymal transition in T47D breast cancer cells." *Mol Biol Rep* 46 (1):355-369. doi: 10.1007/s11033-018-4479-y.

Coker-Gurkan, A., M. Celik, M. Ugur, E. D. Arisan, P. Obakan-Yerlikaya, Z. B. Durdu, and N. Palavan-Unsal. 2018. "Curcumin inhibits autocrine growth hormone-mediated invasion and metastasis by targeting NF-kappaB signaling and polyamine metabolism in breast cancer cells." *Amino Acids* 50 (8):1045-1069. doi: 10.1007/s00726-018-2581-z.

Cuzick, J., J. Forbes, R. Edwards, M. Baum, S. Cawthorn, A. Coates, A. Hamed, A. Howell, T. Powles, and Ibis investigators. 2002. "First results from the International Breast Cancer Intervention Study (IBIS-I): a randomised prevention trial." *Lancet* 360 (9336):817-24. doi: 10.1016/s0140-6736(02)09962-2.

D'Aguanno, S., I. D'Agnano, M. De Canio, C. Rossi, S. Bernardini, G. Federici, and A. Urbani. 2012. "Shotgun proteomics and network analysis of neuroblastoma cell lines treated with curcumin." *Mol Biosyst* 8 (4):1068-77. doi: 10.1039/c2mb05498a.

Da, W., J. Zhu, L. Wang, and Q. Sun. 2015. "Curcumin suppresses lymphatic vessel density in an in vivo human gastric cancer model." *Tumour Biol* 36 (7):5215-23. doi: 10.1007/s13277-015-3178-8.

Davoodvandi, A., M. Farshadi, N. Zare, S. A. Akhlagh, E. Alipour Nosrani, M. Mahjoubin-Tehran, P. Kangari, S. M. Sharafi, H. Khan, M. Aschner, G. Baniebrahimi, and H. Mirzaei. 2021. "Antimetastatic Effects of Curcumin in Oral and Gastrointestinal Cancers." *Front Pharmacol* 12:668567. doi: 10.3389/fphar.2021.668567.

DiMarco-Crook, Christina, KanyasiriRakariyatham, Zhengze Li, Zheyuan Du, Jinkai Zheng, Xian Wu, and Hang Xiao. 2020. "Synergistic anticancer effects of curcumin and 3',4'-didemethylnobiletin in combination on colon cancer cells." *Journal of Food Science,*85 (4):1292-1301. doi: https://doi.org/10.1111/1750-3841.15073.

El-Ashmawy, I. M., K. M. Ashry, A. F. El-Nahas, and O. M. Salama. 2006. "Protection by turmeric and myrrh against liver oxidative damage and genotoxicity induced by lead acetate in mice." *Basic Clin Pharmacol Toxicol* 98 (1):32-7. doi: 10.1111/j.1742-7843.2006.pto_228.x.

Eren, D., and Y. M. Betul. 2016. "Revealing the effect of 6-gingerol, 6-shogaol and curcumin on mPGES-1, GSK-3beta and beta-catenin pathway in A549 cell line." *Chem Biol Interact* 258:257-65. doi: 10.1016/j.cbi.2016.09.012.

Fan, H., Y. Liang, B. Jiang, X. Li, H. Xun, J. Sun, W. He, H. T. Lau, and X. Ma. 2016. "Curcumin inhibits intracellular fatty acid synthase and induces apoptosis in human breast cancer MDA-MB-231 cells." *Oncol Rep* 35 (5):2651-6. doi: 10.3892/or.2016.4682.

Fan, Z., X. Duan, H. Cai, L. Wang, M. Li, J. Qu, W. Li, Y. Wang, and J. Wang. 2015. "Curcumin inhibits the invasion of lung cancer cells by modulating the PKCalpha/Nox-2/ROS/ATF-2/MMP-9 signaling pathway." *Oncol Rep* 34 (2):691-8. doi: 10.3892/or.2015.4044.

Fan, Z., H. Jing, J. Yao, Y. Li, X. Hu, H. Shao, G. Shen, J. Pan, F. Luo, and X. Tian. 2014. "The protective effects of curcumin on experimental acute liver lesion induced by intestinal ischemia-reperfusion through inhibiting the pathway of NF-kappaB in a rat model." *Oxid Med Cell Longev* 2014:191624. doi: 10.1155/2014/191624.

Fathy Abd-Ellatef, G. E., E. Gazzano, D. Chirio, A. R. Hamed, D. C. Belisario, C. Zuddas, E. Peira, B. Rolando, J. Kopecka, M. Assem Said Marie, S. Sapino, S. Ramadan Fahmy, M. Gallarate, A. Z. Abdel-Hamid, and C. Riganti. 2020. "Curcumin-Loaded Solid Lipid Nanoparticles Bypass P-Glycoprotein Mediated Doxorubicin Resistance in Triple Negative Breast Cancer Cells." *Pharmaceutics* 12 (2). doi: 10.3390/pharmaceutics12020096.

Fresno Vara, J. A., E. Casado, J. de Castro, P. Cejas, C. Belda-Iniesta, and M. Gonzalez-Baron. 2004. "PI3K/Akt signalling pathway and cancer." *Cancer Treat Rev* 30 (2):193-204. doi: 10.1016/j.ctrv.2003.07.007.

Fu, H., C. Wang, D. Yang, Z. Wei, J. Xu, Z. Hu, Y. Zhang, W. Wang, R. Yan, and Q. Cai. 2018. "Curcumin regulates proliferation, autophagy, and apoptosis in gastric cancer cells by affecting PI3K and P53 signaling." *J Cell Physiol* 233 (6):4634-4642. doi: 10.1002/jcp.26190.

Galaly, S. R., O. M. Ahmed, and A. M. Mahmoud. 2014. "Thymoquinone and curcumin prevent gentamicin-induced liver injury by attenuating oxidative stress, inflammation and apoptosis." *J Physiol Pharmacol* 65 (6):823-32.

Gandhy, S. U., K. Kim, L. Larsen, R. J. Rosengren, and S. Safe. 2012. "Curcumin and synthetic analogs induce reactive oxygen species and decreases specificity protein (Sp) transcription factors by targeting microRNAs." *BMC Cancer* 12:564. doi: 10.1186/1471-2407-12-564.

Gao, J. Z., J. L. Du, Y. L. Wang, J. Li, L. X. Wei, and M. Z. Guo. 2015. "Synergistic effects of curcumin and bevacizumab on cell signaling pathways in hepatocellular carcinoma." *Oncol Lett* 9 (1):295-299. doi: 10.3892/ol.2014.2694.

Garcia-Nino, W. R., E. Tapia, C. Zazueta, Z. L. Zatarain-Barron, R. Hernandez-Pando, C. C. Vega-Garcia, and J. Pedraza-Chaverri. 2013. "Curcumin pretreatment prevents potassium dichromate-induced hepatotoxicity, oxidative stress, decreased respiratory complex I activity, and membrane permeability transition pore opening." *Evid Based Complement Alternat Med* 2013:424692. doi: 10.1155/2013/424692.

Ghosh, S., S. Dutta, A. Sarkar, M. Kundu, and P. C. Sil. 2021. "Targeted delivery of curcumin in breast cancer cells via hyaluronic acid modified mesoporous silica nanoparticle to enhance anticancer efficiency." *Colloids Surf B Biointerfaces* 197:111404. doi: 10.1016/j.colsurfb.2020.111404.

Giardiello, F. M., S. R. Hamilton, A. J. Krush, S. Piantadosi, L. M. Hylind, P. Celano, S. V. Booker, C. R. Robinson, and G. J. Offerhaus. 1993. "Treatment of colonic and rectal adenomas with sulindac in familial adenomatous polyposis." *N Engl J Med* 328 (18):1313-6. doi: 10.1056/NEJM199305063281805.

Grill, A. E., K. Shahani, B. Koniar, and J. Panyam. 2018. "Chemopreventive efficacy of curcumin-loaded PLGA microparticles in a transgenic mouse model of HER-2-positive breast cancer." *Drug Deliv Transl Res* 8 (2):329-341. doi: 10.1007/s13346-017-0377-4.

Guan, F., Y. Ding, Y. Zhang, Y. Zhou, M. Li, and C. Wang. 2016. "Curcumin Suppresses Proliferation and Migration of MDA-MB-231 Breast Cancer Cells through Autophagy-Dependent Akt Degradation." *PLoS One* 11 (1):e0146553. doi: 10.1371/journal.pone.0146553.

Guo, H., Y. M. Xu, Z. Q. Ye, J. H. Yu, and X. Y. Hu. 2013. "Curcumin induces cell cycle arrest and apoptosis of prostate cancer cells by regulating the expression of IkappaBalpha, c-Jun and androgen receptor." *Pharmazie* 68 (6):431-4.

Haddad, R. I., and D. M. Shin. 2008. "Recent advances in head and neck cancer." *N Engl J Med* 359 (11):1143-54. doi: 10.1056/NEJMra0707975.

Hashemzehi, M., R. Behnam-Rassouli, S. M. Hassanian, M. Moradi-Binabaj, R. Moradi-Marjaneh, F. Rahmani, H. Fiuji, M. Jamili, M. Mirahmadi, N. Boromand, M. Piran, M. Jafari, A. Sahebkar, A. Avan, and M. Khazaei. 2018. "Phytosomal-curcumin antagonizes cell growth and migration, induced by thrombin through AMP-Kinase in breast cancer." *J Cell Biochem* 119 (7):5996-6007. doi: 10.1002/jcb.26796.

Hatcher, H., R. Planalp, J. Cho, F. M. Torti, and S. V. Torti. 2008. "Curcumin: from ancient medicine to current clinical trials." *Cell Mol Life Sci* 65 (11):1631-52. doi: 10.1007/s00018-008-7452-4.

He, B., W. Wei, J. Liu, Y. Xu, and G. Zhao. 2017. "Synergistic anticancer effect of curcumin and chemotherapy regimen FP in human gastric cancer MGC-803 cells." *Oncol Lett* 14 (3):3387-3394. doi: 10.3892/ol.2017.6627.

He, H., W. Zhuang, B. Ma, X. Su, T. Yu, J. Hu, L. Chen, R. Peng, G. Li, and Y. Wang. 2019. "Oxidation-Responsive and Aggregation-Induced Emission Polymeric Micelles with Two-Photon Excitation for Cancer Therapy and Bioimaging." *ACS Biomater Sci Eng* 5 (5):2577-2586. doi: 10.1021/acsbiomaterials.9b00212.

Hong, J. H., G. Lee, and H. Y. Choi. 2015. "Effect of curcumin on the interaction between androgen receptor and Wnt/beta-catenin in LNCaP xenografts." *Korean J Urol* 56 (9):656-65. doi: 10.4111/kju.2015.56.9.656.

Hosseini, S., J. Chamani, M. R. Hadipanah, N. Ebadpour, A. S. Hojjati, M. H. Mohammadzadeh, and H. R. Rahimi. 2019. "Nano-curcumin's suppression of breast cancer cells (MCF7) through the inhibition of cyclinD1 expression." *Breast Cancer (Dove Med Press)* 11:137-142. doi: 10.2147/BCTT.S195800.

Hosseinzadehdehkordi, M., A. Adelinik, and A. Tashakor. 2015. "Dual effect of curcumin targets reactive oxygen species, adenosine triphosphate contents and intermediate steps of mitochondria-mediated apoptosis in lung cancer cell lines." *Eur J Pharmacol* 769:203-10. doi: 10.1016/j.ejphar.2015.11.019.

Hu, B., D. Sun, C. Sun, Y. F. Sun, H. X. Sun, Q. F. Zhu, X. R. Yang, Y. B. Gao, W. G. Tang, J. Fan, A. Maitra, R. A. Anders, and Y. Xu. 2015. "A polymeric nanoparticle formulation of curcumin in combination with sorafenib synergistically inhibits tumor growth and metastasis in an orthotopic model of human hepatocellular carcinoma." *Biochem Biophys Res Commun* 468 (4):525-32. doi: 10.1016/j.bbrc.2015.10.031.

Hu, S., Y. Xu, L. Meng, L. Huang, and H. Sun. 2018. "Curcumin inhibits proliferation and promotes apoptosis of breast cancer cells." *Exp Ther Med* 16 (2):1266-1272. doi: 10.3892/etm.2018.6345.

Hua, W. F., Y. S. Fu, Y. J. Liao, W. J. Xia, Y. C. Chen, Y. X. Zeng, H. F. Kung, and D. Xie. 2010. "Curcumin induces down-regulation of EZH2 expression through the MAPK pathway in MDA-MB-435 human breast cancer cells." *Eur J Pharmacol* 637 (1-3):16-21. doi: 10.1016/j.ejphar.2010.03.051.

Huang, C. S., C. T. Ho, S. H. Tu, M. H. Pan, C. H. Chuang, H. W. Chang, C. H. Chang, C. H. Wu, and Y. S. Ho. 2013. "Long-term ethanol exposure-induced hepatocellular carcinoma cell migration and invasion through lysyl oxidase activation are attenuated by combined treatment with pterostilbene and curcumin analogues." *J Agric Food Chem* 61 (18):4326-35. doi: 10.1021/jf4004175.

Huang, Y. F., D. J. Zhu, X. W. Chen, Q. K. Chen, Z. T. Luo, C. C. Liu, G. X. Wang, W. J. Zhang, and N. Z. Liao. 2017. "Curcumin enhances the effects of irinotecan on colorectal cancer cells through the generation of reactive oxygen species and activation of the endoplasmic reticulum stress pathway." *Oncotarget* 8 (25):40264-40275. doi: 10.18632/oncotarget.16828.

Ide, H., Y. Lu, T. Noguchi, S. Muto, H. Okada, S. Kawato, and S. Horie. 2018. "Modulation of AKR1C2 by curcumin decreases testosterone production in prostate cancer." *Cancer Sci* 109 (4):1230-1238. doi: 10.1111/cas.13517.

Ismail, N. I., I. Othman, F. Abas, H. Lajis N, and R. Naidu. 2019. "Mechanism of Apoptosis Induced by Curcumin in Colorectal Cancer." *Int J Mol Sci* 20 (10). doi: 10.3390/ijms20102454.

James, M. I., C. Iwuji, G. Irving, A. Karmokar, J. A. Higgins, N. Griffin-Teal, A. Thomas, P. Greaves, H. Cai, S. R. Patel, B. Morgan, A. Dennison, M. Metcalfe, G. Garcea, D. M. Lloyd, D. P. Berry, W. P. Steward, L. M. Howells, and K. Brown. 2015. "Curcumin inhibits cancer stem cell phenotypes in ex vivo models of colorectal liver metastases, and is clinically safe and tolerable in combination with FOLFOX chemotherapy." *Cancer Lett* 364 (2):135-41. doi: 10.1016/j.canlet.2015.05.005.

Jee, S. H., S. C. Shen, C. R. Tseng, H. C. Chiu, and M. L. Kuo. 1998. "Curcumin induces a p53-dependent apoptosis in human basal cell carcinoma cells." *J Invest Dermatol* 111 (4):656-61. doi: 10.1046/j.1523-1747.1998.00352.x.

Ji, P., L. Wang, Y. Chen, S. Wang, Z. Wu, and X. Qi. 2020. "Hyaluronic acid hydrophilic surface rehabilitating curcumin nanocrystals for targeted breast cancer treatment with prolonged biodistribution." *Biomater Sci* 8 (1):462-472. doi: 10.1039/c9bm01605h.

Jiang, A., X. Wang, X. Shan, Y. Li, P. Wang, P. Jiang, and Q. Feng. 2015. "Curcumin Reactivates Silenced Tumor Suppressor Gene RARbeta by Reducing DNA Methylation." *Phytother Res* 29 (8):1237-45. doi: 10.1002/ptr.5373.

Jiang, H., D. Geng, H. Liu, Z. Li, and J. Cao. 2016. "Co-delivery of etoposide and curcumin by lipid nanoparticulate drug delivery system for the treatment of gastric tumors." *Drug Deliv* 23 (9):3665-3673. doi: 10.1080/10717544.2016.1217954.

Jiang, M., O. Huang, X. Zhang, Z. Xie, A. Shen, H. Liu, M. Geng, and K. Shen. 2013. "Curcumin induces cell death and restores tamoxifen sensitivity in the antiestrogen-resistant breast cancer cell lines MCF-7/LCC2 and MCF-7/LCC9." *Molecules* 18 (1):701-20. doi: 10.3390/molecules18010701.

Jin, H., J. Pi, Y. Zhao, J. Jiang, T. Li, X. Zeng, P. Yang, C. E. Evans, and J. Cai. 2017. "EGFR-targeting PLGA-PEG nanoparticles as a curcumin delivery system for breast cancer therapy." *Nanoscale* 9 (42):16365-16374. doi: 10.1039/c7nr06898k.

Jin, H., F. Qiao, Y. Wang, Y. Xu, and Y. Shang. 2015. "Curcumin inhibits cell proliferation and induces apoptosis of human non-small cell lung cancer cells through the upregulation of miR-192-5p and suppression of PI3K/Akt signaling pathway." *Oncol Rep* 34 (5):2782-9. doi: 10.3892/or.2015.4258.

Jin, R., Y. Xia, Q. Chen, W. Li, D. Chen, H. Ye, C. Zhao, X. Du, D. Shi, J. Wu, and G. Liang. 2016. "Da0324, an inhibitor of nuclear factor-kappaB activation, demonstrates selective antitumor activity on human gastric cancer cells." *Drug Des Devel Ther* 10:979-95. doi: 10.2147/DDDT.S90081.

Jyoti, K., R. S. Pandey, P. Kush, D. Kaushik, U. K. Jain, and J. Madan. 2017. "Inhalable bioresponsive chitosan microspheres of doxorubicin and soluble curcumin augmented drug delivery in lung cancer cells." *Int J Biol Macromol* 98:50-58. doi: 10.1016/j.ijbiomac.2017.01.109.

Kalashnikova, I., J. Mazar, C. J. Neal, A. L. Rosado, S. Das, T. J. Westmoreland, and S. Seal. 2017. "Nanoparticle delivery of curcumin induces cellular hypoxia and ROS-mediated apoptosis via modulation of Bcl-2/Bax in human neuroblastoma." *Nanoscale* 9 (29):10375-10387. doi: 10.1039/c7nr02770b.

Kanai, M. 2014. "Therapeutic applications of curcumin for patients with pancreatic cancer." *World J Gastroenterol* 20 (28):9384-91. doi: 10.3748/wjg.v20.i28.9384.

Kaur, G., N. Tirkey, S. Bharrhan, V. Chanana, P. Rishi, and K. Chopra. 2006. "Inhibition of oxidative stress and cytokine activity by curcumin in amelioration of endotoxin-induced experimental hepatoxicity in rodents." *Clin Exp Immunol* 145 (2):313-21. doi: 10.1111/j.1365-2249.2006.03108.x.

Kenfield, S. A., M. J. Stampfer, E. Giovannucci, and J. M. Chan. 2011. "Physical activity and survival after prostate cancer diagnosis in the health professionals follow-up study." *J Clin Oncol* 29 (6):726-32. doi: 10.1200/JCO.2010.31.5226.

Kim, K. C., S. H. Baek, and C. Lee. 2015. "Curcumin-induced downregulation of Axl receptor tyrosine kinase inhibits cell proliferation and circumvents chemoresistance in non-small lung cancer cells." *Int J Oncol* 47 (6):2296-303. doi: 10.3892/ijo.2015.3216.

Kim, K., K. H. Kim, H. Y. Kim, H. K. Cho, N. Sakamoto, and J. Cheong. 2010. "Curcumin inhibits hepatitis C virus replication via suppressing the Akt-SREBP-1 pathway." *FEBS Lett* 584 (4):707-12. doi: 10.1016/j.febslet.2009.12.019.

Koo, J. Y., H. J. Kim, K. O. Jung, and K. Y. Park. 2004. "Curcumin inhibits the growth of AGS human gastric carcinoma cells in vitro and shows synergism with 5-fluorouracil." *J Med Food* 7 (2):117-21. doi: 10.1089/1096620041224229.

Lai, H. W., S. Y. Chien, S. J. Kuo, L. M. Tseng, H. Y. Lin, C. W. Chi, and D. R. Chen. 2012. "The Potential Utility of Curcumin in the Treatment of HER-2-Overexpressed Breast Cancer: An In Vitro and In Vivo Comparison Study with Herceptin." *Evid Based Complement Alternat Med* 2012:486568. doi: 10.1155/2012/486568.

Lee, H. Y., S. W. Kim, G. H. Lee, M. K. Choi, H. W. Jung, Y. J. Kim, H. J. Kwon, and H. J. Chae. 2016. "Turmeric extract and its active compound, curcumin, protect against chronic CCl4-induced liver damage by enhancing antioxidation." *BMC Complement Altern Med* 16 (1):316. doi: 10.1186/s12906-016-1307-6.

Lee, Y. H., N. Y. Song, J. Suh, D. H. Kim, W. Kim, J. Ann, J. Lee, J. H. Baek, H. K. Na, and Y. J. Surh. 2018. "Curcumin suppresses oncogenicity of human colon cancer cells by covalently modifying the cysteine 67 residue of SIRT1." *Cancer Lett* 431:219-229. doi: 10.1016/j.canlet.2018.05.036.

Li, F., X. Chen, B. Xu, and H. Zhou. 2015. "Curcumin induces p53-independent necrosis in H1299 cells via a mitochondria-associated pathway." *Mol Med Rep* 12 (5):7806-14. doi: 10.3892/mmr.2015.4395.

Li, L., B. Ahmed, K. Mehta, and R. Kurzrock. 2007. "Liposomal curcumin with and without oxaliplatin: effects on cell growth, apoptosis, and angiogenesis in colorectal cancer." *Mol Cancer Ther* 6 (4):1276-82. doi: 10.1158/1535-7163.MCT-06-0556.

Li, W., Y. Zhou, J. Yang, H. Li, H. Zhang, and P. Zheng. 2017. "Curcumin induces apoptotic cell death and protective autophagy in human gastric cancer cells." *Oncol Rep* 37 (6):3459-3466. doi: 10.3892/or.2017.5637.

Liang, Z., R. Wu, W. Xie, H. Geng, L. Zhao, C. Xie, J. Wu, S. Geng, X. Li, M. Zhu, W. Zhu, J. Zhu, C. Huang, X. Ma, C. Zhong, and H. Han. 2015. "Curcumin Suppresses MAPK Pathways to Reverse Tobacco Smoke-induced Gastric Epithelial-Mesenchymal Transition in Mice." *Phytother Res* 29 (10):1665-71. doi: 10.1002/ptr.5398.

Liao, H., Z. Wang, Z. Deng, H. Ren, and X. Li. 2015. "Curcumin inhibits lung cancer invasion and metastasis by attenuating GLUT1/MT1-MMP/MMP2 pathway." *Int J Clin Exp Med* 8 (6):8948-57.

Lim, T. G., S. Y. Lee, Z. Huang, D. Y. Lim, H. Chen, S. K. Jung, A. M. Bode, K. W. Lee, and Z. Dong. 2014. "Curcumin suppresses proliferation of colon cancer cells by targeting CDK2." *Cancer Prev Res (Phila)* 7 (4):466-74. doi: 10.1158/1940-6207.CAPR-13-0387.

Lippman, S. M., and E. T. Hawk. 2009. "Cancer prevention: from 1727 to milestones of the past 100 years." *Cancer Res* 69 (13):5269-84. doi: 10.1158/0008-5472.CAN-09-1750.

Liu, G., T. Xiang, Q. F. Wu, and W. X. Wang. 2016. "Curcumin suppresses the proliferation of gastric cancer cells by downregulating H19." *Oncol Lett* 12 (6):5156-5162. doi: 10.3892/ol.2016.5354.

Liu, Q., W. T. Loo, S. C. Sze, and Y. Tong. 2009. "Curcumin inhibits cell proliferation of MDA-MB-231 and BT-483 breast cancer cells mediated by down-regulation of NFkappaB, cyclinD and MMP-1 transcription." *Phytomedicine* 16 (10):916-22. doi: 10.1016/j.phymed.2009.04.008.

Llovet, Josep M., Robin Kate Kelley, Augusto Villanueva, Amit G. Singal, Eli Pikarsky, Sasan Roayaie, Riccardo Lencioni, Kazuhiko Koike, Jessica Zucman-Rossi, and Richard S. Finn. 2021. "Hepatocellular carcinoma." *Nature Reviews Disease Primers* 7 (1):6. doi: 10.1038/s41572-020-00240-3.

Loibl, S., P. Poortmans, M. Morrow, C. Denkert, and G. Curigliano. 2021. "Breast cancer." *Lancet* 397 (10286):1750-1769. doi: 10.1016/S0140-6736(20)32381-3.

Lu, Y., C. Wei, and Z. Xi. 2014. "Curcumin suppresses proliferation and invasion in non-small cell lung cancer by modulation of MTA1-mediated Wnt/beta-catenin pathway." *In Vitro Cell Dev Biol Anim* 50 (9):840-50. doi: 10.1007/s11626-014-9779-5.

Luo, Changjiang, Zhixing Du, Xing Wei, Gang Chen, and Zhongxue Fu. 2015. "Bisdemethoxycurcumin attenuates gastric adenocarcinoma growth by inducing mitochondrial dysfunction." *Oncol Lett* 9 (1):270-274. doi: 10.3892/ol.2014.2685.

Lv, L., Y. Guo, Y. Shen, J. Liu, W. Zhang, D. Zhou, and S. Guo. 2015. "Intracellularly Degradable, Self-Assembled Amphiphilic Block Copolycurcumin Nanoparticles for Efficient In Vivo Cancer Chemotherapy." *Adv Healthc Mater* 4 (10):1496-501, 1423. doi: 10.1002/adhm.201500075.

Mahammedi, H., E. Planchat, M. Pouget, X. Durando, H. Cure, L. Guy, I. Van-Praagh, L. Savareux, M. Atger, M. Bayet-Robert, E. Gadea, C. Abrial, E. Thivat, P. Chollet, and J. C. Eymard. 2016. "The New Combination Docetaxel, Prednisone and Curcumin in Patients with Castration-Resistant Prostate Cancer: A Pilot Phase II Study." *Oncology* 90 (2):69-78. doi: 10.1159/000441148.

Maiti, P., A. Plemmons, and G. L. Dunbar. 2019. "Combination treatment of berberine and solid lipid curcumin particles increased cell death and inhibited PI3K/Akt/mTOR pathway of human cultured glioblastoma cells more effectively than did individual treatments." *PLoS One* 14 (12):e0225660. doi: 10.1371/journal.pone.0225660.

Markham, A. 2021. "Naxitamab: First Approval." *Drugs* 81 (2):291-296. doi: 10.1007/s40265-021-01467-4.

Masuelli, L., M. Benvenuto, M. Fantini, L. Marzocchella, P. Sacchetti, E. Di Stefano, I. Tresoldi, V. Izzi, R. Bernardini, C. Palumbo, M. Mattei, F. Lista, F. Galvano, A. Modesti, and R. Bei. 2013. "Curcumin induces apoptosis in breast cancer cell lines and delays the growth of mammary tumors in neutransgenic mice." *J Biol Regul Homeost Agents* 27 (1):105-19.

Mo, N., Z. Q. Li, J. Li, and Y. D. Cao. 2012. "Curcumin inhibits TGF-beta1-induced MMP-9 and invasion through ERK and Smad signaling in breast cancer MDA- MB-231 cells."*Asian Pac J Cancer Prev* 13 (11):5709-14. doi: 10.7314/apjcp.2012.13.11.5709.

Mock, C. D., B. C. Jordan, and C. Selvam. 2015. "Recent Advances of Curcumin and its Analogues in Breast Cancer Prevention and Treatment." *RSC Adv* 5 (92):75575-75588. doi: 10.1039/C5RA14925H.

Moragoda, L., R. Jaszewski, and A. P. Majumdar. 2001. "Curcumin induced modulation of cell cycle and apoptosis in gastric and colon cancer cells." *Anticancer Res* 21 (2A): 873-8.

Mosieniak, G., M. Adamowicz, O. Alster, H. Jaskowiak, A. A. Szczepankiewicz, G. M. Wilczynski, I. A. Ciechomska, and E. Sikora. 2012. "Curcumin induces permanent growth arrest of human colon cancer cells: link between senescence and autophagy." *Mech Ageing Dev* 133 (6):444-55. doi: 10.1016/j.mad.2012.05.004.

Mudduluru, G., J. N. George-William, S. Muppala, I. A. Asangani, R. Kumarswamy, L. D. Nelson, and H. Allgayer. 2011. "Curcumin regulates miR-21 expression and inhibits invasion and metastasis in colorectal cancer." *Biosci Rep* 31 (3):185-97. doi: 10.1042/BSR20100065.

Nakamura, K., Y. Yasunaga, T. Segawa, D. Ko, J. W. Moul, S. Srivastava, and J. S. Rhim. 2002. "Curcumin down-regulates AR gene expression and activation in prostate cancer cell lines." *Int J Oncol* 21 (4):825-30.

Namkaew, J., T. Jaroonwitchawan, N. Rujanapun, J. Saelee, and P. Noisa. 2018. "Combined effects of curcumin and doxorubicin on cell death and cell migration of SH-SY5Y human neuroblastoma cells." *In Vitro Cell Dev Biol Anim* 54 (9):629-639. doi: 10.1007/s11626-018-0288-9.

Notarbartolo, Monica, Paola Poma, Daniela Perri, Luisa Dusonchet, Melchiorre Cervello, and Natale D'Alessandro. 2005. "Antitumor effects of curcumin, alone or in combination with cisplatin or doxorubicin, on human hepatic cancer cells. Analysis of their possible relationship to changes in NF-kB activation levels and in IAP gene expression." *Cancer Letters* 224 (1):53-65. doi: https://doi.org/10.1016/j.canlet.2004.10.051.

Ohashi, Y., Y. Tsuchiya, K. Koizumi, H. Sakurai, and I. Saiki. 2003. "Prevention of intrahepatic metastasis by curcumin in an orthotopic implantation model." *Oncology* 65 (3):250-8. doi: 10.1159/000074478.

Ohtsu, H., Z. Xiao, J. Ishida, M. Nagai, H. K. Wang, H. Itokawa, C. Y. Su, C. Shih, T. Chiang, E. Chang, Y. Lee, M. Y. Tsai, C. Chang, and K. H. Lee. 2002. "Antitumor agents. 217. Curcumin analogues as novel androgen receptor antagonists with potential as anti-prostate cancer agents." *J Med Chem* 45 (23):5037-42. doi: 10.1021/jm020200g.

Paramita, P., B. W. Wardhani, S. I. Wanandi, and M. Louisa. 2018. "Curcumin for the Prevention of Epithelial-Mesenchymal Transition in Endoxifen-Treated MCF-7 Breast Cancer Cel." *Asian Pac J Cancer Prev* 19 (5):1243-1249. doi: 10.22034/APJCP.2018.19.5.1243.

Parandavar, E., and R. Yazdanparast. 2017. "Differential impact of various reactive oxygen species (ROS) on HIF-1alpha/p53 direct interaction in SK-N-MC neuroblastoma cells." *Cell Biosci* 7:52. doi: 10.1186/s13578-017-0180-4.

Park, E. J., C. H. Jeon, G. Ko, J. Kim, and D. H. Sohn. 2000. "Protective effect of curcumin in rat liver injury induced by carbon tetrachloride." *J Pharm Pharmacol* 52 (4):437-40. doi: 10.1211/0022357001774048.

Park, J. R., A. Eggert, and H. Caron. 2008. "Neuroblastoma: biology, prognosis, and treatment." *Pediatr Clin North Am* 55 (1):97-120, x. doi: 10.1016/j.pcl.2007.10.014.

Patial, V., M. S, S. Sharma, K. Pratap, D. Singh, and Y. S. Padwad. 2015. "Synergistic effect of curcumin and piperine in suppression of DENA-induced hepatocellular carcinoma in rats." *Environ Toxicol Pharmacol* 40 (2):445-52. doi: 10.1016/j.etap.2015.07.012.

Picone, P., D. Nuzzo, L. Caruana, E. Messina, V. Scafidi, and M. Di Carlo. 2014. "Curcumin induces apoptosis in human neuroblastoma cells via inhibition of AKT and Foxo3a nuclear translocation." *Free Radic Res* 48 (12):1397-408. doi: 10.3109/10715762.2014.960410.

Pollack, E. S., A. M. Nomura, L. K. Heilbrun, G. N. Stemmermann, and S. B. Green. 1984. "Prospective study of alcohol consumption and cancer." *N Engl J Med* 310 (10):617-21. doi: 10.1056/NEJM198403083101003.

Prasad, S., S. C. Gupta, A. K. Tyagi, and B. B. Aggarwal. 2014. "Curcumin, a component of golden spice: from bedside to bench and back. "*Biotechnol Adv* 32 (6):1053-64. doi: 10.1016/j.biotechadv.2014.04.004.

Rahman, S., S. Cao, K. J. Steadman, M. Wei, and H. S. Parekh. 2012. "Native and beta-cyclodextrin-enclosed curcumin: entrapment within liposomes and their in vitro cytotoxicity in lung and colon cancer." *Drug Deliv* 19 (7):346-53. doi: 10.3109/10717544.2012.721143.

Rajkumar, P., B. S. Mathew, S. Das, R. Isaiah, S. John, R. Prabha, and D. H. Fleming. 2016. "Cisplatin Concentrations in Long and Short Duration Infusion: Implications for the Optimal Time of Radiation Delivery." *J Clin Diagn Res* 10 (7):XC01-XC04. doi: 10.7860/JCDR/2016/18181.8126.

Rechtman, M. M., O. Har-Noy, I. Bar-Yishay, S. Fishman, Y. Adamovich, Y. Shaul, Z. Halpern, and A. Shlomai. 2010. "Curcumin inhibits hepatitis B virus via down-regulation of the metabolic coactivator PGC-1alpha." *FEBS Lett* 584 (11):2485-90. doi: 10.1016/j.febslet.2010.04.067.

Reyes-Gordillo, K., J. Segovia, M. Shibayama, V. Tsutsumi, P. Vergara, M. G. Moreno, and P. Muriel. 2008. "Curcumin prevents and reverses cirrhosis induced by bile duct obstruction or CCl4 in rats: role of TGF-beta modulation and oxidative stress." *Fundam Clin Pharmacol* 22 (4):417-27. doi: 10.1111/j.1472-8206.2008.00611.x.

Sandhu, S., C. M. Moore, E. Chiong, H. Beltran, R. G. Bristow, and S. G. Williams. 2021. "Prostate cancer." *Lancet* 398 (10305):1075-1090. doi: 10.1016/S0140-6736(21)00950-8.

Sesarman, A., L. Tefas, B. Sylvester, E. Licarete, V. Rauca, L. Luput, L. Patras, M. Banciu, and A. Porfire. 2018. "Anti-angiogenic and anti-inflammatory effects of long-circulating liposomes co-encapsulating curcumin and doxorubicin on C26 murine colon cancer cells." *Pharmacol Rep* 70 (2):331-339. doi: 10.1016/j.pharep.2017.10.004.

Shaik, N. A., H. M. Al-Kreathy, G. M. Ajabnoor, P. K. Verma, and B. Banaganapalli. 2019. "Molecular designing, virtual screening and docking study of novel curcumin analogue as mutation (S769L and K846R) selective inhibitor for EGFR." *Saudi J Biol Sci* 26 (3):439-448. doi: 10.1016/j.sjbs.2018.05.026.

Shakibaei, M., P. Kraehe, B. Popper, P. Shayan, A. Goel, and C. Buhrmann. 2015. "Curcumin potentiates antitumor activity of 5-fluorouracil in a 3D alginate tumor microenvironment of colorectal cancer." *BMC Cancer* 15:250. doi: 10.1186/s12885-015-1291-0.

Shao, Z. M., Z. Z. Shen, C. H. Liu, M. R. Sartippour, V. L. Go, D. Heber, and M. Nguyen. 2002. "Curcumin exerts multiple suppressive effects on human breast carcinoma cells." *Int J Cancer* 98 (2):234-40. doi: 10.1002/ijc.10183.

Shapiro, H., M. Ashkenazi, N. Weizman, M. Shahmurov, H. Aeed, and R. Bruck. 2006. "Curcumin ameliorates acute thioacetamide-induced hepatotoxicity." *J Gastroenterol Hepatol* 21 (2):358-66. doi: 10.1111/j.1440-1746.2005.03984.x.

Sharma, M., R. Manoharlal, N. Puri, and R. Prasad. 2010. "Antifungal curcumin induces reactive oxygen species and triggers an early apoptosis but prevents hyphae development by targeting the global repressor TUP1 in Candida albicans." *Biosci Rep* 30 (6):391-404. doi: 10.1042/BSR20090151.

Shlomai, A., N. Paran, and Y. Shaul. 2006. "PGC-1alpha controls hepatitis B virus through nutritional signals." *Proc Natl Acad Sci USA* 103 (43):16003-8. doi: 10.1073/pnas.0607837103.

Sidhar, H., and R. K. Giri. 2017. "Induction of Bex genes by curcumin is associated with apoptosis and activation of p53 in N2a neuroblastoma cells." *Sci Rep* 7:41420. doi: 10.1038/srep41420.

Siegel, R. L., K. D. Miller, H. E. Fuchs, and A. Jemal. 2021. "Cancer Statistics, 2021." *CA Cancer J Clin* 71 (1):7-33. doi: 10.3322/caac.21654.

Siegel, R. L., K. D. Miller, H. E. Fuchs, and A. Jemal. 2022. "Cancer statistics, 2022." *CA Cancer J Clin* 72 (1):7-33. doi: 10.3322/caac.21708.

Silva, Gabriel, Felipe Teixeira Lima, Viviane Seba, Ana Laura Mendes Lourenço, ThaiseGraminha Lucas, Bianca Vieira De Andrade, Guilherme Silva Torrezan, Carlos Roberto Polaquini, Marcelo Engracia Garcia, Lucélio Bernardes Couto, Reinaldo Bulgarelli Bestetti, Suzelei De Castro França, Ana Lúcia Fachin, Luis Octavio Regasini, and Mozart Marins. 2018. "Curcumin Analog CH-5 Suppresses the Proliferation, Migration, and Invasion of the Human Gastric Cancer Cell Line HGC-27." *Molecules,* 23 (2):279.

Sintara, K., D. Thong-Ngam, S. Patumraj, and N. Klaikeaw. 2012. "Curcumin attenuates gastric cancer induced by N-methyl-N-nitrosourea and saturated sodium chloride in rats." *J Biomed Biotechnol* 2012:915380. doi: 10.1155/2012/915380.

Soliman, M. M., A. A. Baiomy, and M. H. Yassin. 2015. "Molecular and Histopathological Study on the Ameliorative Effects of Curcumin Against Lead Acetate-Induced Hepatotoxicity and Nephrototoxicity in Wistar Rats." *Biol Trace Elem Res* 167 (1):91-102. doi: 10.1007/s12011-015-0280-0.

Somers-Edgar, T. J., M. J. Scandlyn, E. C. Stuart, M. J. Le Nedelec, S. P. Valentine, and R. J. Rosengren. 2008. "The combination of epigallocatechin gallate and curcumin suppresses ER alpha-breast cancer cell growth in vitro and in vivo." *Int J Cancer* 122 (9):1966-71. doi: 10.1002/ijc.23328.

Song, H. C., Y. Chen, Y. Chen, J. Park, M. Zheng, Y. J. Surh, U. H. Kim, J. W. Park, R. Yu, H. T. Chung, and Y. Joe. 2020. "GSK-3beta inhibition by curcumin mitigates amyloidogenesis via TFEB activation and anti-oxidative activity in human neuroblastoma cells." *Free Radic Res* 54 (11-12):918-930. doi: 10.1080/10715762.2020.1791843.

Steinbach, G., P. M. Lynch, R. K. Phillips, M. H. Wallace, E. Hawk, G. B. Gordon, N. Wakabayashi, B. Saunders, Y. Shen, T. Fujimura, L. K. Su, B. Levin, L. Godio, S. Patterson, M. A. Rodriguez-Bigas, S. L. Jester, K. L. King, M. Schumacher, J. Abbruzzese, R. N. DuBois, W. N. Hittelman, S. Zimmerman, J. W. Sherman, and G. Kelloff. 2000. "The effect of celecoxib, a cyclooxygenase-2 inhibitor, in familial adenomatous polyposis." *N Engl J Med* 342 (26):1946-52. doi: 10.1056/NEJM200006293422603.

Su, P., Y. Yang, G. Wang, X. Chen, and Y. Ju. 2018. "Curcumin attenuates resistance to irinotecan via induction of apoptosis of cancer stem cells in chemoresistant colon cancer cells." *Int J Oncol* 53 (3):1343-1353. doi: 10.3892/ijo.2018.4461.

Sukumari-Ramesh, S., J. N. Bentley, M. D. Laird, N. Singh, J. R. Vender, and K. M. Dhandapani. 2011. "Dietary phytochemicals induce p53- and caspase-independent cell death in human neuroblastoma cells." *Int J Dev Neurosci* 29 (7):701-10. doi: 10.1016/j.ijdevneu.2011.06.002.

Sun, C., S. Zhang, C. Liu, and X. Liu. 2019. "Curcumin Promoted miR-34a Expression and Suppressed Proliferation of Gastric Cancer Cells." *Cancer Biother Radiopharm* 34 (10):634-641. doi: 10.1089/cbr.2019.2874.

Sun, Q., W. Zhang, Y. Guo, Z. Li, X. Chen, Y. Wang, Y. Du, W. Zang, and G. Zhao. 2016. "Curcumin inhibits cell growth and induces cell apoptosis through upregulation of miR-33b in gastric cancer." *Tumour Biol* 37 (10):13177-13184. doi: 10.1007/s13277-016-5221-9.

Taniguchi, K., and M. Karin. 2018. "NF-kappaB, inflammation, immunity and cancer: coming of age." *Nat Rev Immunol* 18 (5):309-324. doi: 10.1038/nri.2017.142.

Thai, A. A., B. J. Solomon, L. V. Sequist, J. F. Gainor, and R. S. Heist. 2021. "Lung cancer." *Lancet* 398 (10299):535-554. doi: 10.1016/S0140-6736(21)00312-3.

Thaker, P. H., L. Y. Han, A. A. Kamat, J. M. Arevalo, R. Takahashi, C. Lu, N. B. Jennings, G. Armaiz-Pena, J. A. Bankson, M. Ravoori, W. M. Merritt, Y. G. Lin, L. S. Mangala, T. J. Kim, R. L. Coleman, C. N. Landen, Y. Li, E. Felix, A. M. Sanguino, R. A. Newman, M. Lloyd, D. M. Gershenson, V. Kundra, G. Lopez-Berestein, S. K. Lutgendorf, S. W. Cole, and A. K. Sood. 2006. "Chronic stress promotes tumor growth and angiogenesis in a mouse model of ovarian carcinoma." *Nat Med* 12 (8):939-44. doi: 10.1038/nm1447.

Tiwari, G., R. Tiwari, B. Sriwastawa, L. Bhati, S. Pandey, P. Pandey, and S. K. Bannerjee. 2012. "Drug delivery systems: An updated review." *Int J Pharm Investig* 2 (1):2-11. doi: 10.4103/2230-973X.96920.

Toden, S., Y. Okugawa, T. Jascur, D. Wodarz, N. L. Komarova, C. Buhrmann, M. Shakibaei, C. R. Boland, and A. Goel. 2015. "Curcumin mediates chemosensitization to 5-fluorouracil through miRNA-induced suppression of epithelial-to-mesenchymal transition in chemoresistant colorectal cancer." *Carcinogenesis* 36 (3):355-67. doi: 10.1093/carcin/bgv006.

Tong, W., Q. Wang, D. Sun, and J. Suo. 2016. "Curcumin suppresses colon cancer cell invasion via AMPK-induced inhibition of NF-kappaB, uPA activator and MMP9." *Oncol Lett* 12 (5):4139-4146. doi: 10.3892/ol.2016.5148.

Tsai, J. R., P. L. Liu, Y. H. Chen, S. H. Chou, Y. J. Cheng, J. J. Hwang, and I. W. Chong. 2015. "Curcumin Inhibits Non-Small Cell Lung Cancer Cells Metastasis through the Adiponectin/NF-kappab/MMPs Signaling Pathway." *PLoS One* 10 (12):e0144462. doi: 10.1371/journal.pone.0144462.

Tsui, K. H., T. H. Feng, C. M. Lin, P. L. Chang, and H. H. Juang. 2008. "Curcumin blocks the activation of androgen and interlukin-6 on prostate-specific antigen expression in human prostatic carcinoma cells." *J Androl* 29 (6):661-8. doi: 10.2164/jandrol.108.004911.

Tunc, D., E. Dere, D. Karakas, B. Cevatemre, V. T. Yilmaz, and E. Ulukaya. 2017. "Cytotoxic and apoptotic effects of the combination of palladium (II) 5,5-diethylbarbiturate complex with bis(2-pyridylmethyl)amine and curcumin on non small lung cancer cell lines." *Bioorg Med Chem* 25 (5):1717-1723. doi: 10.1016/j.bmc.2017.01.043.

Uehara, Y., M. Inoue, K. Fukuda, H. Yamakoshi, Y. Hosoi, H. Kanda, M. Oshima, Y. Iwabuchi, and H. Shibata. 2015. "Inhibition of beta-catenin and STAT3 with a curcumin analog suppresses gastric carcinogenesis in vivo." *Gastric Cancer* 18 (4):774-83. doi: 10.1007/s10120-014-0434-3.

Vakilinezhad, M. A., A. Amini, T. Dara, and S. Alipour. 2019. "Methotrexate and Curcumin co-encapsulated PLGA nanoparticles as a potential breast cancer therapeutic system: In vitro and in vivo evaluation." *Colloids Surf B Biointerfaces* 184:110515. doi: 10.1016/j.colsurfb.2019.110515.

Van Cutsem, E., X. Sagaert, B. Topal, K. Haustermans, and H. Prenen. 2016. "Gastric cancer." *Lancet* 388 (10060):2654-2664. doi: 10.1016/S0140-6736(16)30354-3.

Wang, K., T. Zhang, L. Liu, X. Wang, P. Wu, Z. Chen, C. Ni, J. Zhang, F. Hu, and J. Huang. 2012. "Novel micelle formulation of curcumin for enhancing antitumor activity and inhibiting colorectal cancer stem cells." *Int J Nanomedicine* 7:4487-97. doi: 10.2147/IJN.S34702.

Wong, K. E., S. C. Ngai, K. G. Chan, L. H. Lee, B. H. Goh, and L. H. Chuah. 2019. "Curcumin Nanoformulations for Colorectal Cancer: A Review." *Front Pharmacol* 10:152. doi: 10.3389/fphar.2019.00152.

Wu, G. Q., K. Q. Chai, X. M. Zhu, H. Jiang, X. Wang, Q. Xue, A. H. Zheng, H. Y. Zhou, Y. Chen, X. C. Chen, J. Y. Xiao, X. H. Ying, F. W. Wang, T. Rui, Y. J. Liao, D. Xie, L. Q. Lu, and D. S. Huang. 2016. "Anti-cancer effects of curcumin on lung cancer through the inhibition of EZH2 and NOTCH1." *Oncotarget* 7 (18):26535-50. doi: 10.18632/oncotarget.8532.

Wu, J., Z. Cai, X. Wei, M. Chen, S. Ying, L. Shi, R. A. Xu, F. He, G. Liang, and X. Zhang. 2015. "Anti-Lung Cancer Activity of the Curcumin Analog JZ534 In Vitro." *Biomed Res Int* 2015:504529. doi: 10.1155/2015/504529.

Xia, Y., B. Weng, Z. Wang, Y. Kang, L. Shi, G. Huang, S. Ying, X. Du, Q. Chen, R. Jin, J. Wu, and G. Liang. 2016. "W346 inhibits cell growth, invasion, induces cycle arrest and potentiates apoptosis in human gastric cancer cells in vitro through the NF-kappaB signaling pathway." *Tumour Biol* 37 (4):4791-801. doi: 10.1007/s13277-015-4277-2.

Xie, M., D. Fan, Y. Li, X. He, X. Chen, Y. Chen, J. Zhu, G. Xu, X. Wu, and P. Lan. 2017. "Supercritical carbon dioxide-developed silk fibroin nanoplatform for smart colon cancer therapy." *Int J Nanomedicine* 12:7751-7761. doi: 10.2147/IJN.S145012.

Xie, Y. H., Y. X. Chen, and J. Y. Fang. 2020. "Comprehensive review of targeted therapy for colorectal cancer." *Signal Transduct Target Ther* 5 (1):22. doi: 10.1038/s41392-020-0116-z.

Xu, X., D. Chen, B. Ye, F. Zhong, and G. Chen. 2015. "Curcumin induces the apoptosis of non-small cell lung cancer cells through a calcium signaling pathway." *Int J Mol Med* 35 (6):1610-6. doi: 10.3892/ijmm.2015.2167.

Yang, H., S. Huang, Y. Wei, S. Cao, C. Pi, T. Feng, J. Liang, L. Zhao, and G. Ren. 2017. "Curcumin Enhances the Anticancer Effect Of 5-fluorouracil against Gastric Cancer through Down-Regulation of COX-2 and NF- kappaB Signaling Pathways." *J Cancer* 8 (18):3697-3706. doi: 10.7150/jca.20196.

Yao, Junchao, Kebin Zheng, Chunhui Li, Haipeng Liu, and Xiaosong Shan. 2015. "Interference of Notch1 inhibits the growth of glioma cancer cells by inducing cell autophagy and down-regulation of Notch1–Hes-1 signaling pathway." *Medical Oncology* 32 (6):174. doi: 10.1007/s12032-015-0610-2.

Yao, Q., M. Lin, Y. Wang, Y. Lai, J. Hu, T. Fu, L. Wang, S. Lin, L. Chen, and Y. Guo. 2015. "Curcumin induces the apoptosis of A549 cells via oxidative stress and MAPK signaling pathways." *Int J Mol Med* 36 (4):1118-26. doi: 10.3892/ijmm.2015.2327.

Yao, Q. Y., B. L. Xu, J. Y. Wang, H. C. Liu, S. C. Zhang, and C. T. Tu. 2012. "Inhibition by curcumin of multiple sites of the transforming growth factor-beta1 signalling pathway ameliorates the progression of liver fibrosis induced by carbon tetrachloride in rats." *BMC Complement Altern Med* 12:156. doi: 10.1186/1472-6882-12-156.

Ye, M., J. Zhang, J. Zhang, Q. Miao, L. Yao, and J. Zhang. 2015. "Curcumin promotes apoptosis by activating the p53-miR-192-5p/215-XIAP pathway in non-small cell lung cancer." *Cancer Lett* 357 (1):196-205. doi: 10.1016/j.canlet.2014.11.028.

Yoshida, Taichi, Takashi Maruyama, Masatomo Miura, Masahiro Inoue, Koji Fukuda, Kazuhiro Shimazu, Daiki Taguchi, Hiroaki Kanda, Masanobu Oshima, Yoshiharu Iwabuchi, and Hiroyuki Shibata. 2018. "Dietary intake of pyrolyzed deketene curcumin inhibits gastric carcinogenesis." *Journal of Functional Foods* 50:192-200. doi: https://doi.org/10.1016/j.jff.2018.09.033.

Yu, J., X. Zhou, X. He, M. Dai, and Q. Zhang. 2011. "Curcumin induces apoptosis involving bax/bcl-2 in human hepatoma SMMC-7721 cells." *Asian Pac J Cancer Prev* 12 (8):1925-9.

Zhang, C., L. J. He, H. Z. Ye, D. F. Liu, Y. B. Zhu, D. D. Miao, S. P. Zhang, Y. Y. Chen, Y. W. Jia, J. Shen, and X. P. Liu. 2018. "Nrf2 is a key factor in the reversal effect of curcumin on multidrug resistance in the HCT8/5Fu human colorectal cancer cell line." *Mol Med Rep* 18 (6):5409-5416. doi: 10.3892/mmr.2018.9589.

Zhang, J. Y., M. T. Lin, M. J. Zhou, T. Yi, Y. N. Tang, S. L. Tang, Z. J. Yang, Z. Z. Zhao, and H. B. Chen. 2015. "Combinational Treatment of Curcumin and Quercetin against Gastric Cancer MGC-803 Cells in Vitro." *Molecules* 20 (6):11524-34. doi: 10.3390/molecules200611524.

Zhang, K., X. Rui, and X. Yan. 2014. "Curcumin inhibits the proliferation and invasiveness of MHCC97-H cells via p38 signaling pathway." *Drug Dev Res* 75 (7):463-8. doi: 10.1002/ddr.21210.

Zhang, Q., H. Qiao, D. Wu, H. Lu, L. Liu, X. Sang, D. Li, and Y. Zhou. 2019. "Curcumin potentiates the galbanic acid-induced anti-tumor effect in non-small cell lung cancer cells through inhibiting Akt/mTOR signaling pathway." *Life Sci* 239:117044. doi: 10.1016/j.lfs.2019.117044.

Zhang, Z., H. Chen, C. Xu, L. Song, L. Huang, Y. Lai, Y. Wang, H. Chen, D. Gu, L. Ren, and Q. Yao. 2016. "Curcumin inhibits tumor epithelialmesenchymal transition by downregulating the Wnt signaling pathway and upregulating NKD2 expression in colon cancer cells." *Oncol Rep* 35 (5):2615-23. doi: 10.3892/or.2016.4669.

Zhao, Y., X. Ma, J. Wang, X. He, Y. Hu, P. Zhang, R. Wang, R. Li, M. Gong, S. Luo, and X. Xiao. 2014. "Curcumin protects against CCl4-induced liver fibrosis in rats by inhibiting HIF-1alpha through an ERK-dependent pathway." *Molecules* 19 (11):18767-80. doi: 10.3390/molecules191118767.

Zhen, L., D. Fan, X. Yi, X. Cao, D. Chen, and L. Wang. 2014. "Curcumin inhibits oral squamous cell carcinoma proliferation and invasion via EGFR signaling pathways." *Int J Clin Exp Pathol* 7 (10):6438-46.

Zhou, G. Z., F. K. Cao, and S. W. Du. 2015. "The apoptotic pathways in the curcumin analog MHMD-induced lung cancer cell death and the essential role of actin polymerization during apoptosis." *Biomed Pharmacother* 71:128-34. doi: 10.1016/j.biopha.2015.02.025.

Zhou, G. Z., Y. Y. Shi, L. L. Wei, and G. C. Sun. 2019. "Autophagy induction and antiproliferative effect of a novel curcumin derivative MOMI-1 on the human lung cancer cells A549." *J Biochem Mol Toxicol* 33 (4):e22280. doi: 10.1002/jbt.22280.

Zhou, G. Z., Q. Q. Wang, P. B. Wang, Z. C. Wang, and G. C. Sun. 2019. "One novel curcumin derivative ZYX01 induces autophagy of human non-small lung cancer cells A549 through AMPK/ULK1/Beclin-1 signaling pathway." *Cell Mol Biol (Noisy-le-grand)* 65 (2):1-6.

Zhou, S., D. Yao, L. Guo, and L. Teng. 2017. "Curcumin suppresses gastric cancer by inhibiting gastrin-mediated acid secretion." *FEBS Open Bio* 7 (8):1078-1084. doi: 10.1002/2211-5463.12237.

Zhu, J. Y., X. Yang, Y. Chen, Y. Jiang, S. J. Wang, Y. Li, X. Q. Wang, Y. Meng, M. M. Zhu, X. Ma, C. Huang, R. Wu, C. F. Xie, X. T. Li, S. S. Geng, J. S. Wu, C. Y. Zhong, and H. Y. Han. 2017. "Curcumin Suppresses Lung Cancer Stem Cells via Inhibiting Wnt/beta-catenin and Sonic Hedgehog Pathways." *Phytother Res* 31 (4):680-688. doi: 10.1002/ptr.5791.

Zhu, J., B. Zhao, P. Xiong, C. Wang, J. Zhang, X. Tian, and Y. Huang. 2018. "Curcumin Induces Autophagy via Inhibition of Yes-Associated Protein (YAP) in Human Colon Cancer Cells." *Med Sci Monit* 24:7035-7042. doi: 10.12659/MSM.910650.

Zou, P., Y. Xia, T. Chen, J. Zhang, Z. Wang, W. Chen, M. Chen, K. Kanchana, S. Yang, and G. Liang. 2016. "Selective killing of gastric cancer cells by a small molecule targeting ROS-mediated ER stress activation." *Mol Carcinog* 55 (6):1073-86. doi: 10.1002/mc.22351.

Chapter 2

Curcumin as a Natural Systemic Disease Modulator

Sohair Aly Hassan[1]
Noha N. Nasr[1]
and Afaf Al Ansary[2]
[1]Therapeutic Chemistry Department, Pharmaceutical & Drug Industries Research Institute, National Research Center, Cairo, Egypt.
[2]Lotus Holistic Alternative Medical Center, URA, Abu Dhabi, United Arab Emirates

Abstract

In the prevention and treatment of various diseases, a variety of preparations based on medicinal plants are now generally acknowledged and well-documented. The main advantages of traditional medicine in underdeveloped nations are safety and affordability. As diferuloyl-methane, curcumin is a naturally occurring polyphenol that is mostly produced in the rhizomes of plant roots. Curcumin has a long history of usage in conventional medicine, although its therapeutic effects and health advantages are still little understood. The therapeutic benefits of curcumin include the treatment of malignancies, neurodegenerative, ocular, and COVID diseases as well as inflammatory and digestive disorders, rheumatic and skin issues, and tumors. Apoptosis-related genes, cytokines, enzymes, and other targets have all been found in certain studies to be modulated by curcumin. Furthermore, little is known about the biological mechanisms that underlie these activities. We will examine some of the known molecular targets and biological processes of curcumin in this chapter. The processes through which curcumin functions in neuroprotection and/or mental health disorders will be

In: Curcumin and Its Role in Health and Disease
Editor: Kathryn Woltjer
ISBN: 979-8-88697-491-1

covered in this chapter. We will also talk about curcumin's protective role in how bone may impact neurological function.

Keywords: neurodegeneration, inflammation, antioxidants, bone, skin, eye disorder, COVID

Abbreviations

AchE	Acetyl choline esterase
PGC1α	Activated receptor gamma co activator
AD	Alzheimer's disease
APP	Amyloid precursor protein
BBB)	Blood brain barrier
BDNE	Brain derived neurotropic factor
COX-2	Cyclooxygenase-2
DHC	Dihydrocurcumin
EV	Endovenously
ER	Estrogen receptor
ERK1	Extracellular signal-regulated kinase
GFAP	Glial fibrillary acidic protein
GSK-3	Glycogen synthase kinase -3
HDL	High density lipoprotein
HER 2	Human epidermal growth factor receptor
ICAM-1	Intercellular adhesion molecule-l
IL-6	Interleukin
IP	Intraperitoneal
MMP-9	Matrix metalloproteinase 9
TFAM	Mitochondrial transcription factor A
NIRF	Near infrared fluorescence
NFT	Neurofibrillary tangles
NSAID	Non-steroidal anti-inflammatory drugs
NrF-2	Nuclear erythroid2-related factor-2
NFkB	Nuclear factor kappa-B
NrF-1	Nuclear respiratory factor-1
PPS	Peroxisome proliferator
PGC-1α	Peroxisome proliferator-activated receptor gamma coactivator
PPARs	Peroxisome proliferator-activated receptors

PET	Positron emission tomography
PSD95	Postsynaptic density protein 95
RNS	Reactive nitrogen species
ROS	Reactive oxygen species
PSD95	Synaptophysin and postsynaptic density protein 95
THC	Tetrahydrocurcumin
TNF-α	Tumor necrosis factor alpha
TK	Tyrosine kinas
VCAM-1	Vascular cell adhesion molecule-l

Introduction

The primary biologically active phytochemical in turmeric, a member of the family, is curcumin. The botanical family Curcuma (Family Zingiberaceae). Numerous research conducted over the past 50 years has shown that curcumin protects against practically all types of bodily illnesses. The chemical is known to have various beneficial effects, including those that are antibacterial, anti-inflammatory, antitumor antihyperlipidemic, antihypertensive, anticancer, antiphlogistic, antidiabetic, antipsoriasis, antihepatotoxic, and antithrombotic. The chemical is known to have neuroprotective effects in addition to its protective impact in peripheral organ diseases (Figure 1) Kulkami et al., (2009). Curcumin's polar shape and low molecular weight make it effective at crossing the blood-brain barrier. Curcumin has been shown to improve adult hippocampus neurogenesis in animal experiments by boosting the number of newly formed cells in the dentate gyrus area of the hippocampus. Additionally, it is a strong inhibitor of reactive astrocyte expression, preventing the death of hippocampal cells brought on by kainic acid. Chen et al. (2008). Low dosages of curcumin have been discovered in one recent study to successfully disaggregate beta amyloid and prevent the production of fibrils and oligomers, making it protective in the treatment of Alzheimer's disease Kulkami et al., (2009). Curcumin has been proven to be protective in animal models of seizures in a number of experimental studies. The chemical prevents rat amygdaloid-induced epileptic convulsions. DU et al. (2009), Jyoti et al. (2009), and electroshock seizures in mice Bharal et al. (2008) are examples of iron-induced experimental models of palatogenesis. Curcumin has also been shown to have antidepressant effects in animal models of depression. Curcumin's potential as an antidepressant has been the subject of exponentially growing recent research. The chemical is helpful in chronic unexpected stress and forced swimming tests. Bhutani et al., (2009). Curcumin has depressive properties through controlling serotonin and dopamine release. The level of neurotrophic substances like brain derived neurotropic factor is increased by curcumin (BDNF) Wang et al., (2008). Curcumin has a fascinating application in the management of diabetic neuropathy. According to Sharma et al. (2007), curcumin increases insulin's ability to reduce blood sugar levels and guards against the development of diabetic neuropathy in animal models of tardive dyskinesia, curcumin has proven to have neuroprotective effects.

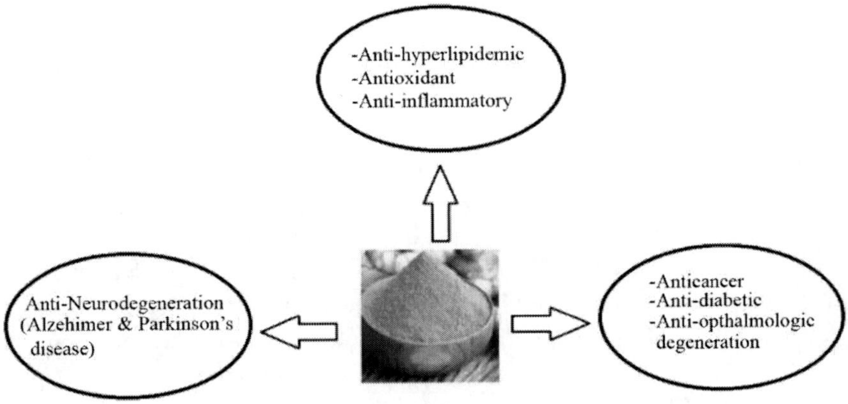

Figure 1. Therapeutic inclusions of curcumin in several human disorders.

Pharmacodynamics, Bio Viability and Formulations of Curcumin

Little has been done to date to utilize Curcumin's medicinal potential because of low oral bioavailability, which is attributed most to its restricted absorption, high digestion and metabolism and also fast body organ exclusion. Second, curcumin does not dissolve well in water (around 11 ng/mL), but it degrades quickly in an acidic milieu. Douglass et al., (2015), Anand et al., (2007) in the intestinal tract, Curcumin undergoes glucuronidation in the intestinal mucosa, inactivating it. Following a first-pass effect reduction to form dihydro-curcumin (DHC), tetrahydrocurcumin (THC), and hexahydro-curcumin, curcumin is subsequently conjugated to glucuronides and sulphates in the liver before being excreted in urine, Purpura et al., (2018). The highest plasma concentrations achieved following oral dose were 0.051 mg/mL from 12 g

Curcumin in humans, 0.22 mg/mL from 1 g/kg in mice, and 1.35 mg/mL from 2 g/kg in rats, according to numerous pharmacokinetic studies carried out in humans and rodents, Stohs et al., (2018). Panda et al. (2018), found that the bioavailability of curcumin when taken orally was just 1%, which is significantly less than what may be accomplished when administered endovenously (EV) and intraperitoneally (IP), Howe et al., (2018). Various formulations are available to promote bioavailability and bio-efficacy. Curcumin delivery mechanisms have been described for micelles, liposomes, phospholipid complexes, microemulsions, nano-emulsions, emulsions, solid lipid nanoparticles, nanostructured lipid carriers, biopolymer nanoparticles, and microgels. They maximize small intestinal penetration and prevent potential gastrointestinal tract degradation, which not only increases effectiveness, but also increases curcumin bioavailability. Yavarpour-Bali et al., (2019), Kharat et al., (2019). The numerous formulations developed to increase curcumin bioavailability can be divided into an expanded categories using specific examples. Taking curcumin along with a fatty meal enhances absorption because curcumin is soluble in fat. Adding turmeric oil (BCM-95®; BioCurcumax®; CurcugreenTM), according to Sunagawa et al., (2015). was one of the earliest ways to improve absorption further to stimulate the digestive system and stop curcumin efflux, a little amount of piperine (Curcumin C3 Complex®) is used, as is turmeric oleoresin (CurcugenTM), which has resulted to minor incremental gains in absorption. In more recent formulations, curcumin has been adsorbing and dispersing onto numerous matrices, including whey protein (CurcuminPro®), rice flour, stearic acid, silica, and magnesium stearate (Curcu FreshTM), and microcrystalline cellulose mixed with soy lecithin phosphatidylcholine (Meriva) (Micronized Curcumin) Purpura et al., (2018). Utilizing widely used excipients that are known to enhance curcumin's solubility and shield it from degradation by the alkaline environment of the small intestine, a novel curcumin formulation was created. Micelles, liposomes, phospholipid complexes, microemulsions, nano-emulsions, emulsions, solid lipid nanoparticles, nanostructured lipid carriers, biopolymer nanoparticles, and microgels are the most promising delivery systems. They increase plasma half-life, decrease possible degradation in the microenvironment, increase small intestine permeability, and enhance curcumin efficacy to increase efficacy and curcumin bioavailability. Yavarpour-Bali et al. (2020), Gera et al., (2017) & Kharat et al. (2019). On the other hand, a number of formulations have made use of various techniques to reduce particle size, including the incorporation of curcumin in liquid droplet nano-micelles containing lauroyl polyoxy 32-glycerides (Gelucire®) and polysorbate 20 (BioCurc®) Stohs et al., (2018), fenugreek-derived galactomannan fibre (CurQfen®) Kumar et al., (2016).

Curcumin's Therapeutic Impact in Oxidative Stress and Inflammation in Different Metabolic and Neurodegenerative Disorder Diseases

Over 18,000 regular papers, reviews, and meta-analyses addressing the possible health benefits of curcumin have been published, with half of them appearing in the previous seven years (after 2014), according to a recent bibliometric analysis of the literature Yeung et al., (2019) towards several chronic illnesses (such as inflammatory and oxidative stress-related diseases, diabetes, cancer, skin, eye, microbiological, cardiovascular, and neurological disorders), as well as other ailments. Although its exact mode of action and bioavailability in different target tissues are still unknown, it has been demonstrated to be active in practically all major organs in vivo. Cardiovascular disease risk is increased by obesity. Kim et al. (2016), and Lee et al. (2013). Patients who are obese emit more pro-inflammatory adipocytokines like TNF-alpha and IL-6, whereas bigger mast cells in visceral adipose tissue limit the release of anti-inflammatory adipocytokines. Schmidt et al., (2015). Numerous mice studies have been conducted to examine the effects of curcumin on obesity models. In a mouse model of obesity brought on by a high-fat diet and a mouse model of hereditary obesity, curcumin decreased macrophage infiltration of adipose tissue, increased production of adiponectin (which has anti-inflammatory and anti-atherosclerotic properties), and suppressed adipose tissue inflammation, Zhao et al., (2017). It highly improved the lipid profile in serum, (including total cholesterol, LDL& HDL – cholesterol and triglycerides levels and free fatty acids) according to Pan et al., (2017), in an experimental obesity model. Additionally, curcumin boosted adipose triglyceride lipase. In obese mice, curcumin also reduced lipids and improved glycolipid metabolism. Zhao et al. (2017). Through percutaneous absorption, curcumin treatment increased serum leptin levels and decreased adipose tissue volume to levels similar to those of normal rats. Reza Ariamoghaddam et al., (2018) reported nonalcoholic steatohepatitis in 84 overweight or obese patients, and Jazayeri-Tehrani et al. (2019) recorded a downregulation in each of the hypersensitivity, TNF-alpha, IL-6, and LDL cholesterol levels as well as an increase in HDL cholesterol levels in the blood.

Additionally, the rate of absorption was raised. Patients taking nanocurcumin had better outcomes than those taking turmeric, according to notable studies.

Curcumin against Cancers, and Neurodegeneration

Cancer cells are identified by faulty signaling pathways regulating proliferation, apoptosis, and. Antiestrogens are frequently used as the main treatment because estrogen receptor (ER) positive breast cancer accounts for more than 70% of cases. However, mounting evidence indicates that the best course of action in a breast cancer scenario is a combination of various medications. NF-B, a transcription factor that promotes inflammation, is important for the growth of breast cancer cells. It regulates more than 500 different genes and influences the expression of proteins participating in cellular signaling pathways, resulting in the progress of malignancies and inflammation. Curcumin displayed the ability to affect the breast cancer cell proliferation and invasion by downregulating the NF-κB inducing genes Liu et al., (2009, Kim, et al., (2012), Curcumin, alone or when combined with its analogues, may affect positively the breast cancer cell lines though inhibiting the human epidermal growth factor receptor 2 (HER2) or tyrosine kinase (TK) receptor (HER2-TK), Yim-im et al., (2014). On the other hand, Catania et al. (2013) claim that Immune-liposome encapsulation boosted the selectivity and specificity of its anti-HER2 activity. Changes (mutation and amplification) in the protein kinase B, known as Akt, are linked to carcinogenesis. Tan et al., (2014) discovered that mTor (kinase) interacted with Akt to regulate cancer cell growth and proliferation. Curcumin inhibited the Akt protein in breast cancer cells in a dose and time-dependent manner, induced autophagy, and may block the ubiquitin-proteasome pathway (Guan et al., (2016). Curcumin is also known to cause apoptosis and autophagy in breast cancer cells by blocking the PI3K/Akt signalling pathway Akkoç et al., (2015). When coupled with a PI3K inhibitor, curcumin has also been found to trigger apoptosis in MCF-7 cells, implying a synergistic effect Jia et al., (2014).

Neurological Diseases (Alzheimer)

Many age-related severe illnesses are characterized by neurodegeneration. Alzheimer's disease (AD) is the most prevalent neurodegenerative disease, accounting for 60-70% of dementia cases, Duthey (2013); Erkkinen et al.,

(2018). Symptoms of Alzheimer's disease include a decline in cognitive ability, followed by a decline in social and behavioral functioning. The major histological characteristics of Alzheimer's disease are amyloid- (A) plaques, which are caused by alterations in the proteolytic processing of amyloid precursor protein (APP), and neurofibrillary tangles (NFTs), which are caused by hyper-phosphorylation of the tau protein (AD) (Hardy and Selkoe, 2002). There are currently no medical treatments available to prevent or cure cognitive deterioration. Even though existing Alzheimer's disease cognitive enhancers, such as donepezil and galantamine, may prevent cognitive decline, many patients do not respond to the treatment, the beneficial effect is ephemeral, and it is accompanied with a number of undesirable side effects. A increasing body of evidence suggests that neuroinflammation, mitochondrial dysfunction, oxidative stress, or autophagy are possible causes of Alzheimer's disease. Amor et al., (2014); Amor et al., (2010); Guo et al., (2018); Kim et al., (2014). It has been discovered that those who regularly use nonsteroidal anti-inflammatory drugs (NSAIDs) have a considerably decreased risk of developing Alzheimer's disease (AD), Stewart et al., (1997). But NSAID toxicity for gastrointestinal seem to be a marked weakness (Lim et al., (2001). As a result, it is widely acknowledged that developing new, safer and more effective pharmaceutical treatments with wide range of biological and pharmacological effects, including anti-inflammatory, antioxidant, neuroprotective, and chemoprotective qualities. Hewlings & Kalman, (2017). Curcumin with its anti-inflammatory activity is associated with the inhibition of inflammatory cytokines such as tumor necrosis factor-alpha (TNF-a) and interleukin (IL) -1, -2, -6, -8, and -12 via nuclear factor kappa B (NF-B) downregulation. Curcumin's antioxidant activity stems from its capacity to scavenge free radicals such as reactive oxygen and nitrogen species (ROS and RNS). Alisi et al., (2018). Curcumin has been shown in multiple studies in rodents and humans to cross the blood brain barrier (BBB). (Reddy et al., 2018; Dende et al., 2017). The main drawback is that it has a low bioavailability due to poor solubility, low absorption, rapid metabolism, and rapid elimination. Different formulations such as liposomal encapsulation, nanoparticles, powder form, micellar form, emulsions, co-administration with other substances, or separate administration of its contents were accepted solutions. According to the Joint Nations and World Health Organization Expert Committee on Food Additives (JECFA), curcumin is safe nutritional food compound and can be consumed on a daily basis. Tello-Franco et al., (2013). Moreover, curcumin has unusual photophysical properties because it includes two phenols linked by a linear -diketone linker. In particular,

Curcumin binds to βA plaques with the emission of a highly fluorescent signal, making it an important diagnostic tool for AD, including in the use of two-photon microscopy, near-infrared fluorescence (NIRF), positron emission tomography (PET) and magnetic resonance imaging (MRI) Goozee et al., (2016), Tu et al., (2015). Curcumin decreases βA levels, deposits, and aggregation by reducing the degree to which it self-assembles and by inducing the disaggregation of fibrillar Aβ40 Garcia-Alloza et al., (2007), Yang et al., (2005), Reddy et al. (2018). It also inhibits the formation of fibrillar βA and destabilizes fibrillar Aβ40 and Aβ42 in vitro, showing a protective effect to βA toxicity, Park and Kim., (2002), Ono et al., (2004). Curcumin also helps in protecting mitochondria from the toxic effects of βA: for instance, it reduces oxidative stress in PC12 caused by βA Kim et al., (2001) and reduces brain IL1β and oxidized proteins in APP mice. Curcumin pretreatment prevents βA-induced toxicity in human neuroblastoma cells (SH-SY5Y), increasing the levels of mRNA and proteins for mitochondria biogenesis genes, such as nuclear respiratory factor 1 (Nrf1), nuclear erythroid 2-related factor 2 (Nrf2), peroxisome proliferator-activated receptor gamma coactivator (PGC)1α, mitochondrial transcription factor A (TFAM) and synaptophysin and postsynaptic density protein 95 (PSD95) Lim et al., (2001). Curcumin can also inhibit glycogen synthase kinase-3 (GSK-3), which regulates the phosphorylation of tau Jope et al., (2007) and protects cells from tau induced neurotoxicity, Di Martino et al., (2016). No NDs (AD included) exist without microglia activation Bottai et al., (2019); indeed, it has been demonstrated that βA reroutes microglia from their neuroprotective phenotype to their neurotoxic phenotype Cai et al., (2014). Because during βA accumulation the microglia and the inflammatory mediators are activated, further βA accumulation and neuroinflammation are induced. Curcumin blocks extracellular signal-regulated kinase 2 (ERK1/2) and p38 kinase signaling in βA-activated microglia in vitro, reducing the synthesis of IL1β, tumor necrosis factor α (TNFα), IL6 mRNAs and proteins Shi et al., (2015). Interestingly, Cur has an inhibitory effect on AChE like many drugs used in AD therapy; however, currently, no studies on Cur inhibition of AChE have been performed in the context of AD cell or animal models Tang et al., (2017). In vivo studies, though, have confirmed the protective effect of Cur in AD. It was demonstrated in a rat model of AD induced by intracerebroventricular injection of streptozotocin (ICV-STZ) that Cur can reduce the deficits in the object recognition test by decreasing neuroinflammation and increasing adult neurogenesis Bassani et al., (2017). Moreover, in a mouse model of AD, Cur treatment caused suppression of the neuroinflammatory response, decreasing the levels of inflammatory molecules such as IL1β, TNFα, cyclooxygenase 2 (COX 2) and nitric oxide (NO) while also decreasing the number of glial fibrillary acidic protein (GFAP) and Iba-1-positive cells, probably because of the promotion of peroxisome proliferator-activated receptor (PPAR)γ activity. Many clinical trials investigating the effects of Cur in Alzheimer's disease are now underway One of the first trials to evaluate the benefits of Cur on Alzheimer's disease patients began in 2004 (NCT00164749); it was pilot research (phase 1) that investigated the effects of Cur in better-absorbed powder or capsule formulations. Liu et al., (2016). It has been shown recently in an animal model of AD that Cur can moderate or reverse memory impairment with no placebo effect which has stimulated the continuation of studies on humans.

Curcumin and Parkinson's Disease (PD)

The second most common neurodegenerative disease Parkinson's disease (PD) comes after Alzheimer's (AD). It was previously known as Shaking Palsy before being renamed Parkinson's disease in 1817 by Jean-Marie Charcot Parkinson. (2002). PD is a multisystem illness rather than a disease, with considerable neuropathological degradation of SNpc dopaminergic neurons and their striatal terminals. There is presently no treatment that can cure or slow the progression of Parkinson's disease. Levodopa (L-3,4-dihydroxyphenylalanine) was launched in the 1960s as a dopamine (DA) prodrug that increases intracerebral DA concentration since the dopaminergic system in the brain is primarily malfunctioning. However, after several months to years of L-dopa medication, patients experience side effects such as dyskinesias, Pandey and Srivanitchapoom (2017). Curcumin's ability to change and interact with a wide range of cell signaling pathways and proteins strongly suggests that it is a multi-targeted pharmacological symptomatic approach). Curcumins have been demonstrated to change the functioning of various signal transduction pathways, which has been linked to a slower course of disease. Curcumin interacts with transcription factors such as transcription factor (STAT) proteins Shishodia et al., (2007), growth factors and their receptors such as epidermal growth factor receptors and HER2, Golonko et al. (2019), cytokines such as interleukin 1b (IL-1b), interleukin 6 (IL-6), Palizgir et al. (2018), enzymes such as hemox (HO-1), Mhillaj, et al. (2019), and some genes that control and regulate cell proliferation and apoptosis.

Curcumin in Ischemic Stroke and Mode of Action

The most common type of stroke is ischemic stroke, which is associated with a high mortality and morbidity rate. Early blood supply restoration to ischemic tissues is a current effective treatment strategy that improves energy metabolism, oxygen supply, and neurological outcomes. Currently, recombinant tissue plasminogen activator (r-TPA) is utilised for thrombolytic therapy; nevertheless, it should be administered within 4.5 hours of the start of stroke; yet, only 3-5% of stroke patients satisfy the criteria and use r-TPA on time. Campbell et al., 2019; Campbell and Khatri, 2020), the damage caused by cerebral ischemia and reperfusion involves oxidative stress, apoptosis, the inflammatory response, BBB destruction, and energy metabolism disorder, among other pathological mechanisms. As a result, curcumin was nominated as a natural element with various targets. In recent years, curcumin has been introduced in various formulations such as liposomes, nanoparticles, and microemulsion as carriers to boost its solubility, stability, and safety, as well as considerably manage its biological activity in treating or lowering diseases, showing great promise for clinical application. Curcumin has recently been found to have neuroprotective properties against a wide range of neurological conditions, including neuropsychiatric disorders, neurodegenerative diseases, spinal cord injury, traumatic brain injury, and epilepsy (Dhir, 2018; Bhat et al., 2019; Yavarpour-Bali et al., 2019; Yuan et al., 2019; Farkhondeh et al., 2020; Nebrisi, 2021; Lamanna-Rama et al., 2022). Neurotransmitter mediation and the hypothalamus-pituitary-adrenal cortical axis, neurotrophic factor release, and nerve regeneration promotion may be engaged, impacting a variety of signaling cascades, promoting neuronal viability and differentiation, and eventually improving neurological functioning.

Curcumin's Mode of Action in Cerebral Ischemia Injury as an Antioxidant and Anti-Inflammatory

Disruption of equilibrium between oxidative and antioxidant systems is a key player mechanism in brain ischemia damage. (Li et al., 2018; Torres Cuevas et al., 2019). Following brain ischemia, reactive oxygen species (ROS) either directly or indirectly induce a variety of pathogenic processes, Fraser, (2011); Orellana-Urzú a et al., (2020). Brain tissues have a higher metabolic rate, a greater requirement for oxygen and polyunsaturated fatty acids, and fewer antioxidant enzymes than other organs, the mater which make the central nervous system more vulnerable to oxidative damage. (Cenini et al., 2019; Torres-Cuevas et al., 2019; Bhatt et al., 2020). As a powerful antioxidant, Curcumin promotes the removal of reactive oxygen species (ROS) by activating antioxidant enzymes and decreasing oxidative stress-induced brain tissue damage. Mukherjee et al., (2019); Zhang et al., (2021). Namgyal et al., (2021). Curcumin pretreatment and post-treatment administration both improved the antioxidative ability of the injured neurons (Wu et al., 2015). Both pretreatment with curcumin and posttreatment with curcumin increased the antioxidative abilities of the damaged neurons. Curcumin treatment, both immediate and delayed (24 h after ischemia), reduced ischemia-induced neuronal damage and oxidative stress, showing the wide time window of curcumin treatment in cerebral ischemia. (Al-Omar et al., 2006). As mentioned Curcumin was found to have the most powerful antioxidant activity in a comparative investigation of three curcuminoids (curcumin, demethoxycurcumin, and bisdemethoxycurcumin) employing a polymeric N-isopropyl acrylamide nanoparticle formulation. (Ahmad et al., 2013).

Further, Curcumin can manage the inflammatory response following brain ischemia via several modes. Curcumin, for example, can inhibit the production and release of inflammatory cytokines such as IL-6, IL-1, TNF-, and COX 2. (Zhang Y. et al., 2017; Wicha et al., 2017). Curcuminoids also reduce neutrophil rolling and adherence to the cerebrovascular endothelium, lower neutrophil numbers, and block neutrophil activation, all of which help to alleviate ischemic brain injury. Funk et al., (2013). NF-B is a transcriptional factor that is activated after cerebral ischemia and contributes in the transcription of important target genes that contribute to the inflammatory response. Numerous studies have shown that curcumin's anti-inflammatory impact in cerebral ischemia is closely related to NF-B regulation. Li et al., (2017); Li et al., (2021). Curcumin, according to Ran et al., (2021), can reduce white matter damage after an ischemic stroke in a rat stroke model by suppressing NF-B and inhibiting the NLRP3 inflammasome. While triblock copolymer nanomicelles containing curcumin have an anti-inflammatory effect following brain ischemia by inhibiting the NF-B pathway, Li et al., (2021). Additional researches recognized the anti-inflammatory impact of curcumin in cerebral ischemia is mediated by the inhibition of the TLR4/MyD88/MAPK/NFκB, TLR2/NF-κB, and PPAR γ/NF-κB pathways (Liu et al., 2013; Wang C. et al., 2020), and tightly associated with the modulation of NF-κB Li et al., (2017) Li et al., (2021) in cerebral ischemia.

Cellular Apoptosis and Autophagy Mechanisms of Curcumin

Cell necrosis and apoptosis coexist in the immediate stage of cerebral ischemia, while apoptosis is the primary kind of delayed cell death post-stroke, according to one study. Indeed, following the commencement of the stroke, necrosis occurs mostly in the ischemic core region, whereas apoptosis occurs primarily in the ischemic penumbra. (Ueda and Fujita, 2004; Radak et al., 2017). The mechanisms that mediate ischemic stroke-induced apoptosis mainly include the mitochondrial and endoplasmic reticulum stress and death receptor pathway, Cao et al., (2001) & (Iurlaro and Muñoz-Pinedo, 2016). Curcumin's particular method for reducing apoptosis following cerebral ischemia is well-established. Exosomes containing curcumin target ischemic brain tissues and reduce ROS-mediated mitochondrial death, (He et al., 2020). Curcumin can also reduce ischemia-induced brain injury and cell death by suppressing CCL3, increasing GLUT1 and GLUT3, inactivating the TLR4/MyD88/MAPK/NF-B and Wnt/JNK1 pathways, and promoting MEK/ERK/CREB and PI3K/Akt pathway activation. Xu L. et al., (2019); Wang C. et al., (2020); Wu et al., (2020); Zhou et al., (2020). demonstrated that a combination of curcumin and vagus nerve stimulation reversed behavioral impairments following brain ischemia by suppressing apoptosis via the Akt/ERK2 pathway. Curcumin, in particular, prevents cellular damage and death by lowering endoplasmic reticulum stress (ERS) (Cheng et al., 2020; Zhou et al., 2022). Curcumin was found to reduce hypoxia-induced ERS-mediated cell death in mouse hippocampus cells by increasing Prdx6 expression and reducing NF-B activation. *In another mechanism through which curcumin can act is autophagy.* Autophagy is a common phenomenon in eukaryotic animals in which cells phagocytose their own cellular components into vesicles, which then fuse with lysosomes to produce autophagolysosomes, which then breakdown to sustain cell metabolism and organelle renewal (Mizushima and Komatsu, 2011). Under extreme conditions such as ischemia and hypoxia, it is essential for cell survival and intracellular homeostasis; nevertheless, excessive autophagy may promote cell death Choi et al., (2018). So far, the researchers have identified more than 30 autophagy-related genes that are involved in autophagy regulation. Autophagy is known to be activated by cerebral ischemia. The role and mechanism of autophagy in cerebral ischemia, however, remain unknown, Wang et al., (2021). Autophagy's influence and effect may be affected by the degree of ischemic injury and the length of ischemia, Hou et al., (2022). Many studies have shown that curcumin reduces brain ischemia injury by promoting autophagy. Curcumin can protect the brain by reducing overactive autophagy, resulting in a lower LC3-II/LC3-I ratio. Zhang et al., (2018). Other studies believe that curcumin reduces cerebral ischemia-reperfusion injury through enhancing mitophagy, as evidenced by an increased LC3-II/LC3-I ratio. (Wang and Xu, 2020).

Curcumin and Microglia Cerebral Ischemia

Under physiological conditions, microglia are working as an immune monitor and defender in the microenvironment of brain cells. In the diseased state, they are rapidly activated and polarized Hu et al., (2015); Ma et al., (2017). Following the incipience of cerebral ischemia, microglia start to perform a differential job dealing with the cerebral insult via M1, M2 polarization as a neuroprotection, Xue et al., (2021). M1 microglia are cytotoxic and generate inflammation in the tissues, whereas M2 microglia are neuroprotective and promote tissue repair and regeneration. During cerebral ischemia, these cells concentrate in the ischemic area and release inflammatory chemicals that boost the inflammatory response. Surprisingly, curcumin has a powerful regulatory effect on microglial responses, altering the microglial phenotype from pro-inflammatory M1 to anti-inflammatory and tissue-reparative M2 and suppressing microglia-mediated pro-inflammatory responses (Hu et al., 2012). Curcumin decreases inflammation through the suppression of M1 microglial activation and by reducing the increase in TNF- and IL-1 in both in vivo MCAO and in vitro OGD models (Liu et al., 2017; Wang et al., 2019).

Curcumin and Integrity of the BBB in Cerebral Ischemia

The BBB is made up mostly of cerebral microvascular endothelial cells, astrocytes, the basal lamina, and pericytes. The major purpose of the BBB is to inhibit macromolecule diffusion into the brain parenchyma and to maintain the stability of the nervous system's internal environment. (Huber et al., 2001; Obermeier et al., 2016; Langen et al., 2019; Alahmari, 2021). Following cerebral ischemia, numerous intermediaries directly produce damage to BBB components, which is amplified by oxidative stress, apoptosis, and inflammatory response, which increase the BBB penetrability and exacerbating brain edoema and neurologic impairment. Jin et al., (2010); Jiang et al., (2018; Kunze and Marti, (2019). After an ischemic stroke Curcumin can protect BBB solidity and reduce brain edoema by upregulating aquaporin 4 and tight junction proteins like zonula occluden 1 (ZO-1), occludin, and claudin-5 while downregulating intercellular adhesion molecule-l (ICAM-1), matrix metalloproteinase 9 (MMP-9), and vascular cell adhesion molecule-l (VCAM-1) (Li et al., (2017); Wang et al., (2019); Wicha et al., (2020); Wu et al., (2021). Curcumin also protects cerebral capillary endothelial cells by suppressing the expression of inducible nitric oxide synthase (iNOS) and the production of NO(x) (nitrites/nitrates contents), preventing BBB damage (Jiang et al., 2007). Shear rate protection can help limit neutrophil adherence to the cerebral microcirculation and avoid early microvascular inflammation (Funk et al., 2013). Curcumin was reported to protect against cerebral ischemia by lowering BBB dysfunction via protein kinase C- (PKC-) signaling by Mo et al. (2021). Furthermore, it has previously been demonstrated that curcumin improves BBB permeability during hypoxia by boosting the expression of Heme oxygenase-1 (HO-1) in microvascular endothelial cells in the brain, Wang et al., (2013).

The Effective Role of Curcumin on Bone

Curcumin looks to be a promising contender for preventing and/or treating osteoporotic fracture development, despite the absence of biological data. Some studies investigated the inhibitory effects of curcumin on enhanced osteoclastic activity in insulin-dependent diabetes mellitus using streptozotocin-induced diabetic rats. Increased TRAP (1.5-fold) and cathepsin K (2.4-fold) activity strongly triggered bone matrix degradation in their diabetic rat model, which lowered the level of hydroxyproline in the distal femur and increased urine excretion of deoxypyridinoline (1.6-fold), a result of collagen breakdown. Curcumin oral therapy (120 mg per day for 14 days) restored cathepsin K and TRAP mRNA levels and activity in diabetic rats. Curcumin also lowered deoxypyridinoline levels in the urine. Furthermore, histochemical analysis demonstrated that the increased number of osteoclasts in the distal femurs of diabetic rats was returned to control levels in the curcumin-supplemented animals. The curcumin supplement had no effect on the reduced levels of ALP and osteocalcin expression in diabetic rats.

Curcumin against Postmenopausal Osteoporosis

Curcumin was delivered orally to bone in a female rat model produced by ovariectomization (OVX). Serum total cholesterol and estrogen levels were examined, as well as bone mass, bone mineral and calcium content, mechanical characteristics, and bone micrometric and histomorphometric parameters. In fact, in rats with normal estrogen levels, curcumin reduced blood estradiol levels while marginally enhancing cancellous bone formation and lowering mineralization. Curcumin (10 mg kg 1 per day for 4 weeks) reduced serum total cholesterol levels and body mass increase in OVX rats, and (ii) enhanced numerous bone histomorphometry parameters, including the breadth of endosteal osteoid in the tibia impacted by estrogen deprivation. The reduction in the breadth of endosteal osteoid in treated OVX rats' tibias could be related to the inhibition of bone matrix synthesis, which results in a reduction in transverse growth. In an in vivo study, French et al. looked at the effects of curcumin on OVX female rats. They examined bone mineral density at the spine and femur before and after ovariectomy in each of the 40 mature rats at 2, 4, and 6 months. They measured bone formation and resorption rates using blood osteocalcin and C-telopeptide levels. After 6 months of treatment, they noticed a significant improvement in femur size at the maximum curcumin dose (15 mg per day Curcumin therapy increased the amount of healing energy needed to fracture in a dose-dependent manner. Riva et al., (2017).

Curcumin in Diabetic Neuropathy

Diabetes-related neuropathic pain, a common consequence, is one of the most challenging types of pain to manage. Sharma et al., (2007). Approximately half of all diabetics will have nerve injury at some point in their lives. This discomfort is caused by nerve damage caused by high blood sugar levels (hyperglycemia). Deep pain, most usually in the feet and legs, loss of sensation of warmth or cold followed by muscular cramps, numbness, tingling, or burning sensation in the extremities, particularly the feet, and weakness are among the symptoms. The most common symptom of neuropathic pain is hyperalgesia. There are numerous medications available to address this problem. Antidepressants (amitriptyline, doxepin, or duloxetine), antiseizure drugs (gabapentin, pregabalin, carbamazepine, and valproate), anti-inflammatory meds, opioids, and capsaicin are examples. However, strict regulation of blood sugar (glucose) is required to avoid symptoms and issues from worsening. A lack of understanding of its genesis, insufficient alleviation, tolerance development, and the possible toxicity of traditional antinociceptives necessitate the research of novel medicines to relieve this pain. The discovery that curcumin has anti-inflammatory capabilities, including an inhibitory influence on the production of interleukin-8 (IL-8), interleukin-1 (IL-1), and TNF- levels, motivated us to investigate its protective function in diabetic neuropathy animal models. To that goal, we administered 200 mg/kg streptozotocin formulated in citrate buffer (pH 4.4, 0.1M) intraperitoneally to mice. Curcumin was injected into one group of mice from the fourth to the eighth week of streptozotocin treatment. Diabetic animals had a lower pain threshold from noxious stimuli at the end of the fourth week than control rats. Daily treatment was found to be effective in tail immersion and hot-plate assays.

Curcumin and Osteosarcoma

Given that malignant cells appear to take up more curcumin than normal cells, curcumin may have a selective effect on tumor tissue over healthy tissue. Chang et al. (2014) evaluated the in vitro cytotoxicity of curcumin at various dosages in MG-63 osteosarcoma cells and healthy human osteoblasts (5, 10, 25, 50, 75 and 100 mM). When compared to the untreated control, curcumin (10 mM) reduced the viability of MG-63 osteosarcoma cells by 50%. Healthy osteoblast cells, on the other hand, kept at least 80% of their viability across all concentrations tested. In terms of cytotoxicity, MG-63 osteosarcoma cells were much more susceptible to curcumin, although healthy human osteoblasts exhibited a higher viability after 24 hours of curcumin therapy. Based on the protective impact of NO in bone tissue, Moran et al. (2012) anticipated that curcumin would modify MG-63 growth and mineralization via a mechanism largely mediated by NO. Moran and colleagues discovered that curcumin can alter the formation and mineralization of MG-63 through a process that is influenced in part by NO. Although the mechanism underlying NO's anti-bone damage impact is not fully known, it appears that NO's influence on osteoblast activity. Low NO levels are an essential second messenger for systemic hormones involved in the control of bone metabolism, such as calcitonin gene-related peptide, parathyroid hormone, and sex steroids, particularly estrogen, under physiological settings.; Yan et al., (2011) It has been proven that osteoblasts' constitutively generated NO enhances both osteoblastic growth and differentiation. Son et al., (2010). In contrast, excessive local NO production promotes cytotoxicity in osteoblastic cells27, which is most likely mediated in part by cGMP. Son et al., (2010) Curcumin have been shown to reduce inducible NO synthase expression and NO production, possibly through interfering with NF-kB activation.

Curcumin and Bone Metastasis

Thyroid cancer is one of the more aggressive cancers, causing severe osteolytic bone lesions (bone destruction). Curcumin's antimetastatic effects on K1 papillary thyroid cancer cells were studied by Zhang et al., (2013), who focused on cancer cell attachment, spreading, migration, and invasion abilities, as well as MMP-9 activity and expression levels. In summary, they discovered that curcumin had a significant impact on the crucial stages of metastasis. Curcumin, for example, promoted mesenchymal-epithelial transition and lowered the migratory rate of K1 papillary thyroid cancer cells by 24-87% at 12.5, 25-, and 50-mM dosages. Curcumin may have anti-metastatic effects via increasing E-cadherin expression levels and decreasing MMP-9 activity and expression.

Curcumin and Bone Metastasis from Breast Cancer

Ganguly et al., (2012), discovered that curcumin reduced bone metastases via modulating FAK and hence MMP-9 synthesis and activity in the well-known estrogen-independent human breast cancer cell line MDA-MB-231. Curcumin also inhibited MDA-MB-231 viability in a dose-dependent manner (IC50 14 82 mM)). Wright et al., 2013 Yamaguchi et al., (2012) recently developed an in vitro model of breast cancer bone metastases. Co-culture with MDA-MB-231 bone metastasis cells reduced osteoblastic mineralization and promoted osteoclast genesis in bone marrow culture. In vivo, they confirmed curcumin's efficacy in decreasing bone loss in a breast cancer bone metastases mouse model. Metastatic cell implantation into the tibia the trabecular bone tissues of the femur and tibia of mice were significantly damaged, resulting in defective and fragmentary bone. Curcumin peros (50 or 150 mg kg 1 body/weight) or i.p. (10 or 20 mg kg 1 bodyweight) given once day for 5 days per week for 7 weeks decreased bone deterioration. Similarly, as reported by Wright et al., (2013), that administering curcumin (25 or 50 mg kg 1) to mice with breast cancer bone metastases for 21 days prevented the development of severe osteolytic bone lesions. While the tumor area within the bone remained unaltered, the number of osteoclasts at the bone-tumor contact was regularly reduced by up to 53%. This activity is connected to the prevention of the osteolytic peptide parathyroid hormone-related protein (PTHrP) release, they discovered (IC50 14 24 mM). Curcumin's inhibitory effect on tumor cell development is independent of its other effects and is mediated through the downregulation of phospho-Smad 2/3 and Ets-1 protein. Wright et al., (2013). Based on the promising results of curcumin treatment in reducing osteolytic bone metastases in breast cancer patients, clinical research was undertaken to investigate the feasibility and tolerability of the combination of docetaxel and curcumin in breast cancer patients. This open-label phase I trial included 14 women with advanced or metastatic breast cancer (Bayet-Robert et al., 2010). The suggested dose for curcumin is 6000 mg per day for 7 days. Every three weeks, in addition to an usual docetaxel dose. According to the authors, a response rate of up to 50% in a population of all evaluable patients treated with the combination of docetaxel/curcumin might be expected. A phase II trial comparing this regimen plus docetaxel to docetaxel alone in advanced and metastatic breast cancer patients is now underway.

Curcumin and Bone Metastasis from Prostate Cancer

Curcumin inhibited the expression of CCL2 CC motif ligand 2 (CCL2; also known as monocyte chemoattractant protein-1 or MCP-1) in PC-3 cells, a human bone-derived androgen-independent PCa cell line. Kocaadam and Şanlier, (2017), (Dorai et al., 2014). Curcumin decreased PC-3 cell adhesion, invasion, and motility as a result. When compared to control cells, a treatment with 30 mM curcumin for 18 hours reduced the invasive characteristics of PC-3 cells by 23%. NFkB, Cbfa1 (an osteoblast transcription factor), and epidermal growth factor receptor. Their preliminary findings strongly suggested that curcumin could significantly influence the formation of bone metastases. They recently confirmed that curcumin suppresses prostate cancer bone metastasis by upregulating the expression of bone morphogenic protein-7 using an adapted in vivo model of C4-2B prostate carcinoma bone metastasis progression. Dorai and colleagues (2014). Curcumin looks to be a viable candidate for preventing and/or treating the formation of bone metastases, regardless of the underlying tumor's origin. (Figure 2).

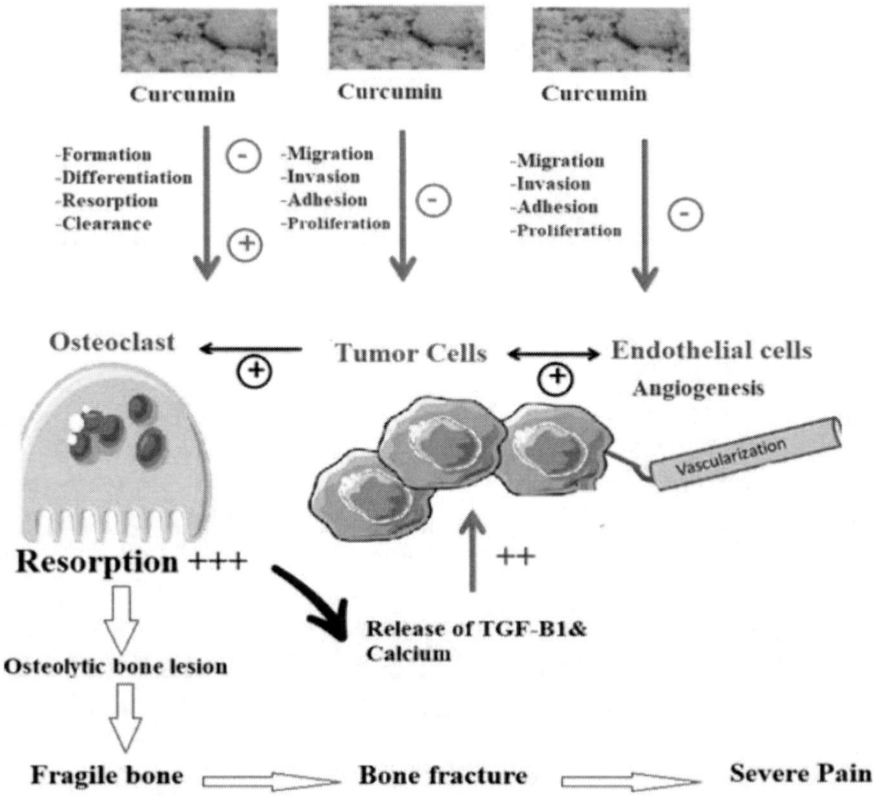

Figure 2. Curcumin (CUR) effects on bone metastases A synopsis of the physiopathology of bone metastases Excessive osteoclastic resorption activity is associated with tumor cells secreting numerous osteolytic agents. This results in the progressive development of serious bone lesions. TGF-b1 is the most implicated in tumor growth and invasion among the growth factors released by bone matrix. Curcumin's effects on osteoclasts, tumor cells, and endothelial cells (in red). Curcumin inhibits TNF-induced expression of adhesion molecules on endothelial cells, such as intracellular adhesion molecule (ICAM)-1, vascular cell adhesion molecule (VCAM)-1, and endothelial leukocyte adhesion molecule (ELAM)-1, which are critical for tumour cell invasion and metastases, in addition to decreasing endothelial cell proliferation and cell colony formation. Curcumin's anti-angiogenic activities may be achieved in part through the suppression of cyclic nucleotide phosphodiesterases, which are important regulators of VEGF-induced endothelial cell activity.

The Role of Curcumin and Curcuminoid Diet in Osteoarthritis (OA) Patients

Osteoarthritis (OA) is a complex chronic illness that is often aggravated by the existence of many comorbidities. Recognizing the dissimilar veiled causes of Knee (KOA) and the presence of comorbidities, numerous studies have focused on identifying distinct phenotypes with distinct features that may assist disease management through molecular targeting. For example, Dell'Isola et al. (2016) recognized six phenotypes: chronic pain, inflammation, metabolic syndrome, bone and cartilage metabolism, mechanical overload, and minimal joint disease. Van der Esch et al., (2015), proposed phenotypes of KOA pain based on lower extremity muscle strength, bodily habitus, and psychological components, on the other hand. There are presently no solid suggestions for grouping KOA patients into specific phenotypes. Despite the lack of agreement, several of these new phenotypic classification systems share the trait of inflammation.

Given the awareness that inflammation may play a significant role in the development and progression of OA, particularly post-traumatic OA, researchers and clinicians have turned to ways to treat this characteristic of the illness as a strategy to manage symptoms and, ideally, halt its progression. A recent review summarizes the current evidence regarding the role of diet and nutrition in OA patients. Interestingly, the American College of Rheumatology [ACR] research did assess various nutraceuticals and concluded that the great majority, including glucosamine, vitamin D, chondroitin sulphate, and fish oil, lacked sufficient evidence. A recent meta-analysis published in the British Journal of Sports Medicine by Liu et al. assessed the use of several nutraceutical supplements, including two randomized controlled trials (RCTs) evaluating turmeric. Though the author highlighted excellent outcomes with turmeric therapy, no recommendations were made due to data constraints. Liu et al., (2018). Turmeric is a ginger family spice that is commonly used in Indo-Asian cuisine and traditional eastern medicine. Curcumin is one of the active ingredients in turmeric, accounting for around 3% to 10% of the turmeric powder that can be extracted. Hewling et al. (2017) Curcumin extract (CE) possesses anti-inflammatory effects comparable to nonsteroidal anti-inflammatories. Kocaadam et al., (2017) Curcumin E has been demonstrated to influence the signaling of pro-inflammatory cytokines such as interleukins, phospholipase A2, 5-lipoxygenase enzyme, and COX-2 via NF kappa Beta activity, Plummer al, (1999). Curcumin has been demonstrated to suppress macrophage inhibitory factor-induced overexpression of matrix metallo-proteinase MMP-1 (interstitial collagenase) and MMP-3 (stromelysin) enzymes, which may be especially relevant at the chondrocyte level. 17 When triggered in synovial fibroblasts, these enzymes accelerate catabolic changes in articular cartilage and the development of OA. The use of paracetamol and NSAID therapy was reduced in the high and low dose turmeric groups, respectively. It is worth mentioning that studies comparing turmeric to placebo found not only an improvement in outcome ratings but also a significant reduction in rescue therapy use. Shep et al., (2019) and Kuptniratsaikul et al., (2014), is a safe addition to regular pharmacological therapy in people with KOA, and it may even allow for lower doses of medications like NSAIDs.

Curcumin and Skin Dermatological Conditions

A skin disease Psoriasis (PsO) is a chronic inflammatory, multisystemic, multifactorial illness that affects around 3% of the world's inhabitants. Keratinocytes proliferate uncontrollably, resulting in the clinically recognized thick, silvery plaques. The activation of mature and inflammatory dendritic cells (DC) is the initial stage in the pathogenesis of psoriasis, leading to hyperproduction of proinflammatory molecules such as cytokines, chemokines, and antimicrobial peptides (AMPs). Cytokines from the IL-23/T-helper-(Th)-17 axis and type I interferons (IFNs) play a critical role, and are targets for various monoclonal antibodies used to treat psoriasis. Krueger et al., (2018). Curcumin suppresses activated macrophages' production of TNF-Jain et al., (2009). Curcumin has been shown to bind directly to TNF- receptor-binding sites via covalent and non-covalent interactions, inhibiting TNF-dependent NF-B activation. Curcumin has also been demonstrated to inhibit lipopolysaccharide (LPS) signaling, which is critical for TNF- production induction, by acting on toll-like receptors (TLRs) 2 and 4. Reuter et al., (2011). Curcumin is also a non-competitive inhibitor of PhK, a serine/threonine protein kinase. PhK levels were found to be directly connected to psoriasis activity in human skin samples from persons with untreated active psoriasis, resolving psoriasis undergoing topical medication, and non-psoriatic participants. Decreased keratinocyte transferrin receptor (TRR) expression, parakeratosis severity, and epidermal CD8+ T cell density were associated with lower PhK levels in plaque samples treated with curcumin 1% alcoholic gel as well as other standard topical therapies, Heng et al., (2000). In animal studies, daily applications of 1% curcumin gel reduced cutaneous psoriasis-like inflammation generated by imiquimod by inhibiting potassium channels (subtypes Kv1.3) expressed in T cells and decreasing IL-17A, IL-17F, IL-22, and other pro-inflammatory cytokines in mouse ear samples, Kang et al. (,2016). Regular applications of a turmeric tonic, when compared to a placebo, significantly decreased cutaneous symptoms and quality of life in patients with scalp psoriasis Bahraini et al., (2018). Meriva, a novel bioavailable lecithin-based curcumin delivery form, was found to have anti-psoriatic effects in a recent randomized, double-blind, placebo-controlled clinical trial, with a reduction in cutaneous symptoms and a decrease in serum levels of IL-22. Furthermore, when used in conjunction, the medication increased the anti-psoriatic effects of topical steroids in patients, Antiga et al., (2015). Curcumin oral therapy (40 mg/kg, for 20 days) was shown in a clinical investigation to reduce serum levels of IL-2, IL-12, IL-22, IL-23, IFN-gamma, and TNF-alpha in psoriatic mice, decreasing psoriasis-associated inflammation as well as keratinocyte hyper-proliferation Kurd et al., (2008), A phase II clinical research confirmed the efficacy of oral curcumin for the symptoms of cutaneous plaque psoriasis, with an excellent safety profile. Singh et al., (1995). Surprisingly, a double-blind, placebo-controlled randomized clinical trial discovered that oral administration of curcumin nanoparticles increased the efficacy of acitretin and resulted in serum cholesterol control in psoriatic patients, implying a role for this compound as adjuvant treatment in moderate-to-severe psoriasis.

Curcumin Therapeutic Effects in Eye Retinal Diseases

As previously mentioned (*Curcuma longa*, Zingiberaceae family), is recognized to have several pharmacological properties, mainly anti-inflammatory, and it is well known that an inflammatory a etiology may be discovered in a wide range of retinal diseases: The retina, which is a component of the central nervous system, is distinguished by the presence of various cell types, including two types of photoreceptors: Cones, which are predominantly found in the macula lutea, and rods, which are mostly found in the retinal periphery. These cells, as well as retinal ganglion cells and retinal pigment epithelial (RPE) cells, are extremely vulnerable to oxidative stress damage. Recent studies have shown that curcumin protects the RPE from oxidative stress and damage caused by the inflammatory process by lowering TNF levels. Recently, these cells, along with retinal ganglion cells and retinal pigment epithelial (RPE) cells, are very susceptible to oxidative stress damage.

Curcumin has been proven in recent research to protect the RPE from oxidative stress and damage induced by the inflammatory process by reducing TNF levels. Recently, Bucolo et al. (2019) revealed that curcumin protects the RPE from oxidative stress damage by activating Nrf2/HO 1 signalling, which requires regulation of the extracellular signal regulated kinase (ERK) pathway, meaning that curcumin protects the RPE from oxidative stress damage. As a result, ROS levels have increased, vascularization has increased, and mitochondria have increased in concentration. The triggering mechanism in a sequence of damaging actions is oxidative stress: A variety of retinal diseases are caused by cell death, angiogenesis, and inflammation. Curcumin's pharmacological properties enable it to prevent the formation of ROS, allowing it to be used effectively in the prevention and treatment of various retinal disorders such as AMD, DR, proliferative vitreoretinopathy (PVR), retinal ischemia reperfusion injury (RIRI), retinitis pigmentosa (RP), and retinal and choroid tumors., Yang et al., (2016).

Role of Curcumin in Diabetic Retinopathy (DR)

DR is frequently recognized as the primary reason of irreversible sight fofeiture in the working-age people all over the world Yau et al., (2011). Clinically, it is classified as a metabolic and microvascular disease characterized by a chronic inflammatory process Bhandarkar and Arbiser, (2007). The most common signs of DR are ischemia, microaneurysms, hemorrhages, retinal edema, neuronal degeneration, and neovascularization, Li et al., (2005). In both circumstances, inflammation and oxidative stress are the underlying causes of DR development and progression, causing photoreceptor and blood vessel damage and the production of cellular mediators capable of stimulating angiogenesis (Aggarwal et al., 2003). Another important element in the aetiology of diabetes is the oxidative damage caused by hyperglycemia: ROS, in particular, contribute to the loss of pericytes, which leads to microaneurysms and, as a result, the vascular syndrome of DR Santibanez et al., (2000), Skopiski et al., (2004). Furthermore, free radicals promote the production of pro-inflammatory mediators such as VEGF and TNF Carmeliet & Jain, (2011) Kim and Byzova, (2014). In one study, curcumin in oral doses of 1 g/kg body weight in Wistar albino rats was evaluated for prevention and treatment in a streptozotocin-induced diabetic paradigm. Curcumin, in particular, demonstrated considerable hypoglycemic efficacy as well as the potential to positively affect the antioxidant system, with an increase in SOD and catalase enzymes. Furthermore, levels of TNF and VEGF levels were reduced Radomska-Leniewska et al., (2015).

Curcumin and Eye Dryness Disease

Dry eye disease is characterised by reduced tear secretion and fast tear evaporation, resulting in ocular surface damage Niederkorn et al., (2006). This process' pathophysiology includes increased tear osmolality and ocular surface irritation. Proinflammatory cytokines such as IL-6, IL-8, and IL-1 are found in corneal cell lines and dry eye patients in a hyperosmotic environment. Li et al., (2006). Curcumin's anti-inflammatory properties may offer some protection. Curcumin, in example, has been demonstrated to suppress the expression of ovalbumin-induced proinflammatory cytokines such as IL-4 and IL-5 in mouse conjunctiva Chung et al., (2012). Curcumin also protected corneal epithelial cells from hyperosmoticity-induced IL-1 overexpression via p38 mitogen activated protein kinase (MAPK/NF-B) pathways, according to an in vitro investigation, Liu et al., (2017) & Chen et al., (2010).

Potential Role of Curcumin in COVID

The mechanism underlying curcuminoids' impact is the inhibition and blockage of free radicals before they grow and spread. Aside from anti-inflammatory and analgesic properties, antibacterial and antiviral properties, hepatoprotective, cholesterol-lowering, and antithrombotic properties have also been reported. In the latter instance, antioxidant activity has been shown to be very efficient in reducing oxidative damage to vessel walls. In fact, oxidation of the vessel membrane structures is one of the primary requirements for the formation of a thrombus. For decades, there has been a link between inflammatory disorders like pneumonia and thrombosis in general (particularly venous thrombosis). Patients with any bacterial or viral pneumonia, not just SARS CoV 2, are routinely given thromboembolic prophylaxis with low molecular weight heparin. The authors recently addressed thrombotic problems in the context of SARS CoV 2, Chen et al., (2010) Burlacu et al., (2020).

Adverse Events of Curcumin

About 2013 study for 26 patients looked at curcumin pharmacokinetics and side effects after a 14-day trial of 2.35 g daily curcumin treatment. This study discovered no major adverse events caused by curcumin, as well as no changes in total activity or general health. There were some minor stomach issues that resolved on their own. Irving et al., (2011), found that two weeks of daily curcumin consumption reduced gastrointestinal disturbances such as nausea, vomiting, constipation, diarrhoea, flatulence, and abdominal discomfort. Given the proclivity of the selected cohorts to adverse events, the gastrointestinal disturbances attributed to curcumin in this investigation and previous studies may not fully reflect the side effect profile. Carroll et al., (2011). The outcomes of the above-mentioned huge number study could imply that curcumin is even therapeutic for gastrointestinal symptoms, which is consistent with earlier clinical trials of IBD and IBS that found curcumin to relieve symptoms in both conditions. This study also discovered no difference in overall health in people who took curcumin, as well as no major harmful side effects. Curcumin has also been linked to a number of negative side effects. Curcumin was discovered in 2013 to have a concentration-dependent suppression of sperm motility in vitro, with a 100% block of motility with higher concentration. Naz et al., (2014). Curcumin has been demonstrated to suppress the synthesis of Hepcidin58, a protein important in iron balance in the body. Curcumin was observed to cause a dose-dependent reduction in hematocrit, hemoglobin, serum iron, and transferrin saturation, particularly in patients with underlying subclinical iron shortage or chronic illness anemia. Curcumin should therefore be used with caution in people who have low iron storage or other iron-related disorders, such as chronic anemia. Curcumin has iron chelator characteristics in cultured cells suggesting that it could cause preclinical or clinical iron deficient anemia. Naz et al., (2014). Other potential curcumin adverse effects include contact dermatitis and urticaria.

Conclusion

Given what has been discussed, it is apparent that curcumin, the principal polyphenolic ingredient in the food flavouring turmeric, has aroused the curiosity of researchers for millennia due to its broad biological activity against numerous health diseases. In addition to its unusual activity, it is non-toxic. As a key active ingredient in turmeric, curcumin has been found to play a great role in management of inflammation activity, oxidative stress neurodegeneration diseases, like Alzheimer, Parkinson, ischemic stroke, bone disorders and cancers, skin disorder and even its potential role in COVID. Curcumin mode of action always was through various mechanisms, such as antioxidant activity, anti-apoptosis, anti-cytokine, and BBB protection. However, there remain several unanswered questions. Curcumin's clinical application is the most difficult. At the moment, the majority of studies are experimental in nature, and associated clinical trials are scarce. Although basic research has yielded promising findings, it should be highlighted that there are considerable differences between animals and humans in terms of therapeutic applications, such as drug dosage and frequency, administration route, and treatment time points. Furthermore, it has a great goal to further demonstrate the usefulness, safety, and stability of curcumin while enhancing bioavailability using appropriate delivery systems such as nano based drug delivery systems. Clinical trials in the body to determine the best treatment plan. Second, the effect of curcumin in combination with other medications and treatment modalities should be investigated in order to determine the potential mechanism of their synergistic effects in boosting curcumin's therapeutic benefit. Herbal therapy, in general, offers intriguing alternatives to existing therapies for neurodegenerative illnesses and other conditions. More human trials investigating curcumin's cognitive boosting effect are also required.

References

Ahmad, N., Umar, S., Ashafaq, M., Akhtar, M., Iqbal, Z., Samim, M. and Ahmad, F.J., 2013. A comparative study of PNIPAM nanoparticles of curcumin, demethoxy-curcumin, and bisdemethoxycurcumin and their effects on oxidative stress markers in experimental stroke. *Protoplasma*, *250*(6), pp.1327-1338.

Akkoç, Y., Berrak, Ö., Arısan, E.D., Obakan, P., Çoker-Gürkan, A. and Palavan-Ünsal, N., 2015. Inhibition of PI3K signaling triggered apoptotic potential of curcumin which is hindered by Bcl-2 through activation of autophagy in MCF-7 cells. *Biomedicine & Pharmacotherapy*, *71*, pp.161-171.

Alahmari, A. (2021). Blood-Brain Barrier Overview: Structural and Functional Correlation. *Neural Plast*. 2021,

Alisi, I.O., Uzairu, A., Abechi, S.E. and Idris, S.O., 2018. Evaluation of the antioxidant properties of curcumin derivatives by genetic function algorithm. *Journal of Advanced Research*, *12*, pp.47-54.

Al-Omar, F.A., Nagi, M.N., Abdulgadir, M.M., Al Joni, K.S. and Al-Majed, A.A., 2006. Immediate and delayed treatments with curcumin prevents forebrain ischemia-induced neuronal damage and oxidative insult in the rat hippocampus. *Neurochemical Research,* 31(5), pp.611-618.

Amor, S., Peferoen, L.A., Vogel, D.Y., Breur, M., van der Valk, P., Baker, D. and van Noort, J.M., 2014. Inflammation in neurodegenerative diseases–an update. *Immunology*, *142*(2), pp.151-166..

Amor, S., Puentes, F., Baker, D. and Van Der Valk, P., 2010. Inflammation in neurodegenerative diseases. *Immunology*, *129*(2), pp.154-169.

Anand, P., Kunnumakkara, A.B., Newman, R.A. and Aggarwal, B.B., 2007. Bioavailability of curcumin: problems and promises. *Molecular Pharmaceutics*, *4*(6), pp.807-818.

Antiga, E., Bonciolini, V., Volpi, W., Del Bianco, E. and Caproni, M., 2015. Oral curcumin (Meriva) is effective as an adjuvant treatment and is able to reduce IL-22 serum levels in patients with psoriasis vulgaris. *BioMed Research International*, 2015.

Bahraini, P., Rajabi, M., Mansouri, P., Sarafian, G., Chalangari, R. and Azizian, Z., 2018. Turmeric tonic as a treatment in scalp psoriasis: A randomized placebo-control clinical trial. *Journal of Cosmetic Dermatology*, *17*(3), pp.461-466.]

Bannuru, R.R., Osani, M.C., Vaysbrot, E.E., Arden, N.K., Bennell, K., Bierma-Zeinstra, S.M.A., Kraus, V.B., Lohmander, L.S., Abbott, J.H., Bhandari, M. and Blanco, F.J., 2019. OARSI guidelines for the non-surgical management of knee, hip, and polyarticular osteoarthritis. *Osteoarthritis and Cartilage*, *27*(11), pp.1578-1589

Barber, Alistair J. "Diabetic retinopathy: recent advances towards understanding neurodegeneration and vision loss." *Science China Life Sciences* 58, no. 6 (2015): 541-549.

Bassani, T.B., Turnes, J.M., Moura, E.L., Bonato, J.M., Cóppola-Segovia, V., Zanata, S.M., Oliveira, R.M. and Vital, M.A., 2017. Effects of curcumin on short-term spatial and recognition memory, adult neurogenesis and neuroinflammation in a streptozotocin-induced rat model of dementia of Alzheimer's type. *Behavioural Brain Research*, *335*, pp.41-54.

Baum, L., Cheung, S.K., Mok, V.C., Lam, L.C., Leung, V.P., Hui, E., Ng, C.C., Chow, M., Ho, P.C., Lam, S. and Woo, J., 2007. Curcumin effects on blood lipid profile in a 6-month human study. *Pharmacological Research*, *56*(6), pp.509-514.

Bhandarkar, S.S. and Arbiser, J.L., 2007. Curcumin as an inhibitor of angiogenesis. *The molecular targets and therapeutic uses of curcumin in health and disease*, pp.185-195.

Bharal, N., Sahaya, K., Jain, S., Mediratta, P.K. and Sharma, K.K., 2008. Curcumin has anticonvulsant activity on increasing current electroshock seizures in mice. *Phytotherapy Research: An International Journal Devoted to Pharmacological and Toxicological Evaluation of Natural Product Derivatives,* 22(12), pp.1660-1664.

Bhat, A., Mahalakshmi, A.M., Ray, B., Tuladhar, S., Hediyal, T.A., Manthiannem, E., et al. (2019). Benefits of Curcumin in Brain Disorders. *Biofactors* 45, 666–689. doi:10.1002/biof.1533

Bhutani, M.K., Bishnoi, M. and Kulkarni, S.K., 2009. Anti-depressant like effect of curcumin and its combination with piperine in unpredictable chronic stress-induced behavioral, biochemical and neurochemical changes. *Pharmacology Biochemistry and Behavior*, *92*(1), pp.39-43.

Blind, 3-Way Crossover Study—. *Journal of Nutritional Science and Vitaminology*, *61*(1), pp.37-44.

Bottai, D., Adami, R., Paroni, R. and Ghidoni, R., 2020. Brain cancer-activated microglia: A potential role for sphingolipids. *Current Medicinal Chemistry*, *27*(24), pp.4039-4061.

Bucolo, C., Drago, F., Maisto, R., Romano, G.L., D'Agata, V., Maugeri, G. and Giunta, S., 2019. Curcumin prevents high glucose damage in retinal pigment epithelial cells through ERK1/2-mediated activation of the Nrf2/HO-1 pathway. *Journal of Cellular Physiology,* 234(10), pp.17295-17304.

Burlacu, A., Genovesi, S., Popa, I.V. and Crisan-Dabija, R., 2020. Unpuzzling COVID-19 prothrombotic state: are preexisting thrombophilic risk profiles responsible for heterogenous thrombotic events? *Clinical and Applied Thrombosis/Hemostasis*, *26*, p.1076029620952884.

Cai, Z., Hussain, M.D. and Yan, L.J., 2014. Microglia, neuroinflammation, and beta-amyloid protein in Alzheimer's disease. *International Journal of Neuroscience,* 124(5), pp.307-321.

Campbell, B.C.V., and Khatri, P. (2020). Stroke. *The Lancet* 396, 129–142. doi:10. 1016/s0140-6736(20)31179-x

Campbell, B.C.V., De Silva, D.A., Macleod, M.R., Coutts, S.B., Schwamm, L.H., Davis, S.M. and Donnan, G.A., 2019. *Ischaemic Stroke Nature Reviews Disease Primers* 5 (1): 70.

Cao, G., Minami, M., Pei, W., Yan, C., Chen, D., O'Horo, C., Graham, S.H. and Chen, J., 2001. Intracellular Bax translocation after transient cerebral ischemia: implications for a role of the mitochondrial apoptotic signaling pathway in ischemic neuronal death. *Journal of Cerebral Blood Flow & Metabolism,* 21(4), pp.321-333.

Carmeliet, P. and Jain, R.K., 2011. Molecular mechanisms and clinical applications of angiogenesis. *Nature*, *473*(7347), pp.298-307.

Catania, A., Barrajón-Catalán, E., Nicolosi, S., Cicirata, F. and Micol, V., 2013. Immunoliposome encapsulation increases cytotoxic activity and selectivity of curcumin and resveratrol against HER2 overexpressing human breast cancer cells. *Breast Cancer Research and Treatment*, *141*(1), pp.55-65.

Cenini, G., Lloret, A. and Cascella, R., 2019. Oxidative stress in neurodegenerative diseases: from a mitochondrial point of view. *Oxidative Medicine and Cellular Longevity*, *2019*.

Chang, R., Sun, L. and Webster, T.J., 2014. Selective cytotoxicity of curcumin on osteosarcoma cells compared to healthy osteoblasts. *International Journal of Nanomedicine*, *9*, p.461.

Chen, L.W., Yung, K.K.L., Chan, Y.S., Shum, D.K.Y. and Bolam, J.P., 2008. The proNGF-p75NTR-sortilin signalling complex as new target for the therapeutic treatment of Parkinson's disease. *CNS & Neurological Disorders-Drug Targets* (Formerly Current Drug Targets-CNS & Neurological Disorders), 7(6), pp.512-523.

Chen, M., Hu, D.N., Pan, Z., Lu, C.W., Xue, C.Y. and Aass, I., 2010. Curcumin protects against hyperosmoticity-induced IL-1β elevation in human corneal epithelial cell via MAPK pathways. *Experimental Eye Research,* 90(3), pp.437-443.

Cheng, T., Zhang, Z., Shen, H., Jian, Z., Li, J., Chen, Y., Shen, Y. and Dai, X., 2020. Topically applicated curcumin/gelatin-blended nanofibrous mat inhibits pancreatic adenocarcinoma by increasing ROS production and endoplasmic reticulum stress mediated apoptosis. *Journal of Nanobiotechnology,* 18(1), pp.1-12.

Choi, Y., Bowman, J.W., and Jung, J.U. (2018). Autophagy during Viral Infection - a Double-Edged Sword. *Nat. Rev. Microbiol.* 16, 341–354.

Chung SH, Choi SH, Choi JA, et al. (2012): Curcumin suppresses ovalbumin-induced allergic conjunctivitis. *Mol Vis* 18: 1966-1972.

Cuomo, A., Bimonte, S., Forte, C.A., Botti, G. and Cascella, M., 2019. Multimodal approaches and tailored therapies for pain management: the trolley analgesic model. *Journal of Pain Research, 12*, p.711.

Dell'Isola, A., Allan, R., Louise, S.S., Marreiros, S.S. and Steultjens, M., 2016. 185 Identification of Clinical Phenotypes in Knee Osteoarthritis: A Systematic Review of the Literature. *Rheumatology, 55*(suppl_1), pp.i137-i137.

Dende, C., Meena, J., Nagarajan, P., Nagaraj, V.A., Panda, A.K., & Padmanaban, G., 2017. Nanocurcumin is superior to native curcumin in preventing degenerative changes in Experimental Cerebral Malaria. *Scientific Reports,* 7(1), 10062-10062

Dhir, A. (2018). Curcumin in Epilepsy Disorders. *Phytother Res.* 32, 1865–1875. doi:10.1002/ptr.6125

Di Martino, R.M.C., De Simone, A., Andrisano, V., Bisignano, P., Bisi, A., Gobbi, S., Rampa, A., Fato, R., Bergamini, C., Perez, D.I. and Martinez, A., 2016. Versatility of the curcumin scaffold: discovery of potent and balanced dual BACE-1 and GSK-3β inhibitors. *Journal of Medicinal Chemistry, 59*(2), pp.531-544.

Dorai, T., Diouri, J., O'Shea, O. and Doty, S.B., 2014. Curcumin inhibits prostate cancer bone metastasis by up-regulating bone morphogenic protein-7 in vivo. *Journal of Cancer Therapy, 5*(4), p.369.

Douglass, B.J.; Clouatre, D.L. Beyond -yellow curry: Assessing commercial curcumin absorption techniques. *J. Am. Coll. Nutr.* 2015, 34, 347–358.

DU, P., Li, X., Lin, H.J., Peng, W.F., Liu, J.Y., Ma, Y., Fan, W. and Wang, X., 2009. Curcumin inhibits amygdaloid kindled seizures in rats. *Chinese Medical Journal, 122*(12), pp.1435-1438

Duthey, B., 2013. Background paper 6.11: Alzheimer disease and other dementias. *A Public Health Approach to Innovation,* 1-74.

Erkkinen, M.G., Kim, M.O. and Geschwind, M.D., 2018. Clinical neurology and epidemiology of the major neurodegenerative diseases. *Cold Spring Harbor Perspectives in Biology, 10*(4), p.a033118.

Farkhondeh, T., Samarghandian, S., Roshanravan, B. and Peivasteh-Roudsari, L., 2020. Impact of curcumin on traumatic brain injury and involved molecular signaling pathways. *Recent Patents on Food, Nutrition & Agriculture, 11*(2), pp.137-144

Fraser, P.A., 2011. The role of free radical generation in increasing cerebrovascular permeability. *Free Radical Biology and Medicine, 51*(5), pp.967-977.

Funk, J.L., Frye, J.B., Davis-Gorman, G., Spera, A.L., Bernas, M.J., Witte, M.H., Weinand, M.E., Timmermann, B.N., McDonagh, P.F. and Ritter, L., 2013. Curcuminoids limit neutrophil-mediated reperfusion injury in experimental stroke by targeting the endothelium. *Microcirculation,* 20(6), pp.544-554.

Ganguly, S.S., Fiore, L.S., Sims, J.T., Friend, J.W., Srinivasan, D., Thacker, M.A., Cibull, M.L., Wang, C., Novak, M., Kaetzel, D.M. and Plattner, R., 2012. c-Abl and Arg are activated in human primary melanomas, promote melanoma cell invasion via distinct pathways, and drive metastatic progression. *Oncogene*, *31*(14), pp.1804-1816.

Garcia-Alloza, M., Borrelli, L.A., Rozkalne, A., Hyman, B.T. and Bacskai, B.J., 2007. Curcumin labels amyloid pathology in vivo, disrupts existing plaques, and partially restores distorted neurites in an Alzheimer mouse model. *Journal of Neurochemistry*, *102*(4), pp.1095-1104.

Gera, M., Sharma, N., Ghosh, M., Lee, S.J., Min, T., Kwon, T. and Jeong, D.K., 2017. Nanoformulations of curcumin: An emerging paradigm for improved remedial application. *Oncotarget*, *8*(39), p.66680.

Golonko, A., Lewandowska, H., Świsłocka, R., Jasińska, U.T., Priebe, W. and Lewandowski, W., 2019. Curcumin as tyrosine kinase inhibitor in cancer treatment. *European Journal of Medicinal Chemistry*, *181*, p.111512.

Goozee, K.G., Shah, T.M., Sohrabi, H.R., Rainey-Smith, S.R., Brown, B., Verdile, G. and Martins, R.N., 2016. Examining the potential clinical value of curcumin in the prevention and diagnosis of Alzheimer's disease. *British Journal of Nutrition*, *115*(3), pp.449-465.

Guan, F., Ding, Y., Zhang, Y., Zhou, Y., Li, M. and Wang, C., 2016. Curcumin suppresses proliferation and migration of MDA-MB-231 breast cancer cells through autophagy-dependent Akt degradation. *PloS One*, *11*(1), p.e0146553.

Guo, F., Liu, X., Cai, H., Le, W., 2018. Autophagy in neurodegenerative diseases: pathogenesis and therapy. *Brain Pathol.* 28 (1), 3–13

Gupta, S.K., Kumar, B., Nag, T.C., Agrawal, S.S., Agrawal, R., Agrawal, P., Saxena, R. and Srivastava, S., 2011. Curcumin prevents experimental diabetic retinopathy in rats through its hypoglycemic, antioxidant, and anti-inflammatory mechanisms. *Journal of Ocular Pharmacology and Therapeutics*, *27*(2), pp.123-130.

Hardy, J. and Selkoe, D.J., 2002. The amyloid hypothesis of Alzheimer's disease: progress and problems on the road to therapeutics. *Science*, *297*(5580), pp.353-356.

He, R., Jiang, Y., Shi, Y., Liang, J. and Zhao, L., 2020. Curcumin-laden exosomes target ischemic brain tissue and alleviate cerebral ischemia-reperfusion injury by inhibiting ROS-mediated mitochondrial apoptosis. *Materials Science and Engineering:* C, 117, p.111314.

Heng, M.C.Y., Song, M.K., Harker, J. and Heng, M.K., 2000. Drug-induced suppression of phosphorylase kinase activity correlates with resolution of psoriasis as assessed by clinical, histological and immunohistochemical parameters. *British Journal of Dermatology*, *143*(5), pp.937-949.

Henrotin, Y., Malaise, M., Wittoek, R., Brasseur, J.P., Luyten, F., Jiangang, Q., Van den Berghe, M., Uhoda, R., Bentin, J., De Vroey, T. and Erpicum, L., 2019. Bio-optimized *Curcuma longa* extract is efficient on knee osteoarthritis pain: a doule-blind multicenter randomized placebo-controlled study. *Osteoarthritis and Cartilage*, *27*, p.S500.

Hewlings, S.J., Kalman, D.S., 2017. Curcumin: a review of its' effects on human health. Retrieved from. *Foods (Basel, Switzerland)* 6 (10), 92

Hou, W., Hao, Y., Sun, L., Zhao, Y., Zheng, X., and Song, L. (2022). The Dual Roles of Autophagy and the GPCRs-Mediating Autophagy Signaling Pathway after Cerebral Ischemic Stroke. *Mol. Brain* 15, 14.

Howes, M.J.R., 2018. Phytochemicals as anti-inflammatory nutraceuticals and phytopharmaceuticals. In *Immunity and Inflammation in Health and Disease* (pp. 363-388). Academic Press.

Hu, X., Leak, R.K., Shi, Y., Suenaga, J., Gao, Y., Zheng, P. and Chen, J., 2015. Microglial and macrophage polarization—new prospects for brain repair. *Nature Reviews Neurology*, 11(1), pp.56-64.

Hu, X., Li, P., Guo, Y., Wang, H., Leak, R.K., Chen, S., Gao, Y. and Chen, J., 2012. Microglia/macrophage polarization dynamics reveal novel mechanism of injury expansion after focal cerebral ischemia. *Stroke,* 43(11), pp.3063-3070.

Huber, J.D., Egleton, R.D. and Davis, T.P., 2001. Molecular physiology and pathophysiology of tight junctions in the blood–brain barrier. *Trends in Neurosciences*, *24*(12), pp.719-725.

Irving GR, Howells LM, Sale S, et al. Prolonged biologically active colonic tissue levels of curcumin achieved after oral administrationda clinical pilot study including assessment of patient acceptability. *Cancer Prev Res (Phila).* 2013;6: 119e128

Irving GR, Karmokar A, Berry DP, Brown K, Steward WP. Curcumin: the potential for efficacy in gastrointestinal diseases. *Best Pract Res Clin Gastroenterol.* 2011; 25:519e534

Iurlaro, R. and Muñoz-Pinedo, C., 2016. Cell death induced by endoplasmic reticulum stress. *The FEBS Journal*, *283*(14), pp.2640-2652.

Jain, S.K., Rains, J., Croad, J., Larson, B. and Jones, K., 2009. Curcumin supplementation lowers TNF-α, IL-6, IL-8, and MCP-1 secretion in high glucose-treated cultured monocytes and blood levels of TNF-α, IL-6, MCP-1, glucose, and glycosylated hemoglobin in diabetic rats. *Antioxidants & Redox Signaling*, *11*(2), pp.241-249.

Jazayeri-Tehrani, S.A., Rezayat, S.M., Mansouri, S., Qorbani, M., Alavian, S.M., Daneshi-Maskooni, M. and Hosseinzadeh-Attar, M.J., 2019. Nano-curcumin improves glucose indices, lipids, inflammation, and Nesfatin in overweight and obese patients with non-alcoholic fatty liver disease (NAFLD): a double-blind randomized placebo-controlled clinical trial. *Nutrition & Metabolism*, *16*(1), pp.1-13.

Jia, T., Zhang, L., Duan, Y., Zhang, M., Wang, G., Zhang, J. and Zhao, Z., 2014. The differential susceptibilities of MCF-7 and MDA-MB-231 cells to the cytotoxic effects of curcumin are associated with the PI3K/Akt-SKP2-Cip/Kips pathway. *Cancer Cell International*, *14*(1), pp.1-14.

Jiang, J., Wang, W., Sun, Y.J., Hu, M., Li, F. and Zhu, D.Y., 2007. Neuroprotective effect of curcumin on focal cerebral ischemic rats by preventing blood–brain barrier damage. *European Journal of Pharmacology,* 561(1-3), pp.54-62.

Jiang, X., Andjelkovic, A.V., Zhu, L., Yang, T., Bennett, M.V.L., Chen, J., et al. (2018). Blood-brain Barrier Dysfunction and Recovery after Ischemic Stroke. *Prog. Neurobiol.* 163-164, 144–171

Jin, R., Yang, G. and Li, G., 2010. Molecular insights and therapeutic targets for blood–brain barrier disruption in ischemic stroke: critical role of matrix metalloproteinases and tissue-type plasminogen activator. *Neurobiology of Disease*, *38*(3), pp.376-385.

Jope, R.S., Yuskaitis, C.J. and Beurel, E., 2007. Glycogen synthase kinase-3 (GSK3): inflammation, diseases, and therapeutics. *Neurochemical Research*, *32*(4), pp.577-595.

Jyoti, A., Sethi, P. and Sharma, D., 2009. Curcumin protects against electrobehavioral progression of seizures in the iron-induced experimental model of epileptogenesis. *Epilepsy & Behavior*, *14*(2), pp.300-308.

Kalaycıoğlu, Z., Gazioğlu, I. and Erim, F.B., 2017. Comparison of antioxidant, anticholinesterase, and antidiabetic activities of three curcuminoids isolated from *Curcuma longa* L. *Natural Product Research*, *31*(24), pp.2914-2917.

Kang, D., Li, B., Luo, L., Jiang, W., Lu, Q., Rong, M. and Lai, R., 2016. Curcumin shows excellent therapeutic effect on psoriasis in mouse model. *Biochimie*, *123*, pp.73-80.

Kharat, M. and McClements, D.J., 2019. Recent advances in colloidal delivery systems for nutraceuticals: a case study–delivery by design of curcumin. *Journal of Colloid and Interface Science*, *557*, pp.506-518.

Kim Y-W, Byzova TV (2014): Oxidative stress in angiogenesis and vascular disease. *Blood* 123: 625-631.

Kim, D.S., Park, S.Y. and Kim, J.Y., 2001. Curcuminoids from *Curcuma longa* L. (Zingiberaceae) that protect PC12 rat pheochromocytoma and normal human umbilical vein endothelial cells from βA (1–42) insult. *Neuroscience Letters*, *303*(1), pp.57-61.

Kim, J.M., Noh, E.M., Kwon, K.B., Kim, J.S., You, Y.O., Hwang, J.K., Hwang, B.M., Kim, B.S., Lee, S.H., Lee, S.J. and Jung, S.H., 2012. Curcumin suppresses the TPA-induced invasion through inhibition of PKCα-dependent MMP-expression in MCF-7 human breast cancer cells. *Phytomedicine*, *19*(12), pp.1085-1092.

Kim, S.H., Després, J.P. and Koh, K.K., 2016. Obesity and cardiovascular disease: friend or foe? *European Heart Journal*, *37*(48), pp.3560-3568.

Kim, S.J., Son, T.G., Park, H.R., Park, M., Kim, M.S., Kim, H.S., Chung, H.Y., Mattson, M.P. and Lee, J., 2008. Curcumin stimulates proliferation of embryonic neural progenitor cells and neurogenesis in the adult hippocampus. *Journal of Biological Chemistry*, *283*(21), pp.14497-14505.

Kocaadam, B. and Şanlier, N., 2017. Curcumin, an active component of turmeric (*Curcuma longa*), and its effects on health. *Critical Reviews in Food Science and Nutrition*, 57(13), pp.2889-2895.

Kolasinski, S.L., Neogi, T., Hochberg, M.C., Oatis, C., Guyatt, G., Block, J., Callahan, L., Copenhaver, C., Dodge, C., Felson, D. and Gellar, K., 2020. 2019 American College of Rheumatology/Arthritis Foundation guideline for the management of osteoarthritis of the hand, hip, and knee. *Arthritis & Rheumatology*, *72*(2), pp.220-233.

Krueger, J.G. and Brunner, P.M., 2018. Interleukin-17 alters the biology of many cell types involved in the genesis of psoriasis, systemic inflammation and associated comorbidities. *Experimental Dermatology*, *27*(2), pp.115-123.

Kubisch, J., Türei, D., Földvári-Nagy, L., Dunai, Z.A., Zsákai, L., Varga, M., Vellai, T., Csermely, P. and Korcsmáros, T., 2013, August. Complex regulation of autophagy in cancer–integrated approaches to discover the networks that hold a double-edged sword. In *Seminars in cancer biology* (Vol. 23, No. 4, pp. 252-261). Academic Press.

Kulkami S, Dhir A, Akula KK 2009. Potentials of curcumin as an antidepressant. *Scientific World Journal,* 9:1233-41.

Kulkarni, S.K., Bhutani, M.K. and Bishnoi, M., 2008. Antidepressant activity of curcumin: involvement of serotonin and dopamine system. *Psychopharmacology*, *201*(3), pp.435-442.

Kumar, D., Jacob, D., Subash, P.S., Maliakkal, A., Johannah, N.M., Kuttan, R., Maliakel, B., Konda, V. and Krishnakumar, I.M., 2016. Enhanced bioavailability and relative distribution of free (unconjugated) curcuminoids following the oral administration of a food-grade formulation with fenugreek dietary fibre: A randomised double-blind crossover study. *Journal of Functional Foods*, *22*, pp.578-587.

Kunze, R. and Marti, H.H., 2019. Angioneurins–Key regulators of blood–brain barrier integrity during hypoxic and ischemic brain injury. *Progress in neurobiology*, *178*, p.101611.

Küpeli Akkol, E., Bardakcı, H., Yücel, Ç., Şeker Karatoprak, G., Karpuz, B. and Khan, H., 2022. A New Perspective on the Treatment of Alzheimer's Disease and Sleep Deprivation-Related Consequences: Can Curcumin Help? *Oxidative Medicine and Cellular Longevity*, *2022*.

Kuptniratsaikul, V., Dajpratham, P., Taechaarpornkul, W., Buntragulpoontawee, M., Lukkanapichonchut, P., Chootip, C., Saengsuwan, J., Tantayakom, K. and Laongpech, S., 2014. Efficacy and safety of Curcuma domestica extracts compared with ibuprofen in patients with knee osteoarthritis: a multicenter study. *Clinical Interventions in Aging*, *9*, p.451.

Kurd, S.K., Smith, N., VanVoorhees, A., Troxel, A.B., Badmaev, V., Seykora, J.T. and Gelfand, J.M., 2008. Oral curcumin in the treatment of moderate to severe psoriasis vulgaris: A prospective clinical trial. *Journal of the American Academy of Dermatology*, *58*(4), pp.625-631.

Lamanna-Rama, N., Romero-Miguel, D., Desco, M. and Soto-Montenegro, M.L., 2022. An Update on the Exploratory Use of Curcumin in Neuropsychiatric Disorders. *Antioxidants*, *11*(2), p.353.

Langen, U.H., Ayloo, S. and Gu, C., 2019. Development and cell biology of the blood-brain barrier. *Annual Review of Cell and Developmental Biology*, 35, p.591.

Lee, H., Lee, I.S. and Choue, R., 2013. Obesity, inflammation and diet. *Pediatric Gastroenterology, Hepatology & Nutrition*, *16*(3), pp.143-152.

Li, D.Q., Luo, L., Chen, Z., Kim, H.S., Song, X.J. and Pflugfelder, S.C., 2006. JNK and ERK MAP kinases mediate induction of IL-1β, TNF-α and IL-8 following hyperosmolar stress in human limbal epithelial cells. *Experimental Eye Research*, *82*(4), pp.588-596.

Li, F., Xu, Y., Li, X., Wang, X., Yang, Z., Li, W., Cheng, W. and Yan, G., 2021. Triblock Copolymer Nanomicelles Loaded with Curcumin Attenuates Inflammation via Inhibiting the NF-Kb Pathway in the Rat Model of Cerebral Ischemia. *International Journal of Nanomedicine*, *16*, p.3173.

Li, H., Soria, C., Griscelli, F., Opolon, P., Soria, J., Yeh, P., Legrand, C., Vannier, J.P., Belin, D., Perricaudet, M. and Lu, H., 2005. Amino-terminal fragment of urokinase inhibits tumor cell invasion in vitro and in vivo: respective contribution of the urokinase plasminogen activator receptor-dependent or-independent pathway. *Human Gene Therapy*, *16*(10), pp.1157-1167.

Li, P., Stetler, R.A., Leak, R.K., Shi, Y., Li, Y., Yu, W., Bennett, M.V. and Chen, J., 2018. Oxidative stress and DNA damage after cerebral ischemia: Potential therapeutic targets to repair the genome and improve stroke recovery. *Neuropharmacology*, *134*, pp.208-217.

Li, W., Suwanwela, N.C. and Patumraj, S., 2017. Curcumin prevents reperfusion injury following ischemic stroke in rats via inhibition of NF-κB, ICAM-1, MMP-9 and caspase-3 expression. *Molecular Medicine Reports*, *16*(4), pp.4710-4720.

Lim, G.P., Chu, T., Yang, F., Beech, W., Frautschy, S.A. and Cole, G.M., 2001. The curry spice curcumin reduces oxidative damage and amyloid pathology in an Alzheimer transgenic mouse. *Journal of Neuroscience*, *21*(21), pp.8370-8377.

Limoli, P.G., Vingolo, E.M., Limoli, C. and Nebbioso, M., 2019. Stem cell surgery and growth factors in retinitis pigmentosa patients: pilot study after literature review. *Biomedicines*, *7*(4), p.94.

Liu, D. and Chen, Z., 2013. The effect of curcumin on breast cancer cells. *Journal of Breast Cancer*, *16*(2), pp.133-137.

Liu, Q., Loo, W.T., Sze, S.C.W. and Tong, Y., 2009. Curcumin inhibits cell proliferation of MDA-MB-231 and BT-483 breast cancer cells mediated by down-regulation of NFκB, cyclinD and MMP-1 transcription. *Phytomedicine*, *16*(10), pp.916-922.

Liu, W., Zhai, Y., Heng, X., Che, F.Y., Chen, W., Sun, D. and Zhai, G., 2016. Oral bioavailability of curcumin: problems and advancements. *Journal of Drug Targeting*, *24*(8), pp.694-702.

Liu, X., Machado, G.C., Eyles, J.P., Ravi, V. and Hunter, D.J., 2018. Dietary supplements for treating osteoarthritis: a systematic review and meta-analysis. *British Journal of Sports Medicine*, *52*(3), pp.167-175.

Liu, X.F., Hao, J.L., Xie, T., Mukhtar, N.J., Zhang, W., Malik, T.H., Lu, C.W. and Zhou, D.D., 2017. Curcumin, a potential therapeutic candidate for anterior segment eye diseases: a review. *Frontiers in Pharmacology*, *8*, p.66

Liu, Z.J., Li, Z.H., Liu, L., Tang, W.X., Wang, Y., Dong, M.R. and Xiao, C., 2016. Curcumin attenuates beta-amyloid-induced neuroinflammation via activation of peroxisome proliferator-activated receptor-gamma function in a rat model of Alzheimer's disease. *Frontiers in Pharmacology*, *7*, p.261.

López-Malo, D., Villarón-Casares, C.A., Alarcón-Jiménez, J., Miranda, M., Díaz-Llopis, M., Romero, F.J. and Villar, V.M., 2020. Curcumin as a therapeutic option in retinal diseases. *Antioxidants*, *9*(1), p.48.

Ma, L., Li, M., Ma, X., Cheng, L., Du, P. and Liu, Y., 2017. A review of supervised object-based land-cover image classification. *ISPRS Journal of Photogrammetry and Remote Sensing,* 130, pp.277-293.

Mhillaj, E., Tarozzi, A., Pruccoli, L., Cuomo, V., Trabace, L. and Mancuso, C., 2019. Curcumin and heme oxygenase: neuroprotection and beyond. *International Journal of Molecular Sciences*, *20*(10), p.2419.

Mizushima, N., and Komatsu, M. (2011). Autophagy: Renovation of Cells and Tissues. *Cell* 147, 728–741

Mo, Y., Yue, E., Shi, N. and Liu, K., 2021. The protective effects of curcumin in cerebral ischemia and reperfusion injury through PKC-θ signaling. *Cell Cycle,* 20(5-6), pp.550-560.

Mobasheri, A., Henrotin, Y., Biesalski, H.K. and Shakibaei, M., 2012. Scientific evidence and rationale for the development of curcumin and resveratrol as nutraceutricals for joint health. *International Journal of Molecular Sciences*, *13*(4), pp.4202-4232.

Moran, J.M., Roncero-Martin, R., Rodriguez-Velasco, F.J., Calderon-Garcia, J.F., Rey-Sanchez, P., Vera, V., Canal-Macias, M.L. and Pedrera-Zamorano, J.D., 2012. Effects of curcumin on the proliferation and mineralization of human osteoblast-like cells: implications of nitric oxide. *International Journal of Molecular Sciences*, *13*(12), pp.16104-16118.

Muangnoi, C. and Sharif, U., 2019. Ratnatilaka Na Bhuket, P.; Rojsitthisak, P.; Paraoan, L. Protective effects of curcumin ester prodrug, curcumin diethyl disuccinate against H2O2-induced oxidative stress in human retinal pigment epithelial cells: Potential therapeutic avenues for age-related macular degeneration. *Int. J. Mol. Sci*, *20*, p.3367.

Mukherjee, A., Sarkar, S., Jana, S., Swarnakar, S. and Das, N., 2019. Neuro-protective role of nanocapsulated curcumin against cerebral ischemia-reperfusion induced oxidative injury. *Brain Research,* 1704, pp.164-173.

Namgyal, D., Ali, S., Hussain, M.D., Kazi, M., Ahmad, A. and Sarwat, M., 2021. Curcumin Ameliorates the Cd-Induced Anxiety-like Behavior in Mice by Regulating Oxidative Stress and Neuro-Inflammatory Proteins in the Prefrontal Cortex Region of the Brain. *Antioxidants*, *10*(11), p.1710.

Naz RK, Lough ML. Curcumin as a potential non-steroidal contraceptive with spermicidal and microbicidal properties. *Eur J Obstet Gynecol Reprod Biol.* 2014; 176:142e148.

Nebrisi, E.E. (2021). Neuroprotective Activities of Curcumin in Parkinson's Disease: A Review of the Literature. *Int. J. Mol. Sci*. 22, 11248. doi:10.3390/ijms222011248

Niederkorn, J.Y., Stern, M.E., Pflugfelder, S.C., De Paiva, C.S., Corrales, R.M., Gao, J. and Siemasko, K., 2006. Desiccating stress induces T cell-mediated Sjögren's syndrome-like lacrimal keratoconjunctivitis. *The Journal of Immunology*, *176*(7), pp.3950-3957.

Obermeier, B., Verma, A. and Ransohoff, R.M., 2016. The blood–brain barrier. *Handbook of Clinical Neurology,* 133, pp.39-59.

Ono, K., Hasegawa, K., Naiki, H. and Yamada, M., 2004. Curcumin has potent anti-amyloidogenic effects for Alzheimer's β-amyloid fibrils in vitro. *Journal of Neuroscience Research*, *75*(6), pp.742-750.

Orellana-Urzúa, S., Rojas, I., Líbano, L. and Rodrigo, R., 2020. Pathophysiology of ischemic stroke: role of oxidative stress. *Current Pharmaceutical Design*, *26*(34), pp.4246-4260.

Palizgir, M.T., Akhtari, M., Mahmoudi, M., Mostafaei, S., Rezaiemanesh, A. and Shahram, F., 2018. Curcumin reduces the expression of interleukin 1 β and the production of interleukin 6 and tumor necrosis factor alpha by M1 macrophages from patients with Behcet's disease. *Immunopharmacology and Immunotoxicology*, *40*(4), pp.297-302.

Pan, Y., Zhao, D., Yu, N., An, T., Miao, J., Mo, F., Gu, Y., Zhang, D., Gao, S. and Jiang, G., 2017. Curcumin improves glycolipid metabolism through regulating peroxisome proliferator activated receptor γ signalling pathway in high-fat diet-induced obese mice and 3T3-L1 adipocytes. *Royal Society Open Science*, *4*(11), p.170917.

Panda, S.K., Nirvanashetty, S., Missamma, M. and Jackson-Michel, S., 2021. The enhanced bioavailability of free curcumin and bioactive-metabolite tetrahydrocurcumin from a dispersible, oleoresin-based turmeric formulation. *Medicine*, *100*(27).

Pandey, S. and Srivanitchapoom, P., 2017. Levodopa-induced dyskinesia: clinical features, pathophysiology, and medical management. *Annals of Indian Academy of Neurology*, *20*(3), p.190.

Park, S.Y. and Kim, D.S., 2002. Discovery of natural products from Curcuma l onga that protect cells from beta-amyloid insult: A drug discovery effort against Alzheimer's disease. *Journal of Natural Products*, *65*(9), pp.1227-1231.

Parkinson, J., 2002. An essay on the shaking palsy. *The Journal of Neuropsychiatry and Clinical Neurosciences*, *14*(2), pp.223-236.

Pawar, Y.B., Munjal, B., Arora, S., Karwa, M., Kohli, G., Paliwal, J.K. and Bansal, A.K., 2012. Bioavailability of a lipidic formulation of curcumin in healthy human volunteers. *Pharmaceutics*, *4*(4), pp.517-530.

Plummer, S.M., Holloway, K.A., Manson, M.M., Munks, R.J., Kaptein, A., Farrow, S. and Howells, L., 1999. Inhibition of cyclo-oxygenase 2 expression in colon cells by the chemopreventive agent curcumin involves inhibition of NF-κB activation via the NIK/IKK signalling complex. *Oncogene*, *18*(44), pp.6013-6020.

Purpura, M., Lowery, R.P., Wilson, J.M., Mannan, H., Münch, G. and Razmovski-Naumovski, V., 2018. Analysis of different innovative formulations of curcumin for improved relative oral bioavailability in human subjects. *European Journal of Nutrition*, *57*(3), pp.929-938.

Radak, D., Katsiki, N., Resanovic, I., Jovanovic, A., Sudar-Milovanovic, E., Zafirovic, S., A Mousad, S. and R Isenovic, E., 2017. Apoptosis and acute brain ischemia in ischemic stroke. *Current Vascular Pharmacology*, 15(2), pp.115-122.

Radomska-Leśniewska, D.M., Skopiński, P., Bałan, B.J., Białoszewska, A., Jóźwiak, J., Rokicki, D., Skopińska-Różewska, E., Borecka, A. and Hevelke, A., 2015. Angiomodulatory properties of Rhodiola spp. and other natural antioxidants. *Central European Journal of Immunology*, *40*(2), pp.249-262.

Ran, Y., Su, W., Gao, F., Ding, Z., Yang, S., Ye, L., Chen, X., Tian, G., Xi, J. and Liu, Z., 2021. Curcumin ameliorates white matter injury after ischemic stroke by inhibiting microglia/macrophage pyroptosis through NF-κB suppression and NLRP3 inflammasome inhibition. *Oxidative Medicine and Cellular Longevity*, *2021*.

Reddy, P.H., Manczak, M., Yin, X., Grady, M.C., Mitchell, A., Kandimalla, R. and Kuruva, C.S., 2016. Protective effects of a natural product, curcumin, against amyloid β induced mitochondrial and synaptic toxicities in Alzheimer's disease. *Journal of Investigative Medicine*, *64*(8), pp.1220-1234.

Reddy, P.H., Manczak, M., Yin, X., Grady, M.C., Mitchell, A., Tonk, S., Kuruva, C.S., Bhatti, J.S., Kandimalla, R., Vijayan, M. and Kumar, S., 2018. Protective effects of Indian spice curcumin against amyloid-β in Alzheimer's disease. *Journal of Alzheimer's Disease*, *61*(3), pp.843-866.

Reuter, S., Gupta, S.C., Park, B., Goel, A. and Aggarwal, B.B., 2011. Epigenetic changes induced by curcumin and other natural compounds. *Genes & Nutrition*, *6*(2), pp.93-108.

reza Ariamoghaddam, A., Ebrahimi-Hosseinzadeh, B., Hatamian-Zarmi, A. and Sahraeian, R., 2018. In vivo anti-obesity efficacy of curcumin loaded nanofibers transdermal patches in high-fat diet induced obese rats. *Materials Science and Engineering: C*, *92*, pp.161-171.

Riva, A., Togni, S., Giacomelli, L., Franceschi, F., Eggenhoffner, R., Feragalli, B., Belcaro, G., Cacchio, M., Shu, H. and Dugall, M., 2017. Effects of a curcumin-based supplementation in asymptomatic subjects with low bone density: a preliminary 24-week supplement study. *Eur Rev Med Pharmacol Sci*, *21*(7), pp.1684-1689.

Roy, S., Maiello, M. and Lorenzi, M., 1994. Increased expression of basement membrane collagen in human diabetic retinopathy. *The Journal of Clinical Investigation*, *93*(1), pp.438-442.

Santibanez, J.F., Quintanilla, M. and Martinez, J., 2000. Genistein and curcumin block TGF-β1-induced u-PA expression and migratory and invasive phenotype in mouse epidermal keratinocytes. *Nutrition and Cancer*, *37*(1), pp.49-54.

Schmidt, F.M., Weschenfelder, J., Sander, C., Minkwitz, J., Thormann, J., Chittka, T., Mergl, R., Kirkby, K.C., Faßhauer, M., Stumvoll, M. and Holdt, L.M., 2015. Inflammatory cytokines in general and central obesity and modulating effects of physical activity. *PloS One*, *10*(3), p.e0121971.

Sharma, S., Chopra, K. and Kulkarni, S.K., 2007. Effect of insulin and its combination with resveratrol or curcumin in attenuation of diabetic neuropathic pain: participation of nitric oxide and TNF-alpha. *Phytotherapy Research*, *21*(3), pp.278-283.

Shep, D., Khanwelkar, C., Gade, P. and Karad, S., 2019. Safety and efficacy of curcumin versus diclofenac in knee osteoarthritis: a randomized open-label parallel-arm study. *Trials*, *20*(1), pp.1-11.

Shi, X., Zheng, Z., Li, J., Xiao, Z., Qi, W., Zhang, A., Wu, Q. and Fang, Y., 2015. Curcumin inhibits Aβ-induced microglial inflammatory responses in vitro: Involvement of ERK1/2 and p38 signaling pathways. *Neuroscience Letters*, *594*, pp.105-110.

Shishodia, S., Singh, T. and Chaturvedi, M.M., 2007. Modulation of transcription factors by curcumin. *The molecular targets and therapeutic uses of curcumin in health and disease*, pp.127-148. [CrossRef] [PubMed]

Singh, S.; Aggarwal, B.B. 1995. Activation of transcription factor NF-kappa B is suppressed by curcumin (diferuloylmethane) [corrected]. *J. Biol. Chem.,* 270, 24995–25000.

Skopinski, P., Szaflik, J., Duda-Król, B., Nartowska, J., Sommer, E., Chorostowska-Wynimko, J., Demkow, U. and Skopinska-Rózewska, E., 2004. Suppression of angiogenic activity of sera from diabetic patients with non-proliferative retinopathy by compounds of herbal origin and sulindac sulfone. *International Journal of Molecular Medicine*, *14*(4), pp.707-718.

Son, M.J., Lee, S.B., Byun, Y.J., Lee, H.O., Kim, H.S., Kwon, O.J., Nam, S.W. and Jeong, S.W., 2010. Sodium nitroprusside induces autophagic cell death in glutathione-depleted osteoblasts. *Molecular & Cellular Toxicology*, *6*(1), pp.41-49.

Stewart, W.F., Kawas, C., Stewart, W.F., Kawas, C., Corrada, M. and Metter, E.J., 1997. Risk of Alzheimer's disease and duration of NSAID use. *Neurology*, *48*(3), pp.626-632.

Stohs, S.J.; Ray, S.D. Issues with human bioavailability determinations of bioactive curcumin. *Biomed. J. Sci. Tech. Res.* 2019, 12, 9417–9419.

Sunagawa, Y., Hirano, S., Katanasaka, Y., Miyazaki, Y., Funamoto, M., Okamura, N., Hojo, Y., Suzuki, H., Doi, O., Yokoji, T. and Morimoto, E., 2015. *Colloidal Submicron-Particle Curcumin Exhibits High Absorption Efficiency—A Double.*

Tan, H.K., Moad, A.I.H. and Tan, M.L., 2014. The mTOR signalling pathway in cancer and the potential mTOR inhibitory activities of natural phytochemicals. *Asian Pacific Journal of Cancer Prevention*, *15*(16), pp.6463-6475.

Tang, M. and Taghibiglou, C., 2017. The mechanisms of action of curcumin in Alzheimer's disease. *Journal of Alzheimer's Disease*, *58*(4), pp.1003-1016.

Tello-Franco V, Lozada-García MC, Soriano-García M,.2013. Experimental and computational studies on the inhibition of acetylcholinesterase by curcumin and some of its derivatives. *Curr Comput Aided Drug Des.* 9:289-298 866

Torres-Cuevas, I., Corral-Debrinski, M. and Gressens, P., 2019. Brain oxidative damage in murine models of neonatal hypoxia/ischemia and reoxygenation. *Free Radical Biology and Medicine*, *142*, pp.3-15.

Tu, P., Fu, H. and Cui, M., 2015. Compounds for imaging amyloid-β deposits in an Alzheimer's brain: a patent review. *Expert Opinion on Therapeutic Patents*, *25*(4), pp.413-423.

Ueda, H. and Fujita, R., 2004. Cell death mode switch from necrosis to apoptosis in brain. *Biological and Pharmaceutical Bulletin,* 27(7), pp.950-955.

Van der Esch, M., Knoop, J., Van der Leeden, M., Roorda, L.D., Lems, W.F., Knol, D.L. and Dekker, J., 2015. Clinical phenotypes in patients with knee osteoarthritis: a study in the Amsterdam osteoarthritis cohort. *Osteoarthritis and cartilage*, *23*(4), pp.544-549.

Wang, L.L., Sun, Y., Huang, K. and Zheng, L., 2013. Curcumin, a potential therapeutic candidate for retinal diseases. *Molecular Nutrition & Food Research*, *57*(9), pp.1557-1568.

Wang, R., Li, Y.B., Li, Y.H., Xu, Y., Wu, H.L. and Li, X.J., 2008. Curcumin protects against glutamate excitotoxicity in rat cerebral cortical neurons by increasing brain-derived neurotrophic factor level and activating TrkB. *Brain Research*, *1210*, pp.84-91.

Wang, W. and Xu, J., 2020. Curcumin attenuates cerebral ischemia-reperfusion injury through regulating mitophagy and preserving mitochondrial function. *Current Neurovascular Research*, *17*(2), pp.113-122.

Wang, X., Fang, Y., Huang, Q., Xu, P., Lenahan, C., Lu, J., Zheng, J., Dong, X., Shao, A. and Zhang, J., 2021. An updated review of autophagy in ischemic stroke: from mechanisms to therapies. *Experimental Neurology,* 340, p.113684.

Wang, Y., Luo, J. and Li, S.Y., 2019. Nano-curcumin simultaneously protects the blood–brain barrier and reduces M1 microglial activation during cerebral ischemia–reperfusion injury. *ACS Applied Materials & Interfaces*, *11*(4), pp.3763-3770.

Wicha, P., Tocharus, J., Janyou, A., Jittiwat, J., Changtam, C., Suksamrarn, A. and Tocharus, C., 2017. Hexahydrocurcumin protects against cerebral ischemia/ reperfusion injury, attenuates inflammation, and improves antioxidant defenses in a rat stroke model. *PloS One,* 12(12), p.e0189211.

Wright E, L., Frye B, J., Gorti, B., Timmermann N, B. and Funk L, J., 2013. Bioactivity of turmeric-derived curcuminoids and related metabolites in breast cancer. *Current Pharmaceutical Design, 19*(34), pp.6218-6225.

Wright, L.E., Frye, J.B., Lukefahr, A.L., Timmermann, B.N., Mohammad, K.S., Guise, T.A. and Funk, J.L., 2013. Curcuminoids block TGF-β signaling in human breast cancer cells and limit osteolysis in a murine model of breast cancer bone metastasis. *Journal of Natural Products,* 76(3), pp.316-321.

Wu, J.X., Zhang, L.Y., Chen, Y.L., Yu, S.S., Zhao, Y. and Zhao, J., 2015. Curcumin pretreatment and post-treatment both improve the antioxidative ability of neurons with oxygen-glucose deprivation. *Neural Regeneration Research*, 10(3), p.481.

Wu, L., Jiang, C., Kang, Y., Dai, Y., Fang, W. and Huang, P., 2020. Curcumin exerts protective effects against hypoxia-reoxygenation injury via the enhancement of apurinic/apyrimidinic endonuclease 1 in SH-SY5Y cells: involvement of the PI3K/ AKT pathway. *International Journal of Molecular Medicine,* 45(4), pp.993-1004.

Wu, S., Guo, T., Qi, W., Li, Y., Gu, J., Liu, C., Sha, Y., Yang, B., Hu, S. and Zong, X., 2021. Curcumin ameliorates ischemic stroke injury in rats by protecting the integrity of the blood-brain barrier. *Experimental and Therapeutic Medicine*, *22*(1), pp.1-8.

Xu, H., Nie, B., Liu, L., Zhang, C., Zhang, Z., Xu, M. and Mei, Y., 2019. Curcumin prevents brain damage and cognitive dysfunction during ischemic-reperfusion through the regulation of miR-7-5p. *Current Neurovascular Research,* 16(5), pp.441-454.

Xue, Y., Nie, D., Wang, L.J., Qiu, H.C., Ma, L., Dong, M.X., Tu, W.J. and Zhao, J., 2021. Microglial polarization: novel therapeutic strategy against ischemic stroke. *Aging and Disease,* 12(2), p.466.

Yamaguchi M, Moore TW, Sun A, Snyder JP, Shoji M. Novel curcumin analogue UBS109 potently stimulates osteoblastogenesis and suppresses osteoclastogenesis: involvement in Smad activation and NF-kappaB inhibition. *Integr Biol* (Camb) 2012; 4: 905–913

Yan, L., Yinghui, T., Bo, Y., Gang, Z., Xian, X. and Lu, Z., 2011. Effect of calcitonin gene-related peptide on nitric oxide production in osteoblasts: an experimental study. *Cell Biology International*, *35*(8), pp.757-765.

Yang, F., Lim, G.P., Begum, A.N., Ubeda, O.J., Simmons, M.R., Ambegaokar, S.S., Chen, P.P., Kayed, R., Glabe, C.G., Frautschy, S.A. and Cole, G.M., 2005. Curcumin inhibits formation of amyloid β oligomers and fibrils, binds plaques, and reduces amyloid in vivo. *Journal of Biological Chemistry*, *280*(7), pp.5892-5901.

Yang, Y., Qin, Y.J., Yip, Y.W., Chan, K.P., Chu, K.O., Chu, W.K., Ng, T.K., Pang, C.P. and Chan, S.O., 2016. Green tea catechins are potent anti-oxidants that ameliorate sodium iodate-induced retinal degeneration in rats. *Scientific Reports*, *6*(1), pp.1-10.

Yavarpour-Bali, H. and Ghasemi-Kasman, M., 2020. Update on neurological manifestations of COVID-19. *Life Sciences,* 257, p.118063.

Yavarpour-Bali, H., Ghasemi-Kasman, M. and Pirzadeh, M., 2019. Curcumin-loaded nanoparticles: A novel therapeutic strategy in treatment of central nervous system disorders. *International Journal of Nanomedicine,* 14, p.4449.

Yeung, A.W.K., Horbańczuk, M., Tzvetkov, N.T., Mocan, A., Carradori, S., Maggi, F., Marchewka, J., Sut, S., Dall'Acqua, S., Gan, R.Y. and Tancheva, L.P., 2019. Curcumin: total-scale analysis of the scientific literature. *Molecules, 24*(7), p.1393.

Yim-Im, W., Sawatdichaikul, O., Semsri, S., Horata, N., Mokmak, W., Tongsima, S., Suksamrarn, A. and Choowongkomon, K., 2014. Computational analyses of curcuminoid analogs against kinase domain of HER2. *BMC Bioinformatics, 15*(1), pp.1-13. [CrossRef]

Yuan, J., Botchway, B.O. A., Zhang, Y., Tan, X., Wang, X., and Liu, X. (2019). Curcumin Can Improve Spinal Cord Injury by Inhibiting TGF-β-SOX9 Signaling Pathway. *Cell Mol Neurobiol* 39, 569–575. doi:10.1007/s10571-019- 00671-x

Zhang U., Duan D., Song Z., Liu T., Hou Y., Fang J. 2021. Small molecules regulating reactive oxygen species homeostasis for cancer therapy. *Med Res Rev*. 2021; 41:342–394.

Zhang, M., Bian, F., Wen, C. and Hao, N., 2007. Inhibitory effect of curcumin on proliferation of human pterygium fibroblasts. *Journal of Huazhong University of Science and Technology*, 27(3), pp.339-342.

Zhang, Y., Chen, P., Hong, H., Wang, L., Zhou, Y. and Lang, Y., 2017. JNK pathway mediates curcumin-induced apoptosis and autophagy in osteosarcoma MG63 cells. *Experimental and Therapeutic Medicine, 14*(1), pp.593-599.

Zhang, Y., Fang, M., Sun, Y., Zhang, T., Shi, N., Li, J., Jin, L., Liu, K. and Fu, J., 2018. Curcumin attenuates cerebral ischemia injury in Sprague–Dawley rats and PC12 cells by suppressing overactivated autophagy. *Journal of Photochemistry and Photobiology B: Biology*, *184*, pp.1-6.

Zhao Y, Chen B, Shen J, et al. The beneficial effects of quercetin, curcumin, and resveratrol in obesity. *Oxid Med Cell Longev* 2017; 2017:1459497.

Zhao, S.C., Ma, L.S., Chu, Z.H., Xu, H., Wu, W.Q., and Liu, F. (2017). Regulation of Microglial Activation in Stroke. *Acta Pharmacol. Sin* 38, 445–458. doi:10. 1038/aps.2016.162

Zhou, H.Y., Sun, Y.Y., Chang, P. and Huang, H.C., 2022. Curcumin Inhibits Cell Damage and Apoptosis Caused by Thapsigargin-Induced Endoplasmic Reticulum Stress Involving the Recovery of Mitochondrial Function Mediated by Mitofusin-2. *Neurotoxicity Research*, *40*(2), pp.449-460.

Zhou, Y., Shao, A., Yao, Y., Tu, S., Deng, Y. and Zhang, J., 2020. Dual roles of astrocytes in plasticity and reconstruction after traumatic brain injury. *Cell Communication and Signaling*, *18*(1), pp.1-16.

Chapter 3

Effects of Curcumin Supplantation and Exercise Training on Alzheimer's Disease and Age-Associated Cognitive Decline

S. Amani-Shalamzari[1,*], PhD
M. Molanouri Shamsi[2,†], PhD
S. Agha-Mohammadi[2,‡]
and C. D. Paton[3,§], PhD

[1]Department of Exercise Physiology, Faculty of Physical Education and Sport Sciences, Kharazmi University, Tehran, Iran
[2]Department of Physical Education and Sport Sciences, Faculty of Humanities, Tarbiat Modares University, Tehran, Iran
[3]School of Health and Sport Science, The Eastern Institute of Technology, Napier, New Zealand

Abstract

Aging is associated with cognitive impairment and is a major risk factor for neurological disorders, including dementia and Alzheimer's disease (AD). AD is a progressive neurodegenerative disease characterised by gradual loss of memory and motor activity. Although the exact pathogenesis of AD is not fully understood, there is ample evidence that oxidative stress and inflammation may play a critical role in the underlying mechanisms of cognitive impairment and AD. Curcumin is a

* Corresponding Author's Email: amani_sadegh@khu.ac.ir.
† Corresponding Author's Email: molanouri@modares.ac.ir.
‡ Corresponding Author's Email: samaneaghamohammadi@modares.ac.ir.
§ Corresponding Author's Email: cpaton@eit.ac.nz.

In: Curcumin and Its Role in Health and Disease
Editor: Kathryn Woltjer
ISBN: 979-8-88697-491-1

chemical component of turmeric (*Curcuma longa*), a natural compound with antioxidant and anti-inflammatory properties proposed to combat neurological dysfunction, reduce neurodegenerative diseases such as AD, protect the hippocampus, and treat cognitive dysfunction. Epidemiological evidence links regular physical exercise to improved age-related cognitive function, lower risk for dementia, reduced pathological changes in the central nervous system, and reduced atrophy of brain executive function. Regular physical exercise reduces inflammatory cytokines and increases the production of brain-derived neurotrophic factors, especially in the hippocampus, which is the main center of learning and memory formation. Exercise can also enhance the antioxidant protection of the hippocampus and induce positive effects of brain-derived neurotrophic factor (BDNF) on neurons. Therefore, the synergic effects of regular exercise training and curcumin supplementation may be considered an effective strategy for dealing with neurological and cognitive disorders. In this chapter, we assess the combined effects of physical exercise and curcumin supplementation on the reduction in cognitive function due to aging and AD.

Keywords: Alzheimer, curcumin, aging, regular physical exercise, cognitive impairment

Abbreviations

AD	Alzheimer's disease
ALT	Alanine aminotransferase
AST	Aspartate aminotransferase
Aβ	Beta-amyloid
BDNF	Brain-derived neurotrophic factor
cAMP	Cyclic adenosine monophosphate
CBF	Cerebral blood flow
CK	Creatine kinase
CNS	Central nervous system
COX-2	Cyclooxygenase-2
DNA	Deoxyribonucleic acid
EIMD	Exercise-induced muscle damage
ER	Endoplasmic reticulum
GSH	Glutathione
IL-1β	Interleukin-1β
LDH	Lactate dehydrogenase

LDL	Low-density lipoprotein
MBE	Mind-body exercise
MCI	Mild cognitive impairment
MMSE	Mini-Mental State Examination
MoCA	Montreal cognitive assessment
MVC	Maximal voluntary contraction
NF-kB	Nuclear factor kappa-light-chain-enhancer of activated B cells
NO	Nitric oxide
Nrf2	Nuclear factor erythroid 2–related factor 2
PI3K	Phosphoinositide 3-kinase
QoL	Quality of life
ROM	Range of motion
ROS	Reactive oxygen species
SOD	Superoxide dismutase
T2D	Type 2 diabetes
TNF-α	Tumor necrosis factor-α

Introduction

Cellular senescence is a process that is related to various cellular mechanisms. Cells undergo senescence due to different factors, including telomere erosion, reactive oxygen species (ROS) production, DNA damage, endoplasmic reticulum (ER) stress, and chromatin structure dysfunction (de Magalhães and Passos 2018, Naylor, Baker, and van Deursen 2013). One particular change during the aging process is nervous system atrophy which leads to sensory, motor, and cognitive impairments and eventually manifests as neurodegenerative diseases (Schirinzi et al. 2020). Additionally, chronic inflammation and oxidative stress, obesity, alterations in diversity and numbers of intestinal microbiota, autophagy disorders, and prothrombotic state are associated with cognitive impairment in aging (Bielak-Zmijewska et al. 2019).

Alzheimer's disease (AD) is the most common form of neurodegenerative disease in the world, accounting for 60%–80% of all dementia cases in the United States (Association 2021). Furthermore, ~95% of all AD patients in the United States are aged over 65 years. Prior to the year 2000, AD was the eighth leading cause of death ;ten years later, it became the sixth leading cause of death in the USA (Murphy, Xu, and Kochanek 2013). AD can impose a heavy psychological and economic burden on family members and caregivers during the disease course. AD affects brain regions involved in memory and learning and causes the progressive destruction of neurons in the hippocampus and the neocortex. The neuropathogenesis of AD is related to the accumulation of two proteins, senile plaques like beta-amyloid (Aβ) and neurofibrillary tangles like tau protein (Lansbury and Lashuel 2006).

Scientific and medical developments have led to an increase in human lifespan, which in turn has lead to a rise in diseases related to old age. Research shows that nutritional interventions with particular food compounds, and physical activity can delay aging related disorders (Benameur et al. 2021a). Curcumin is a safe and inexpensive polyphenolic antixoxidant with proposed anti-aging properties. Curcumin ingestion has been associated with anti-inflammatory (immune system) effects and may also provide beneficial cardiovascular effects, and positive effects on diseases such as AD and arthritis (Thiyagarajan and Sharma 2004, Shishodia, Sethi, and Aggarwal 2005). However, curcumin's low absorption in the intestinal cells and its rapid metabolism in the liver causes it to be excreted from the body rapidly (Gupta, Kismali, and Aggarwal 2013). It also seems that curcumin's beneficial effects depend on the dosage taken. This dose phenomenon, known as the hormetic effect (Moghaddam et al. 2019), indicates possible stimulatory effects at low doses and inhibitory effects at higher doses. It has been shown that curcumin has a possible cytostatic, cytotoxic, and genotoxic at high doses (Bielak-Zmijewska et al. 2019).

It has been demonstrated that curcumin may play a role in the possible prevention and treatment of brain-related diseases with potential effects on specific target proteins, creating anti-inflammatory and antioxidant effects and regulating microglia (Benameur et al. 2021). However, a recent systematic review did not fully confirm curcumin's effects in treating and preventing cognitive decline symptoms in human samples (Seddon et al. 2019). Considering risk factors related to cognitive dysfunction, such as hypertension, dyslipidemia, obesity at midlife, diabetes mellitus, smoking, physical inactivity, and depression, multimodal lifestyle interventions should be recommended for older populations.

Regular physical exercise along with positive nutritional interventions may prevent many diseases, including disorders related to cognitive function (Dominguez et al. 2021). Physical activity combats diseases related to conditions such as diabetes, high blood pressure, and obesity. Regular exercise also provides positive effects on some indicators related to cognitive performance. The direct effects of exercise on physiological and immunological indicators in the brain may effectively prevent mental disorders (Phillips and Fahimi 2018, Mokhtarzade et al. 2022a). Various studies have been conducted assessing the type, intensity, and repetition of physical exercises required to create positive changes in the brain in old age (Jonasson et al. 2017). This study examines the effects of regular physical exercise combined with curcumin supplementation on AD and cognitive disorders related to aging.

Exercise Training and Alzheimer's Disease and Age-Associated Cognitive Decline

Considerable evidence exists to support that regular exercise promotes the health and functionality of the central nervous system (CNS), reduces the cognitive decline associated with aging, and risk of cognitive impairment and dementia. Regular physical exercise has been reported to delay the onset of memory loss and reduce the risk of developing AD, so it is possible that exercise training could be considered a preventive strategy against age-related memory loss and neurodegeneration (Erickson et al. 2011). It has been reported that exercise training can delay the transition from mild cognitive impairment (MCI) to dementia (Nuzum et al. 2020); this is valuable when it is reported that 10-15% of individuals with MCI develop dementia within a year. In healthy older individuals, long-term exercise training has many beneficial effects, including improvements in reaction time, motor function, and cognitive processing speed, indicating that exercise is effective in slowing the age-related declines in cognitive processing (Rikli and Edwards 1991).

Regular physical exercise can improve cognition in people with dementia. This improvement is probably due to several pathways at the molecular and cellular levels. Physical exercise triggers cascades of cellular and molecular processes, including synaptogenesis, angiogenesis, and neurogenesis, and stimulates the release of neurotrophic factors that enhance learning, memory, and brain plasticity (De la Rosa et al. 2020, Deslandes et al. 2009). Exercise training also increases cerebral blood flow (CBF) in cortical and subcortical regions and decreases the formation of Aβ plaques(Moore et al. 2016). The phosphorylation of the tau protein in the hippocampus has been accompanied by improvements in learning and spatial memory (Ohia-Nwoko et al. 2014, Tapia-Rojas et al. 2016).

Moreover, increased size of the hippocampus and spatial memory (Erickson et al. 2011) and increased gray and white matter in the anterior cingulate cortex (Colcombe et al. 2006) were reported following moderate exercise training. It is apparent that exercise training in the early stages of the disease has more positive effects than in the advanced stages of AD. Exercise training cannot hinder the formation of Aβ plaques and cognitive deterioration if the intervention is carried out in progressive stages after plaques appear (Tabei et al. 2018).

One of the characteristics of AD is inflammation in the brain. Inflammaging is a prodrome to AD and microglial dysfunction, a common event during aging (Giunta et al. 2008). Inflammation alone inhibits neurogenesis, leading to progressive cognitive decline; therefore, preventing inflammation through pharmacological and non-pharmacological methods may restore neurogenesis and retrieve cognitive function. There is growing evidence that neuroinflammation and peripheral immune system activation are associated with cognitive dysfunction (Barrientos et al. 2015). In the early stages of the disease, the immune response removes the Aβ plaques and relieves the symptoms (Chakrabarty et al. 2010); however, in the advanced stages, prolonged stimulation of the immune response leads to a decrease in the efficiency of the microglia to degrade Aβ plaques (Hickman, Allison, and El Khoury 2008). The advanced stages are accompanied by the release of pro-inflammatory cytokines, and free radicals (reactive oxygen and nitrogen species), which cause an increase in the production of Aβ and the hyperphosphorylation of tau protein, leading to devastating neuronal cells, and a further decline in cognitive function and the development of AD. Microglia, the primary mediators of the immune response in the CNS, are typically quiescent; however, they activate and generate pro-inflammatory cytokines, interleukin-1β (IL-1β) and tumor necrosis factor-α (TNF-α), when a pathogen threaten the immune system (Colton 2009). When the threat is removed, microglia produce anti-inflammatory cytokines to re-establish homeostasis.

Exercise training has anti-inflammatory effects and counteracts the effects of long-term systemic inflammation. In rodents, it was shown that short-term exercise training was sufficient to decrease the levels of Aβ and the pro-inflammatory cytokines such as IL-1β and TNF-α, interferon-Y in the hippocampus (Nichol et al. 2008). Additionally, the anti-inflammatory effects of physical exercise on the CNS have also been confirmed in older animals. After only ten days of running on the treadmill, higher concentrations of hippocampal IL-10 and lower IL-1β/IL-10, IL-6/IL-10, and TNF-α/IL-10 ratios have been reported in rats (Gomes da Silva et al. 2013). Overall, these findings indicate that exercise training modulates inflammatory responses in the CNS and suggest that regular physical exercise has the potential to minimize the risk of neuroinflammation diseases, such as AD.

Neurotrophins are growth factors that regulate axonal growth, neurotransmission, synaptic plasticity, synaptic protein expression, hippocampal neurogenesis, and long-term potentiation (Huang and Reichardt 2001). Additionally, exercise training increases neuronal spine density and the number of neurons produced in the hippocampus in animal models, which correlates with increased spatial memory performance (Liu and Nusslock 2018). Low concentrations of brain-derived neurotrophic factor (BDNF) have been found in the brains of individuals with AD, which that increasing the production of this cytokine is an effective way to delay the onset of the disease. The brain produces more than 70% of resting-state BDNF levels. Following prolonged exercise training, the circulating BDNF levels are increased by 2- to 3-fold; there is evidence indicating that serum BDNF levels correlate with brain tissue BDNF levels (Kim, Choi, and Chung 2016). Circulating BDNF released by acute physical exercise may be transported back to, and used in, the brain. High levels of BDNF produced with moderate exercise training are associated with improved recognition memory in older rodents (Maejima et al. 2018). Moreover, exercise-induced increments in hippocampal volume were associated with greater circulating BDNF levels in healthy older individuals (Weinstein et al. 2014). Overall, higher serum BDNF levels are associated with a lower risk of developing AD.

Aging and AD lead to decreased cerebral blood flow (CBF) and arterial stiffness, which cause an accelerated decline in cognitive function and an increased risk of dementia (de la Torre 2002, Laurent et al. 2006). Aortic stiffening and dysfunction of the vascular endothelium are considered primary features of normal aging and are likely reasons for the increased risk of age-related cardiovascular disease. There appears an inverse relationship between arterial stiffness and cognitive performance, and therefore arterial stiffness may predict the rate of cognitive decline. The neural and vascular systems are inextricably linked. The "vascular hypothesis" proposes that vascular dysfunction affects the heart and brain, and has destructive consequences on cognitive function. The capacity of the vascular endothelium to release and respond to vasodilators, particularly nitric oxide (NO), declines with increasing age, thereby reducing CBF as well as the capacity of the endothelium to react efficiently to changing conditions (Virdis et al. 2010).

Table 1. Summary of systematic reviews and meta-analyses exploring the effect of exercise on cognitive function in people with dementia

First author	Subjects	Sample size (n)	Exercise intervention	Results
(Gates et al. 2013)	Older adults with MCI	1695	Mixed exercise intervention, three times per week, 40 min duration	– Limited evidence that exercise improves cognitive function
(Öhman et al. 2014)	Patients with MCI and Dementia	1699	Mixed exercise intervention	– Positive effects of physical exercise on cognition, mainly on global cognition, executive function, attention, and delayed recall
(Zheng et al. 2016)	Patients with MCI	1479	Aerobic exercise. 2-3 times per week; Mean duration 53 min	– Improved global cognitive ability – Improved memory with a small effect size
(Groot et al. 2016)	Patients with dementia	802	Aerobic exercise, combined exercise	– Both interventions positively influence cognitive function
(Learner and Williams 2016)	Patients with dementia	423	Mixed exercise; 3-4 times per week, 35 min duration	– All interventions had a favorable effect on cognition. – Prolonged aerobic exercise may be most effective for those with mild-to-moderate cognitive impairment; while multimodal programs may be most effective for moderate-to-severe dementia
(Cammisuli et al. 2017)	MCI patients	768	Aerobic exercise. Mean frequency 2.55 times per week; Mean duration 57 min	– Aerobic exercise improves cognition – Moderate effects on global cognition, logical memory, inhibitory control, and divided attention
(Cammisuli et al. 2018)	AD patients	554	Aerobic exercise	– Positive effects on patient's global cognition after aerobic intervention
(Song et al. 2018)	People with MCI	929	Aerobic, resistance, and combined exercises	– Physical exercise, aerobic exercise, in particular, has positive effects on global cognition
(Jia et al. 2019)	Patients with AD	673	Mixed exercise training; 2 times per week, 40 min duration	– Improved cognition with exercise interventions

First author	Subjects	Sample size (n)	Exercise intervention	Results
(Ojagbemi and Akin-Ojagbemi 2019)	Persons with dementia	903	Mixed Physical activity	– Exercise interventions led to small and no significant improvements in quality of life (QoL)
(Wang et al. 2019)	People with MCI	1088	Aerobic, resistance, and mind-body exercises	– Resistance exercises were the most effective exercise type, followed by exergames, aerobic exercises, and mind-body exercises to improve global cognition
(Li et al. 2019)	Dementia patients	2051	Exercise programs	– Exercise programs increased cognitive levels and activities of daily living
(Lim et al. 2019)	Older adults with dementia	325	Tai Chi. Mean frequency three times per week; Mean duration 46 min	– Tai Chi has positive impacts on global cognitive functions, visuospatial skills, semantic memory, verbal learning/memory, and self-perception of memory
(Zou et al. 2019)	People with MCI	1298	Mind-body exercise (MBE) (Tai Chi, yoga, qigong) Mean frequency 3.8 times per week; Mean duration 60 min	– Improved various cognitive functions (attention, short-term memory, executive function, visual-spatial/executive function, global cognitive function)
(de Almeida, Gomes da Silva, and Marques 2020)	People with dementia	1129	Home-based physical activity	– A home-based exercise is a good option for delaying cognitive function decline and improving changes in behavioural and psychological symptoms of dementia. – Intervention improves the activities of daily living, health-related physical fitness, and the career's burden
(Demurtas et al. 2020)	Participants with MCI/Dementia	28205	Mixed exercise interventions	– Mixed physical activity interventions had a negligible effect on global cognition – Exercise had positive effects on non-cognitive outcomes
(Zhu et al. 2020)	Older adults with MCI	842	Aerobic exercise/dance	– Improved global cognitive function, executive function, and memory

Table 1. (Continued)

First author	Subjects	Sample size (n)	Exercise intervention	Results
(Biazus-Sehn et al. 2020)	Older persons with MCI	2077	Physical exercise mixed, mid-body exercise	– Physical exercise can ameliorate cognitive deficits of older adults with MCI. The marked effects were obtained from moderate exercise and mind-body exercises.
(Law et al. 2020)	People with MCI or dementia	5099	Aerobic exercise	– Physical exercise can reduce global cognitive decline – Aerobic exercise at moderate intensity or above can produce a more pronounced effect on global cognition.
(López-Ortiz et al. 2021)	Patients with AD	1337	Aerobic, strength, or combined training	– Improved global cognition, physical function, functional independence, and neuropsychiatric symptoms – Aerobic exercise was the most effective exercise model
(Pisani et al. 2021)	Participants with MCI/AD	1793	Mixed exercise interventions	– Improved cognition in both AD and MCI groups the effect size for physical exercise was generally comparable to donepezil
(Huang et al. 2022)	Patients with MCI or dementia	5606	Aerobic, strength, or combined training	– All exercise types were effective in slowing cognitive decline, – Resistance exercise was the most effective intervention – Multicomponent exercise tends to be most effective in protecting global cognition and executive function
(Salzman et al. 2022)	Older adults with MCI	2711	Cognitive and physical components; multiple exercise or cognitive components; mind-body; combined cognitive training	– Short-term multidomain interventions (<1 year) were associated with improvements in global cognition, executive function, memory, and verbal fluency
(Meng et al. 2022)	Patients with MCI	1337	Combined exercise intervention	– Positive effects on global cognition
(Zhou et al. 2022)	Older adults with MCI	1290	Traditional Chinese exercises	– The effect size on global cognitive and multiple domains of cognitive function was small when compared to the active control and was moderate compared to the inactive control

Decreased production capacity of NO causes the increased production of cytotoxic amyloid-β (Aβ) peptides, both in the cerebral micro-vessels and in the brain (Katusic and Austin 2014), a process closely associated with AD. Regular exercise has been shown to improve the vascular system, arterial stiffness, endothelial function, and CBF (Kennedy et al. 2017). Regular aerobic and resistance exercises prevent the decline of and restore or improve the process of the vascular endothelium in middle-aged and older healthy males (Ashor et al. 2015). Stimulation of the endothelial cells through shear stress and increased localized blood flow, increased levels of circulating catecholamines, and lower resting heart rate reducing mechanical stress are proposed mechanisms for improved age-related endothelial function following exercise.

Regular physical exercise can improve both cognitive and non-cognitive consequences in people with dementia. Exercise training can also increase the health of the nervous system through synaptogenesis, angiogenesis, neurogenesis, and the release of neurotrophic factors (Erickson et al. 2011, Vecchio et al. 2018). These benefits could enhance learning, memory, and cognitive functions in people with dementia. In addition, exercise training can decrease the risk of disability, falls, and neuropsychiatric symptoms and improve quality of life (Du et al. 2018, De la Rosa et al. 2020). Table 1 reports studies on the effect of exercise interventions on the cognitive function of individuals with mild cognitive impairment (MCI) or dementia. Briefly, all exercise modalities appear to increase or maintain the global cognitive function in patients with diagnosed MCI or dementia. The effect size reported for resistance and high-intensity exercise training ($d>1.1$) was greater than that of low-intensity interventions (Wang et al. 2019, Huang et al. 2022). In addition, combined exercise training seems to have a more substantial protective effect (Learner and Williams 2016, Jia et al. 2019, Pisani et al. 2021).

Excessive exercise could be associated with negative metabolic changes, disruption of mitochondrial function, and increased production of ROS. In the long term, this may disrupt the positive adaptations associated with exercise training and may lead to local or systemic inflammation, muscle damage, oxidative stress, and skeletal muscle dysfunction (Murray et al. 1985, Murray et al. 1980, Gallagher et al. 1997). In the conditions of old age, high-intensity exercise activities can also play a role in causing other complications such as muscle mass loss (Receno et al. 2019, Lee et al. 2021, Cheragh-Birjandi et al. 2020, Sugawara et al. 2012). Some studies suggest using anti-inflammatory and antioxidant compounds to prevent the mentioned complications and promote the desired adaptations from exercise training (Fernández-Lázaro et al. 2020, Tanabe et al. 2015). The aging process will be accompanied by oxidative stress and inflammation (Yu and Chung 2006), so combining antioxidant and anti-inflammatory agents with higher-intensity exercises may prove beneficial.

Numerous medicinal herbs and plants have been proposed to possess antioxidant and anti-inflammatory effects (Ferguson, Abbott, and Garg 2021). Curcumin has been used in many exercise studies for preventing muscle injuries, modulating immune system responses and intestinal microbiota and reducing gastrointestinal side effects, and as an effective anti-inflammatory (Rolfe et al. 2020). The following section examines the effects of curcumin on indicators of cognitive function, especially in old age; we discuss the possible effects of combining curcumin with exercise activities in relation to age-related cognitive decline and AD.

Effect of Curcumin Supplementation on Alzheimer's Disease and Age-Related Cognitive Function

Evidence suggests that polyphenols may have potential health-promoting properties (Spagnuolo et al. 2016). It has also been reported that polyphenols may counteract nerve damage. Therefore polyphenols have a potential role in preventing or treating cognitive disorders and neurological diseases, especially dementia. Table 2 summarizes the finding of systematic reviews and meta-analyses examining the effect of curcumin on cognitive function in people with and without dementia. Curcumin has been shown to inhibit the formation of Aβ fibrils, destroy preformed fibrils, and inhibit tau phosphorylation in vivo and in vitro animal models (Lim GP 2001). The intake of 100 mg/d for 12 weeks or 400 mg/d of curcumin supplement improved symptoms of cognitive impairment, modified blood biomarkers, and enhanced cognitive functions like attention and memory in adults (Hishikawa et al. 2012, Cox, Pipingas, and Scholey 2014). In one study, taking 750 mg/d of curcumin for nine months improved overall beta cell function and blood sugar levels (Chuengsamarn S 2012).

Additionally, treatment with 100 mg/d of curcumin and donepezil for 12 weeks significantly improved cognitive performance in three patients with dementia and severe behavioural and psychological symptoms (Hishikawa et al. 2012). In an RCT, 400 mg/d of curcumin supplementation improved cognitive function, mood, and blood biomarkers in 60 healthy adults and enhanced sustained attention and working memory (Cox, Pipingas, and Scholey 2014). Conversely, in another RCT study with 96 participants, 1500 mg/d of curcumin supplement per day for 12 months provided no improvement in cognitive function compared to the placebo group (Rainey-Smith et al. 2016). In a study, the short-term and long-term effects of curcumin (480 mg/kg of feed) in aged male Sprague-Dawley rats evaluated both behavioural and physiological effects. Curcumin did not affect motor behaviour but both treatment periods had significant cognitive effects. Both short and long-term interventions improved the social recognition index, a measurement for non-spatial learning; however, only those who underwent more extended treatment had a better spatial understanding (Dong et al. 2012). Further, the mice with the more extended treatment also had enhanced cell proliferation in the dentate gyrus indicating neurogenesis. (Dong S 2012). In a study that examined the different dosages of the curcumin supplement (1 g/d or 4 g/d), there was no difference in Mini-Mental State Examination (MMSE) between the interventions at a 6-month follow-up (Baum et al. 2008).

Aging and brain atrophy is associated with increased free radicals production, and this is notable in AD. This chronic neurological disorder leads to progressive synapses, memory loss, and speech and behaviour changes (Fusco D 2007). In addition, curcumin is a lipophilic compound that makes it an efficient scavenger of peroxyl radicals. Curcumin can modulate the activity of GSH, catalase, and SOD enzymes, which neutralizes free radicals (Nakmareong et al. 2011). Another common feature of aging is sarcopenia in the skeletal muscles, which can impair the ability to perform everyday activities and negatively affect the quality of life. Sarcopenia is independently related to cognitive impairment (Lee et al. 2018). As an antioxidant, curcumin has anti-aging properties that are important for older people in preventing muscle breakdown and inhibiting nuclear factor kappa-light-chain-enhancer of activated B cells (NF-kB) levels which are typically responsible for the onset of sarcopenia. Curcumin enhances antioxidant defence, potentially precludes the onset of sarcopenia, and prevents the development of pro-inflammatory cytokines (Franceschi F 2016).

Diabetes is a disorder in which dysregulation of the insulin signalling pathway leads to insulin resistance (Biessels and Reijmer 2014). Clinical studies have shown that glucose intolerance and insulin dysfunction can negatively affect brain function (Biessels et al. 2014). In addition, several studies have shown that diabetes is a risk factor for cognitive function-related diseases such as dementia and AD (Riederer et al. 2017). Diabetes is also associated with cerebral atrophy, neurological disabilities, cognitive decline, and psychomotor dysfunction (Chen et al. 2018). Evidence suggests that low-grade inflammation and oxidative stress contribute to insulin resistance (Ferroni et al. 2004).

Chronic inflammation is a significant contributor to the development of non-communicable diseases. Curcumin is a known natural anti-inflammatory that reduces the inflammatory response in T2D through the Nrf2 and PI3K/AKT signalling pathways (Biswas et al. 2019, Yan et al. 2018, Rashid et al. 2017). In addition, the finding of a review showed a reduction in C-reactive protein, interleukin-6, TNF-α, IL-8, monocyte chemoattractant protein-1, and an increase in IL-10, with no effect on intracellular adhesion molecule-1. These data provide evidence for the anti-inflammatory effects of curcumin (Ferguson, Abbott, and Garg 2021). Curcumin has also been shown to reduce the expression of the insulin receptor gene and insulin receptor substrate 1 in the hippocampus (Feng et al. 2016, Wang and Holsinger 2018). In one study, mice fed curcumin at 5 g/kg reported weight loss, improved glucose homeostasis and lipid profiles, and enhanced diabetes-related cognitive function (Jin Ah Cho, Se Hwan Park. 2020). In addition, curcumin supplementation has been shown to increase vascular function by improving endothelium-dependent vasodilation (Santos-Parker et al. 2017).

The ability to develop cognitive-behavioural communication between the gut microbiome and the so-called brain-gut axis in neurological diseases has been extensively studied (Mokhtarzade et al. 2022b). Intestinal microbiomes alter intestinal hormone secretion and immune response, block the intestinal mucosa, control the blood-brain barrier and create and break down neurotransmitters, so they interact closely with the central nervous system, which affects the brain. A new working hypothesis that could explain the neuroprotective role of curcumin, is that curcumin indirectly affects the central nervous system by affecting the "intestinal and brain microbiota axis" (Peluso 2019). Despite the positive effects of the curcumin supplement, its effects depend on the dosage, so gastrointestinal symptoms were the most common side effects of high dosages (Nathan Seddon 2019). However, the critical point is that curcumin has not shown any significant toxicity in most pre-clinical and clinical studies, and few studies have reported any adverse effects (Sharma et al. 2004, Lao et al. 2006). In addition, natural supplements like curcumin may be a safe and inexpensive source of drugs to control or prevent diseases.

Table 2. Summary of systematic reviews and meta-analyses exploring the effect of curcumin on cognitive function in people with and without dementia

First author	Target population	Sample size (n)	Curcumin intervention	Results
(Zhu et al. 2019) Six studies N = 289	Elderly population, Elderly population Elderly population Patient with AD Patient with AD Schizophrenia	N = 60 (63-75yrs.) N = 96 (60-74yrs.) N = 40 (60-74yrs.) N = 30 (60-78yrs) N = 27 (60-80yrs.) N = 36 (18-65 yrs.)	4 W; 80 mg/day 12 M; 1.3 g/day 18 M; 180 mg/day 24 W; 1.9-3.9 g/day 6 M; 1-4 g/day 8 W; 360 mg/day	- Improve cognitive functions in older adults (memory performance, cognitive process) - No significant improvement in cognition status of the patient with AD or schizophrenia - The occurrence of adverse events was similar to those who received a placebo
(Seddon et al. 2019) Five studies N = 292	Adults with AD Patient with AD Healthy adults Healthy adults Healthy and MCI	N = 34 (73.4 yrs.) N = 36 (65-80yrs.) N = 60 (60-75yrs) N = 96 (60-75yrs.) N = 40 (55-75yrs.)	24 W; 1-4 g/day 48 W; 2-4 g/day 4 W; 400 mg/day 52 W; 1500 mg/day 78 W; 2×90 mg/day	- Improvements in cognitive indicators, reminding, visual memory, and attention - Improvement in MoCA test - Improvement in serial three subtraction task responses - Adverse events were reported (n = 58), and gastrointestinal symptoms were the most common
(Sarraf et al. 2019) Four studies N = 155	Healthy Adult Healthy Adult Healthy Adult Healthy Adult	N = 20 (50-65yrs.) N = 45 (18-65yrs.) N = 20 (40-55yrs.) N = 70 (18-50yrs.)	8 W; 1480 mg/day 8 W;360 mg/day 8 W; 1820 mg/day 12W;200 mg/day	- Significantly increased serum BDNF levels - Significant heterogeneity among the studies (sex, mean age of participants, curcumin dosage, and trial duration were potential sources of heterogeneity)
(Voulgaropoulou et al. 2019) Five clinical studies N = 253	Healthy elderly Healthy elderly patient with MCI Patient with AD Non- demented	N = 96 (40-90yrs.) N = 60 (60-85yrs.) N = 27(>50yrs.) N = 49 (>49yrs.) N = 40 (51-84yrs.)	12M;1500 mg/day 4 W; 400mg/day 6 M;1-4 g/day 24 W;2-4 g/day 18 M; 90mg/day	- Improved working memory and attention. - Downregulation in total and LDL cholesterol. - Improved memory and attention performance and prevented neuropathological deposition in the amygdala and hypothalamus - Non-significant change/decline in MMSE

Table 2. (Continued)

First author	Target population	Sample size (n)	Curcumin intervention	Results
(Tsai et al. 2021) Eight studies N = 389	Overweight older Healthy Elderly Schizophrenia Schizophrenia Non-demented Older adults Patient with AD Patient with AD	N = 63 (63-68yrs.) N = 85 (60-75yrs.) N = 12 (27-55 yrs.) N = 36 (18-65yrs.) N = 40 (51-75yrs.) N = 96 (60-74yrs.) N = 30 (63-85yrs.) N = 27 (60-80yrs.)	16W; 160 mg/day 12 W; 80 mg/day 8 W; 180 mg/day 8 W; 360 mg/day 18 M; 180 mg/day 12 M; 1.3 g/day 24 W; 2-4 g/day 6 M; 1-4 g/day	- An improvement in working memory and processing speed - No effect on domains of language: episodic memory, verbal memory, cognitive flexibility/problem solving, and overall cognitive function - The curcumin group had a significantly higher risk of gastrointestinal adverse events than the placebo group
(Mehrabadi, Alinaghpour, and Zahedi 2021) Three studies N = 96	patient with AD Healthy Elderly patient with AD	N = 30 (63-85yrs.) N = 38 (40-55yrs.) N = 27 (60-80yrs.)	24 W; 2-4 mg/day 4 W; 80 mg/day 6 M; 1-4 g/day	- No significant change in serum Aβ level

Studies have shown that natural products or nutrients may have anti-aging properties, and their consumption has been recommended as a preventive measure. In addition, other lifestyle factors, such as regular exercise training, play a critical role in aging. Considering some of the same effects of regular exercise training and supplementation on cognition, especially in older adults, combining exercise training and curcumin supplementation may be more effective in preventing age-related cognitive impairment and AD. Previous studies suggest that a healthy diet and exercise training can stimulate brain plasticity and help individuals cope with neurological disorders (Gomez-Pinilla 2011). In the following section, we examine the potential benefits of combining exercise training and curcumin supplementation on preventing age-related cognitive impairment and AD.

Combined Effects of Curcumin Supplantation and Exercise Training on Age-Associated Cognitive Decline and Alzheimer's Disease

Regular physical exercise and nutritional interventions have been promoted as critical interventions in controlling the age-related decline in cognitive performance. Curcumin supplementation reduces the subjective perception of the severity of muscle pain; reduces muscle damage through the diminution of creatine kinase (CK), and may enhance muscle performance. Additionally, curcumin provides an anti-inflammatory effect by lowering the level of the pro-inflammatory cytokines and may have an antioxidant effect. The administration of curcumin at a dose between 150-1500 mg/day before, during and up until 72 h post-exercise improved performance by reducing exercise-induced muscle damage (EIMD) and modulating the inflammation caused by physical activity (Fernández-Lázaro et al. 2020, Hewlings and Kalman 2017). However, adverse side effects of high doses (>500 mg) have been reported including diarrhoea, headache, rash, and yellow stool. The metabolic effects of exercise training may help to tolerate these high doses of curcumin.

Aging is an inevitable and progressive process that leads to deterioration in the quality of life and an increasing incidence of age-related chronic diseases through deterioration in morphological, functional, hemodynamic, and psychological systems, (Roubenoff 2000). Pathological changes in the brain generally occur at older ages. Age-related cognitive decline is one of the significant public health concerns (Fink et al. 2018). Increased risk factors for cognitive decline include heart disease, stroke, hypertension, high cholesterol, and diabetes. However, aging remains the most significant risk factor due to increases in oxidative stress which exacerbates cognitive decline through hemostatic imbalance (Heneka et al. 2015). Research shows that aging has a negative relationship with the volume of white and gray matter in the hippocampus and amygdala, as well as other areas of the brain, including the frontal cortex, temporal lobe, parietal and occipital cortex (Raz and Rodrigue 2006). Because these cortical and subcortical regions are involved in cognition, their atrophy is often accompanied by cognitive decline. Aging inhibits several mental functions, including information processing speed, reasoning, attention, and memory formation (Murman 2015). Factors such as increased LDL cholesterol, homocysteine, hypertension, history of stroke, depressive symptoms, interleukin-6, Alpha-1-antichymotrypsin, alcohol use, and smoking have been associated with the decline of age-related cognitive function (Sabia et al. 2012, van Vliet 2012, Mansukhani, Kolla, and Somers 2019). Population-based studies show that regular physical activity and managing cardiovascular risk factors such as diabetes, obesity, hypertension, and smoking are strongly associated with reduced risk of dementia. In addition, a healthy diet and using functional nutrients may lower the risk of cognitive function decline (Smyth et al. 2015).

The beneficial effects of regular physical exercise in reducing age-related cognitive performance have been reported in various studies (Table 1). Physical activity can modulate the cardiovascular risk factors related to dementia. Also, appropriate exercise training can modulate blood lipid profiles, blood pressure, metabolic indicators and pathways, inflammatory responses, and factors related to immune system function. Regular physical exercise is one of the primary interventions recommended for managing diabetes and obesity, along with other weight control methods (Westerterp 2018). In addition, herbal medicines are recommended as complementary treatments, especially in the prevention of chronic diseases. The effect of curcumin on age-related cognitive disease risk indicators such as hypertension, lipid profiles, and inflammatory status has also been considered (Benameur et al. 2021b). The use of curcumin to combat conditions such as obesity, metabolic syndrome, and hypertension has also received attention in recent years. Also, polyphenol compounds have been considered due to their special antioxidant effects on controlling cellular aging (Ferguson, Abbott, and Garg 2021).

Considering the potential effects of exercise training and curcumin supplementation in reducing cognitive function, combining these two may provide a synergic effect in controlling age-related risk factors. Few studies have investigated the simultaneous impacts of curcumin and exercise training interventions on the risk indicators of cognitive deficits. In rodents, the combination of regular physical exercise and curcumin supplementation provided neuroprotection through antioxidant effects, which could lead to improved brain health (Gallagher et al. 1997). It has been reported that the combination of moderate-intensity exercise training and curcumin supplementation increases BDNF concentration in rats (Gallagher et al. 1997). In addition, a short period of aerobic exercise training with curcumin was effective in controlling inflammatory indices, glycemic indices, and oxidative stress while increasing BDNF levels in aged women with metabolic syndrome (Murray et al. 1980). A review article suggests that curcumin also potentially affects the prevention and treatment of AD (Mishra and Palanivelu 2008). Curcumin, an antioxidant, and anti-inflammatory with lipophilic action, improves the cognitive functions of patients with AD (Mishra and Palanivelu 2008). The combination of exercise and curcumin also improves mental processes through the modulation of indirect factors involved in cognitive impairments. The literature indicates that increases in oxidative stress, free radicals, beta-amyloid, and proinflammatory cytokines contribute to AD pathology. It has been shown the combination of curcumin and exercise results in reduced beta-amyloid plaques, delaying the degradation of neurons, metal-chelation, anti-inflammatory, antioxidant, and decreasing microglia formation, improving chronic glycosylation and lipid peroxidation (Miller et al. 2012). In addition, it could improve flow-mediated endothelial dilation (Luhtala et al. 1994) whereby the overall memory in patients with AD would improve (Fernández-Lázaro et al. 2020).

Exercise intensity can affect the age-related cognitive decline in AD (Wang et al. 2019). High-intensity exercises can increase local or systemic inflammation, muscle damage, oxidative stress, and skeletal muscle dysfunction, especially in older populations (Cerqueira et al. 2020). Taking curcumin along with intense exercises may moderate the harmful effects of such exercises due to curcumin antioxidant and anti-inflammatory effects. Additionally, some inflammatory and oxidative indicators have been reduced following exercise training and curcumin supplementation in young and athletic subjects (Fernández-Lázaro et al. 2020, Ferguson, Abbott, and Garg 2021). Intense exercise increases circulating levels of muscle damage markers such as lactate dehydrogenase (LDH), creatine kinase (CK), myoglobin, transaminases, alanine aminotransferase (ALT), and aspartate amino-transferase (AST). Research shows that a dose of 150 mg of curcumin, when administered immediately after exercise, is associated with a significant reduction in the levels of three circulating muscle damage markers (CK, AST, and ALT) (Yoon, Lee, and Kim 2020). Potentially, the reduction in CK after curcumin supplementation can be attributed to the neutralising of oxygen free radicals (ROS) produced during the electron transport chain of oxidative phosphorylation, which is necessary for the energy required in physical exercise. Another possible mechanism for reduced CK activity may be the inhibition of the production of histamine and prostaglandins which suppress the upregulation of cyclooxygenase-2 (COX-2), a pathway involved in vascular permeability (Moriyuki et al. 2010).

The mechanical stress-induced muscle damage produced during eccentric exercise and subsequent inflammatory responses leads to deterioration of muscle performance, such as maximal voluntary contraction (MVC), range of motion (ROM), and isokinetic strength. Isokinetic strength, MVC, and ROM are reduced by the activation of the NF-kB signalling pathway under the high mechanical stress caused by overuse of joints in exercise, which produces fragments of the extracellular matrix of the bone or cartilage (Fernández-Lázaro et al. 2020). These fragments are recognised by receptors of innate immunity, which signal recognition receptors, called toll-like receptors. Cell activation mediated by the NF-kB signalling stimulates the release of inflammatory cytokines, chemokines, and metalloproteases, all of which cause tissue damage (Daily, Yang, and Park 2016). Curcumin can diminish these tissue-damaging factors as it blocks the NF-kB signalling pathway (Alamdari, O'Neal, and Hasselgren 2009). In addition, curcumin reduces the adhesion and migration of leukocytes thus relieving pain and swelling and improving joint mobility and stiffness (Alamdari, O'Neal, and Hasselgren 2009). It has been shown that 150 mg of curcumin taken before and 12 hours after 50 eccentric contractions of the elbow flexors produced a significantly smaller decrease in MVC (Tanabe et al. 2015). These studies suggest that taking a dose of curcumin (90 to 200 mg) after exercise may enhance muscle function and improve recovery.

Also, combining curcumin supplementation with higher training intensities can prevent the decline of cognitive function with direct benefits on skeletal muscle. A positive correlation between sarcopenia and impaired cognitive function has been reported (Lee et al. 2018). Sarcopenia is the loss of muscle mass related to old age and can lead to impaired muscle strength, reduced physical activity, and individual independence. Exercise training in elderly populations can prevent sarcopenia. Lee et al. (2021) showed that curcumin has anti-apoptotic, anti-inflammatory effects and regulates the antioxidation-mediated modulation of gene expressions related to muscle degradation and protein synthesis. Therefore, curcumin may be effective in controlling sarcopenia and act as an adjunct therapy with high-intensity exercise training to mitigate muscle disorders (Lee et al. 2021). Similarly curcumin treatment during high-intensity swimming training in rats has been associated with mitochondrial biogenesis by increasing cAMP levels (Ray Hamidie et al. 2015). It has also been suggested that the possible cross-talk between skeletal muscle and the brain through myokines released following exercise activities can play a role in maintaining brain function and preventing cognitive decline (Isaac, Lima-Filho, and Lourenco 2021).

In addition, prolonged periods of curcumin use, especially in higher doses, can improve the responses related to metabolic indicators related to cognitive impairment. The recommended amount of curcumin is 0-3 mg per kilogram of body weight. However, adverse side effects of high doses (>500) have been reported, including diarrhoea, headache, rash, and yellow stool (Hewlings and Kalman 2017). Higher doses of curcumin, in some cases, have been associated with limited toxic effects in animal models (Jantawong et al. 2021). In a study, A study by (Sharma et al. 2004) reported that taking 0.45 to 3.6 grams per day of curcumin for four months caused nausea and diarrhoea and increased serum alkaline phosphatase and lactate dehydrogenase content. Chronic use of curcumin can cause liver toxicity, especially in long-term supplementation. Thus, it is recommended that individuals who consume a lot of alcohol or drugs that are metabolized in the liver should avoid using turmeric products (Mishra and Palanivelu 2008). However, metabolic effects observed during physical exercise in older adults can effectively diminish the side effects of curcumin supplementation. Well-designed exercise training with increased energy expenditure can modulate metabolic responses in the liver (Smart et al. 2018). In addition, exercise training can reverse the age-associated decrease in the hepatic free radical scavenging system (Mallikarjuna et al. 2010).

Moreover, one concern that should be considered by athletes who are susceptible to iron deficiencies when taking curcumin supplements is the interaction between high doses of curcumin and the change of iron metabolism by the chelation of iron and the rise of hepcidin, which could be one of the potential causes of decreased iron levels. For this reason, it is recommended to take a low dose of curcumin with piperine to increase the bioavailability of curcumin. Regular exercise increases iron absorption from the intestine (Schmid et al. 1996) and therefore, may partially mitigate the harmful effects of high doses of curcumin supplementation.

Conclusion

Combining exercise training and curcumin supplementation may ameliorate risk factors related to cognitive diseases by creating synergistic effects. It seems that higher intensities of physical exercise may be an optimal method for improving cognitive indicators. However, high-intensity exercise training can increase inflammatory indices, muscle damage, and fatigue. The use of curcumin supplementation can be effective in improving the physiological and psychological responses to exercise training. At the same time, the metabolic regulatory effects of physical exercise can effectively increase people's tolerance to higher doses and prolonged use of curcumin. However, more studies are needed, especially in the elderly with different metabolic conditions (obesity and diabetes), to investigate the combined effects of different types of physical exercise and different doses of curcumin on age-related risk factors in cognitive function. Also, the combined effects of exercise activities and curcumin on cognitive performance in Alzheimer's patients should be considered in more studies.

Acknowledgment

We wish to thank the Research Center of Tarbiat Modares University (TMU).

Conflict of Interest

All authors declare they have no conflict of interest.

Ethical Approval for Studies Involving Humans

This article does not contain any studies with human participants performed by any authors.

Ethical Approval for Studies Involving Animals

This article does not contain any studies with animals performed by any of the authors.

References

Alamdari, N., P. O'Neal, and P. O. Hasselgren. 2009. "Curcumin and muscle wasting: a new role for an old drug?" *Nutrition* 25 (2):125-9. doi: 10.1016/j.nut. 2008.09.002.

Alzheimer's Association. "2015 Alzheimer's disease facts and figures." *Alzheimers Dement* 11 (3):332-84. doi: 10.1016/j.jalz.2015.02.003.

Alzheimer's Association. 2021. "2021 Alzheimer's disease facts and figures." *Alzheimers Dement* 17 (3):327-406. doi: 10.1002/alz.12328.

Benameur, T., R. Soleti, M. A. Panaro, M. E. La Torre, V. Monda, G. Messina, and C. Porro. 2021a. "Curcumin as Prospective Anti-Aging Natural Compound: Focus on Brain." *Molecules* 26 (16). doi: 10.3390/molecules26164794.

Benameur, Tarek, Raffaella Soleti, Maria Antonietta Panaro, Maria Ester La Torre, Vincenzo Monda, Giovanni Messina, and Chiara Porro. 2021b. "Curcumin as Prospective Anti-Aging Natural Compound: Focus on Brain." *Molecules (Basel, Switzerland)* 26 (16):4794. doi: 10.3390/molecules26164794.

Biazus-Sehn, L. F., F. B. Schuch, J. Firth, and F. S. Stigger. 2020. "Effects of physical exercise on cognitive function of older adults with mild cognitive impairment: A systematic review and meta-analysis." *Arch Gerontol Geriatr* 89:104048. doi: 10.1016/j.archger.2020.104048.

Bielak-Zmijewska, A., W. Grabowska, A. Ciolko, A. Bojko, G. Mosieniak, Ł Bijoch, and E. Sikora. 2019. "The Role of Curcumin in the Modulation of Ageing." *Int J Mol Sci* 20 (5). doi: 10.3390/ijms20051239.

Cammisuli, D. M., A. Innocenti, F. Franzoni, and C. Pruneti. 2017. "Aerobic exercise effects upon cognition in Mild Cognitive Impairment: A systematic review of randomized controlled trials." *Arch Ital Biol* 155 (1-2):54-62. doi: 10.12871/000398292017126.

Cammisuli, D. M., A. Innocenti, J. Fusi, F. Franzoni, and C. Pruneti. 2018. "Aerobic exercise effects upon cognition in Alzheimer's Disease: A systematic review of randomized controlled trials." *Arch Ital Biol* 156 (1-2):54-63. doi: 10.12871/00039829201816.

Cerqueira, Érica, Daniel A. Marinho, Henrique P. Neiva, and Olga Lourenço. 2020. "Inflammatory Effects of High and Moderate Intensity Exercise-A Systematic Review." *Frontiers in Physiology* 10:1550-1550. doi: 10.3389/fphys.2019.01550.

Daily, J. W., M. Yang, and S. Park. 2016. "Efficacy of Turmeric Extracts and Curcumin for Alleviating the Symptoms of Joint Arthritis: A Systematic Review and Meta-Analysis of Randomized Clinical Trials." *J Med Food* 19 (8):717-29. doi: 10.1089/jmf.2016.3705.

de Almeida, S. I. L., M. Gomes da Silva, and Aspd Marques. 2020. "Home-Based Physical Activity Programs for People With Dementia: Systematic Review and Meta-Analysis." *Gerontologist* 60 (8):600-608. doi: 10.1093/geront/gnz176.

De la Rosa, Adrian, Gloria Olaso-Gonzalez, Coralie Arc-Chagnaud, Fernando Millan, Andrea Salvador-Pascual, Consolacion García-Lucerga, Cristina Blasco-Lafarga, Esther Garcia-Dominguez, Aitor Carretero, Angela G. Correas, Jose Viña, and Mari Carmen Gomez-Cabrera. 2020. "Physical exercise in the prevention and treatment of

Alzheimer's disease." *Journal of Sport and Health Science* 9 (5):394-404. doi: https://doi.org/10.1016/j.jshs.2020.01.004.

Demurtas, J., D. Schoene, G. Torbahn, A. Marengoni, G. Grande, L. Zou, M. Petrovic, S. Maggi, M. Cesari, S. Lamb, P. Soysal, W. Kemmler, C. Sieber, C. Mueller, S. D. Shenkin, L. Schwingshackl, L. PhD Smith, and N. Veronese. 2020. "Physical Activity and Exercise in Mild Cognitive Impairment and Dementia: An Umbrella Review of Intervention and Observational Studies." *J Am Med Dir Assoc* 21 (10):1415-1422.e6. doi: 10.1016/j.jamda.2020.08.031.

Dominguez, L. J., N. Veronese, L. Vernuccio, G. Catanese, F. Inzerillo, G. Salemi, and M. Barbagallo. 2021. "Nutrition, Physical Activity, and Other Lifestyle Factors in the Prevention of Cognitive Decline and Dementia." *Nutrients* 13 (11). doi: 10.3390/nu13114080.

Dong, S., Q. Zeng, E. S. Mitchell, J. Xiu, Y. Duan, C. Li, J. K. Tiwari, Y. Hu, X. Cao, and Z. Zhao. 2012. "Curcumin enhances neurogenesis and cognition in aged rats: implications for transcriptional interactions related to growth and synaptic plasticity." *PLoS One* 7 (2):e31211. doi: 10.1371/journal.pone.0031211.

Du, Z., Y. Li, J. Li, C. Zhou, F. Li, and X. Yang. 2018. "Physical activity can improve cognition in patients with Alzheimer's disease: a systematic review and meta-analysis of randomized controlled trials." *Clin Interv Aging* 13:1593-1603. doi: 10.2147/cia.s169565.

Erickson, K. I., M. W. Voss, R. S. Prakash, C. Basak, A. Szabo, L. Chaddock, J. S. Kim, S. Heo, H. Alves, S. M. White, T. R. Wojcicki, E. Mailey, V. J. Vieira, S. A. Martin, B. D. Pence, J. A. Woods, E. McAuley, and A. F. Kramer. 2011. "Exercise training increases size of hippocampus and improves memory." *Proc Natl Acad Sci U S A* 108 (7):3017-22. doi: 10.1073/pnas.1015950108.

Ferguson, J. J. A., K. A. Abbott, and M. L. Garg. 2021. "Anti-inflammatory effects of oral supplementation with curcumin: a systematic review and meta-analysis of randomized controlled trials." *Nutr Rev* 79 (9):1043-1066. doi: 10.1093/nutrit/ nuaa114.

Fernández-Lázaro, D., J. Mielgo-Ayuso, J. Seco Calvo, A. Córdova Martínez, A. Caballero García, and C. I. Fernandez-Lazaro. 2020. "Modulation of Exercise-Induced Muscle Damage, Inflammation, and Oxidative Markers by Curcumin Supplementation in a Physically Active Population: A Systematic Review." *Nutrients* 12 (2). doi: 10.3390/nu12020501.

Ferroni, Patrizia, Stefani Basili, Angela Falco, and Giovanni Davì. 2004. "Inflammation, insulin resistance, and obesity." *Current atherosclerosis reports* 6 (6):424-431.

Fink, H. A., E. Jutkowitz, J. R. McCarten, L. S. Hemmy, M. Butler, H. Davila, E. Ratner, C. Calvert, T. R. Barclay, M. Brasure, V. A. Nelson, and R. L. Kane. 2018. "Pharmacologic Interventions to Prevent Cognitive Decline, Mild Cognitive Impairment, and Clinical Alzheimer-Type Dementia: A Systematic Review." *Ann Intern Med* 168 (1):39-51. doi: 10.7326/m17-1529.

Gallagher, D., M. Visser, R. E. De Meersman, D. Sepúlveda, R. N. Baumgartner, R. N. Pierson, T. Harris, and S. B. Heymsfield. 1997. "Appendicular skeletal muscle mass: effects of age, gender, and ethnicity." *J Appl Physiol (1985)* 83 (1):229-39. doi: 10.1152/jappl.1997.83.1.229.

Gates, N., M. A. Fiatarone Singh, P. S. Sachdev, and M. Valenzuela. 2013. "The effect of exercise training on cognitive function in older adults with mild cognitive impairment: a meta-analysis of randomized controlled trials." *Am J Geriatr Psychiatry* 21 (11):1086-97. doi: 10.1016/j.jagp.2013.02.018.

Groot, C., A. M. Hooghiemstra, P. G. Raijmakers, B. N. van Berckel, P. Scheltens, E. J. Scherder, W. M. van der Flier, and R. Ossenkoppele. 2016. "The effect of physical activity on cognitive function in patients with dementia: A meta-analysis of randomized control trials." *Ageing Res Rev* 25:13-23. doi: 10.1016/j.arr.2015.11. 005.

Hamidie, Ray D. R., T. Yamada, R. Ishizawa, Y. Saito, and K. Masuda. 2015. "Curcumin treatment enhances the effect of exercise on mitochondrial biogenesis in skeletal muscle by increasing cAMP levels." *Metabolism* 64 (10):1334-47. doi: 10.1016/j.metabol.2015.07.010.

Heneka, Michael T., Monica J. Carson, Joseph El Khoury, Gary E. Landreth, Frederic Brosseron, Douglas L. Feinstein, Andreas H. Jacobs, Tony Wyss-Coray, Javier Vitorica, Richard M. Ransohoff, Karl Herrup, Sally A. Frautschy, Bente Finsen, Guy C. Brown, Alexei Verkhratsky, Koji Yamanaka, Jari Koistinaho, Eicke Latz, Annett Halle, Gabor C. Petzold, Terrence Town, Dave Morgan, Mari L. Shinohara, V. Hugh Perry, Clive Holmes, Nicolas G. Bazan, David J. Brooks, Stéphane Hunot, Bertrand Joseph, Nikolaus Deigendesch, Olga Garaschuk, Erik Boddeke, Charles A. Dinarello, John C. Breitner, Greg M. Cole, Douglas T. Golenbock, and Markus P. Kummer. 2015. "Neuroinflammation in Alzheimer's disease." *The Lancet Neurology* 14 (4):388-405. doi: https://doi.org/10.1016/S1474-4422(15)70016-5.

Hewlings, Susan J., and Douglas S. Kalman. 2017. "Curcumin: A Review of Its Effects on Human Health." *Foods (Basel, Switzerland)* 6 (10):92. doi: 10.3390/ foods6100092.

Huang, X., X. Zhao, B. Li, Y. Cai, S. Zhang, Q. Wan, and F. Yu. 2022. "Comparative efficacy of various exercise interventions on cognitive function in patients with mild cognitive impairment or dementia: A systematic review and network meta-analysis." *J Sport Health Sci* 11 (2):212-223. doi: 10.1016/j.jshs. 2021.05.003.

Isaac, A. R., R. A. S. Lima-Filho, and M. V. Lourenco. 2021. "How does the skeletal muscle communicate with the brain in health and disease?" *Neuropharmacology* 197:108744. doi: 10.1016/j.neuropharm.2021.108744.

Jantawong, Chanakan, Aroonsri Priprem, Kitti Intuyod, Chawalit Pairojkul, Porntip Pinlaor, Sakda Waraasawapati, Itnarin Mongkon, Yaovalux Chamgramol, and Somchai Pinlaor. 2021. "Curcumin-loaded nanocomplexes: Acute and chronic toxicity studies in mice and hamsters." *Toxicology Reports* 8:1346-1357. doi: 10.1016/j.toxrep.2021.06.021.

Jia, R. X., J. H. Liang, Y. Xu, and Y. Q. Wang. 2019. "Effects of physical activity and exercise on the cognitive function of patients with Alzheimer disease: a meta-analysis." *BMC Geriatr* 19 (1):181. doi: 10.1186/s12877-019-1175-2.

Jonasson, Lars S, Lars Nyberg, Arthur F Kramer, Anders Lundquist, Katrine Riklund, and Carl-Johan Boraxbekk. 2017. "Aerobic exercise intervention, cognitive performance, and brain structure: results from the physical influences on brain in aging (PHIBRA) study." *Frontiers in Aging Neuroscience* 8:336.

Lao, C. D., M. T. th Ruffin, D. Normolle, D. D. Heath, S. I. Murray, J. M. Bailey, M. E. Boggs, J. Crowell, C. L. Rock, and D. E. Brenner. 2006. "Dose escalation of a curcuminoid formulation." *BMC Complement Altern Med* 6:10. doi: 10.1186/ 1472-6882-6-10.

Law, C. K., F. M. Lam, R. C. Chung, and M. Y. Pang. 2020. "Physical exercise attenuates cognitive decline and reduces behavioural problems in people with mild cognitive impairment and dementia: a systematic review." *J Physiother* 66 (1):9-18. doi: 10.1016/j.jphys.2019.11.014.

Learner, Nicole A., and Jonathan M. Williams. 2016. "Can physical activity be used to maintain cognitive function in nursing home residents with dementia? A literature review." *Physical Therapy Reviews* 21 (3-6):184-191. doi: 10.1080/10833196.2016. 1266138.

Lee, D. Y., Y. S. Chun, J. K. Kim, J. O. Lee, S. K. Ku, and S. M. Shim. 2021. "Curcumin Attenuates Sarcopenia in Chronic Forced Exercise Executed Aged Mice by Regulating Muscle Degradation and Protein Synthesis with Antioxidant and Anti-inflammatory Effects." *J Agric Food Chem* 69 (22):6214-6228. doi: 10.1021/ acs.jafc.1c00699.

Lee, Inhwan, Jinkyung Cho, Haeryun Hong, Youngyun Jin, Donghyun Kim, and Hyunsik Kang. 2018. "Sarcopenia Is Associated with Cognitive Impairment and Depression in Elderly Korean Women." *Iranian journal of public health* 47 (3):327-334.

Li, Xudong, Rui Guo, Zhenhong Wei, Jing Jia, and Chaojun Wei. 2019. "Effectiveness of Exercise Programs on Patients with Dementia: A Systematic Review and Meta-Analysis of Randomized Controlled Trials." *BioMed Research International* 2019:2308475. doi: 10.1155/2019/2308475.

Lim, K. H., A. Pysklywec, M. Plante, and L. Demers. 2019. "The effectiveness of Tai Chi for short-term cognitive function improvement in the early stages of dementia in the elderly: a systematic literature review." *Clin Interv Aging* 14:827-839. doi: 10.2147/cia.s202055.

Liu, Patrick Z., and Robin Nusslock. 2018. "Exercise-Mediated Neurogenesis in the Hippocampus via BDNF." *Frontiers in Neuroscience* 12 (52). doi: 10.3389/fnins. 2018.00052.

López-Ortiz, S., P. L. Valenzuela, M. M. Seisdedos, J. S. Morales, T. Vega, A. Castillo-García, R. Nisticò, N. B. Mercuri, S. Lista, A. Lucia, and A. Santos-Lozano. 2021. "Exercise interventions in Alzheimer's disease: A systematic review and meta-analysis of randomized controlled trials." *Ageing Res Rev* 72:101479. doi: 10.1016/j.arr.2021.101479.

Luhtala, T. A., E. B. Roecker, T. Pugh, R. J. Feuers, and R. Weindruch. 1994. "Dietary restriction attenuates age-related increases in rat skeletal muscle antioxidant enzyme activities." *J Gerontol* 49 (5):B231-8. doi: 10.1093/geronj/49.5.b231.

Mallikarjuna, K., K. R. Shanmugam, K. Nishanth, Ming-Chieh Wu, Chien-Wen Hou, Chia-Hua Kuo, and K. Sathyavelu Reddy. 2010. "Alcohol-induced deterioration in primary antioxidant and glutathione family enzymes reversed by exercise training in the liver of old rats." *Alcohol* 44 (6):523-529. doi: https://doi.org/10.1016/j.alcohol. 2010.07.004.

Mansukhani, Meghna P., Bhanu Prakash Kolla, and Virend K. Somers. 2019. "Hypertension and Cognitive Decline: Implications of Obstructive Sleep Apnea." *Frontiers in Cardiovascular Medicine* 6. doi: 10.3389/fcvm.2019.00096.

Mehrabadi, Shima, Azam Alinaghpour, and Elham Zahedi. 2021. "Effect of curcumin on beta-amyloid plasma level in alzheimer disease: a systematic review and meta-analysis." *International Clinical Neurosciences Journal* 8 (2):55-59.

Meng, Q., H. Yin, S. Wang, B. Shang, X. Meng, M. Yan, G. Li, J. Chu, and L. Chen. 2022. "The effect of combined cognitive intervention and physical exercise on cognitive function in older adults with mild cognitive impairment: a meta-analysis of randomized controlled trials." *Aging Clin Exp Res* 34 (2):261-276. doi: 10.1007/s40520-021-01877-0.

Miller, C. J., S. S. Gounder, S. Kannan, K. Goutam, V. R. Muthusamy, M. A. Firpo, J. D. Symons, R. Paine, 3rd, J. R. Hoidal, and N. S. Rajasekaran. 2012. "Disruption of Nrf2/ARE signaling impairs antioxidant mechanisms and promotes cell degradation pathways in aged skeletal muscle." *Biochim Biophys Acta* 1822 (6):1038-50. doi: 10.1016/j.bbadis.2012.02.007.

Mishra, S., and K. Palanivelu. 2008. "The effect of curcumin (turmeric) on Alzheimer's disease: An overview." *Ann Indian Acad Neurol* 11 (1):13-9. doi: 10.4103/0972-2327.40220.

Mokhtarzade, Motahare, Mahdieh Molanouri Shamsi, Maryam Abolhasani, Bita Bakhshi, Mohamad Ali Sahraian, and Sara Soudi. 2022a. "Lifetime physical activity is associated with gut bacteria and brain health in people with multiple sclerosis: Focus on physical activity intensity." *Multiple Sclerosis and Related Disorders* 59.

Mokhtarzade, Motahare, Mahdieh Molanouri Shamsi, Maryam Abolhasani, Bita Bakhshi, Mohamad Ali Sahraian, and Sara Soudi. 2022b. "Lifetime physical activity is associated with gut bacteria and brain health in people with multiple sclerosis: Focus on physical activity intensity." *Multiple Sclerosis and Related Disorders* 59:103639.

Moore, Kaitlin M, Renee E Girens, Sara K Larson, Maria R Jones, Jessica L Restivo, David M Holtzman, John R Cirrito, Carla M Yuede, Scott D Zimmerman, and Benjamin F Timson. 2016. "A spectrum of exercise training reduces soluble Aβ in a dose-dependent manner in a mouse model of Alzheimer's disease." *Neurobiology of disease* 85:218-224.

Moriyuki, K., F. Sekiguchi, K. Matsubara, H. Nishikawa, and A. Kawabata. 2010. "Curcumin Inhibits the proteinase-activated receptor-2-triggered prostaglandin E2 production by suppressing cyclooxygenase-2 upregulation and Akt-dependent activation of nuclear factor-κB in human lung epithelial cells." *J Pharmacol Sci* 114 (2):225-9. doi: 10.1254/jphs.10126sc.

Murman, D. L. 2015. "The Impact of Age on Cognition." *Semin Hear* 36 (3):111-21. doi: 10.1055/s-0035-1555115.

Murphy, S. L., J. Xu, and K. D. Kochanek. 2013. "Deaths: final data for 2010." *Natl Vital Stat Rep* 61 (4):1-117.

Murray, M. P., G. M. Gardner, L. A. Mollinger, and S. B. Sepic. 1980. "Strength of isometric and isokinetic contractions: knee muscles of men aged 20 to 86." *Phys Ther* 60 (4):412-9. doi: 10.1093/ptj/60.4.412.

Öhman, H., N. Savikko, T. E. Strandberg, and K. H. Pitkälä. 2014. "Effect of physical exercise on cognitive performance in older adults with mild cognitive impairment or dementia: a systematic review." *Dement Geriatr Cogn Disord* 38 (5-6):347-65. doi: 10.1159/000365388.

Ojagbemi, A., and N. Akin-Ojagbemi. 2019. "Exercise and Quality of Life in Dementia: A Systematic Review and Meta-Analysis of Randomized Controlled Trials." *J Appl Gerontol* 38 (1):27-48. doi: 10.1177/0733464817693374.

Phillips, Cristy, and Atoossa Fahimi. 2018. "Immune and Neuroprotective Effects of Physical Activity on the Brain in Depression." *Frontiers in Neuroscience* 12. doi: 10.3389/fnins.2018.00498.

Pisani, S., C. Mueller, J. Huntley, D. Aarsland, and M. J. Kempton. 2021. "A meta-analysis of randomised controlled trials of physical activity in people with Alzheimer's disease and mild cognitive impairment with a comparison to donepezil." *Int J Geriatr Psychiatry* 36 (10):1471-1487. doi: 10.1002/gps.5581.

Raz, N., and K. M. Rodrigue. 2006. "Differential aging of the brain: patterns, cognitive correlates and modifiers." *Neurosci Biobehav Rev* 30 (6):730-48. doi: 10.1016/j.neubiorev.2006.07.001.

Rolfe, Vivien, Marion Mackonochie, Simon Mills, and Euan MacLennan. 2020. "Turmeric/curcumin and health outcomes: A meta-review of systematic reviews." *European Journal of Integrative Medicine* 40:101252. doi: https://doi.org/10.1016/j.eujim.2020.101252.

Roubenoff, R. 2000. "Sarcopenia and its implications for the elderly." *European Journal of Clinical Nutrition* 54 (3):S40-S47. doi: 10.1038/sj.ejcn.1601024.

Sabia, Séverine, Alexis Elbaz, Aline Dugravot, Jenny Head, Martin Shipley, Gareth Hagger-Johnson, Mika Kivimaki, and Archana Singh-Manoux. 2012. "Impact of smoking on cognitive decline in early old age: the Whitehall II cohort study." *Archives of general psychiatry* 69 (6):627-635. doi: 10.1001/archgenpsychiatry. 2011.2016.

Salzman, T., Y. Sarquis-Adamson, S. Son, M. Montero-Odasso, and S. Fraser. 2022. "Associations of Multidomain Interventions With Improvements in Cognition in Mild Cognitive Impairment: A Systematic Review and Meta-analysis." *JAMA Netw Open* 5 (5):e226744. doi: 10.1001/jamanetworkopen.2022.6744.

Santos-Parker, Jessica R, Talia R Strahler, Candace J Bassett, Nina Z Bispham, Michel B Chonchol, and Douglas R Seals. 2017. "Curcumin supplementation improves vascular endothelial function in healthy middle-aged and older adults by increasing nitric oxide bioavailability and reducing oxidative stress." *Aging (Albany NY)* 9 (1):187.

Sarraf, P., M. Parohan, M. H. Javanbakht, S. Ranji-Burachaloo, and M. Djalali. 2019. "Short-term curcumin supplementation enhances serum brain-derived neurotrophic factor in adult men and women: a systematic review and dose-response meta-analysis of randomized controlled trials." *Nutr Res* 69:1-8. doi: 10.1016/j.nutres.2019.05.001.

Schirinzi, T., M. Canevelli, A. Suppa, M. Bologna, and L. Marsili. 2020. "The continuum between neurodegeneration, brain plasticity, and movement: a critical appraisal." *Rev Neurosci* 31 (7):723-742. doi: 10.1515/revneuro-2020-0011.

Schmid, A., E. Jakob, A. Berg, T. Russmann, D. König, M. Irmer, and J. Keul. 1996. "Effect of physical exercise and vitamin C on absorption of ferric sodium citrate." *Med Sci Sports Exerc* 28 (12):1470-3. doi: 10.1097/00005768-199612000-00005.

Seddon, Nathan, Nathan M D'Cunha, Duane D Mellor, Andrew J McKune, Ekavi N Georgousopoulou, Demosthenes B Panagiotakos, Jane Kellett, and Nenad Naumovski. 2019. "fects of Curcumin on Cognitive Function—A Systematic Review of Randomized Controlled Trials." *Exploratory Research and Hypothesis in Medicine* 4 (1):1-11. doi: 10.14218/ERHM.2018.00024.

Sharma, R. A., S. A. Euden, S. L. Platton, D. N. Cooke, A. Shafayat, H. R. Hewitt, T. H. Marczylo, B. Morgan, D. Hemingway, S. M. Plummer, M. Pirmohamed, A. J. Gescher, and W. P. Steward. 2004. "Phase I clinical trial of oral curcumin: biomarkers of systemic activity and compliance." *Clin Cancer Res* 10 (20):6847-54. doi: 10.1158/1078-0432.ccr-04-0744.

Smart, N. A., N. King, J. R. McFarlane, P. L. Graham, and G. Dieberg. 2018. "Effect of exercise training on liver function in adults who are overweight or exhibit fatty liver disease: a systematic review and meta-analysis." *Br J Sports Med* 52 (13):834-843. doi: 10.1136/bjsports-2016-096197.

Smyth, Andrew, Mahshid Dehghan, Martin O'Donnell, Craig Anderson, Koon Teo, Peggy Gao, Peter Sleight, Gilles Dagenais, Jeffrey L. Probstfield, Andrew Mente, Salim Yusuf, Ontarget, and Transcend Investigators. 2015. "Healthy eating and reduced risk of cognitive decline: A cohort from 40 countries." *Neurology* 84 (22):2258-2265. doi: 10.1212/WNL.0000000000001638.

Song, D., D. S. F. Yu, P. W. C. Li, and Y. Lei. 2018. "The effectiveness of physical exercise on cognitive and psychological outcomes in individuals with mild cognitive impairment: A systematic review and meta-analysis." *Int J Nurs Stud* 79:155-164. doi: 10.1016/j.ijnurstu.2018.01.002.

Tanabe, Y., S. Maeda, N. Akazawa, A. Zempo-Miyaki, Y. Choi, S. G. Ra, A. Imaizumi, Y. Otsuka, and K. Nosaka. 2015. "Attenuation of indirect markers of eccentric exercise-induced muscle damage by curcumin." *Eur J Appl Physiol* 115 (9):1949-57. doi: 10.1007/s00421-015-3170-4.

Tsai, I. C., C. W. Hsu, C. H. Chang, P. T. Tseng, and K. V. Chang. 2021. "The Effect of Curcumin Differs on Individual Cognitive Domains across Different Patient Populations: A Systematic Review and Meta-Analysis." *Pharmaceuticals (Basel)* 14 (12). doi: 10.3390/ph14121235.

van Vliet, P. 2012. "Cholesterol and late-life cognitive decline." *J Alzheimers Dis* 30 Suppl 2:S147-62. doi: 10.3233/jad-2011-111028.

Vecchio, Laura M., Ying Meng, Kristiana Xhima, Nir Lipsman, Clement Hamani, and Isabelle Aubert. 2018. "The Neuroprotective Effects of Exercise: Maintaining a Healthy Brain Throughout Aging." *Brain plasticity (Amsterdam, Netherlands)* 4 (1):17-52. doi: 10.3233/BPL-180069.

Voulgaropoulou, S. D., T. A. M. J. van Amelsvoort, J. Prickaerts, and C. Vingerhoets. 2019. "The effect of curcumin on cognition in Alzheimer's disease and healthy aging: A systematic review of pre-clinical and clinical studies." *Brain Research* 1725:146476. doi: https://doi.org/10.1016/j.brainres.2019.146476.

Wang, S., H. Yin, X. Wang, Y. Jia, C. Wang, L. Wang, and L. Chen. 2019. "Efficacy of different types of exercises on global cognition in adults with mild cognitive impairment: a network meta-analysis." *Aging Clin Exp Res* 31 (10):1391-1400. doi: 10.1007/s40520-019-01142-5.

Westerterp, Klaas R. 2018. "Exercise, energy balance and body composition." *European Journal of Clinical Nutrition* 72 (9):1246-1250. doi: 10.1038/s41430-018-0180-4.

Yoon, Wan-Young, Kihyuk Lee, and Jooyoung Kim. 2020. "Curcumin supplementation and delayed onset muscle soreness (DOMS): effects, mechanisms, and practical considerations." *Physical Activity and Nutrition* 24 (3):39-43. doi: 10.20463/pan.2020.0020.

Zheng, G., R. Xia, W. Zhou, J. Tao, and L. Chen. 2016. "Aerobic exercise ameliorates cognitive function in older adults with mild cognitive impairment: a systematic review and meta-analysis of randomised controlled trials." *Br J Sports Med* 50 (23):1443-1450. doi: 10.1136/bjsports-2015-095699.

Zhou, K., M. Liu, D. Bao, and J. Zhou. 2022. "Effects of Traditional Chinese Exercises on Cognitive Function in Older Adults With Mild Cognitive Impairment: A Systematic Review and Meta-Analysis." *Front Hum Neurosci* 16:849530. doi: 10.3389/fnhum.2022.849530.

Zhu, L. N., X. Mei, Z. G. Zhang, Y. P. Xie, and F. Lang. 2019. "Curcumin intervention for cognitive function in different types of people: A systematic review and meta-analysis." *Phytother Res* 33 (3):524-533. doi: 10.1002/ptr.6257.

Zhu, Y., Q. Zhong, J. Ji, J. Ma, H. Wu, Y. Gao, N. Ali, and T. Wang. 2020. "Effects of Aerobic Dance on Cognition in Older Adults with Mild Cognitive Impairment: A Systematic Review and Meta-Analysis." *J Alzheimers Dis* 74 (2):679-690. doi: 10.3233/jad-190681.

Zou, L., P. D. Loprinzi, A. S. Yeung, N. Zeng, and T. Huang. 2019. "The Beneficial Effects of Mind-Body Exercises for People With Mild Cognitive Impairment: a Systematic Review With Meta-analysis." *Arch Phys Med Rehabil* 100 (8):1556-1573. doi: 10.1016/j.apmr.2019.03.009.

Chapter 4

Antiviral Effect of Curcumin: A Special Emphasis on COVID-19 Virus

Shivangini R. Desai
Manni J. Vishwakarma
and Sonal S. Desai*

Department of Quality Assurance, SSR College of Pharmacy, Sayli, Silvassa, Union Territory of Dadra Nagar Haveli and Daman Diu, India

Abstract

Plant derived biomolecules are said to possess various pharmacological actions. Curcumin obtained from rhizomes of *Curcuma longa*, is the primary bioactive molecule which exhibits antiviral, antinociceptive, anti-inflammatory, antipyretic and anti-fatigue effects. Recent studies reveal that curcumin also shows antiviral activity against many viruses such as dengue, hepatitis, zika, chikungunya, etc. Few research studies revealed that curcumin has binding potential to target a variety of SARS-Cov-2 proteins. This chapter covers antiviral activity of curcumin with special focus on its role in inhibiting COVID-19 virus. These findings will be utilized to develop therapeutic lead using curcumin against COVID-19.

Keywords: antiviral, curcumin, *Curcuma longa*, COVID-19, SARS-CoV-2

---

* Corresponding Author's Email: sdesai6381@gmail.com.

In: Curcumin and Its Role in Health and Disease
Editor: Kathryn Woltjer
ISBN: 979-8-88697-491-1

Abbreviations

4EWA	It is a protein of HCV NS5B, considered to be involved in the replication step of Hepatitis C virus life cycle
A549 cells	Adenocarcinomic Human Alveolar Basal Epithelial Cells
ACE	Angiotensin Converting Enzyme
ADAM17	A Disintegrin and Metalloprotease 17
AIDS	Acquired Immunodeficiency Syndrome
Akt-SREBP-1	Akt (protein kinase B) Sterol Regulatory Element-Binding Transcription Factor 1
AMPK	Activated protein kinase
AP-1	Activator Protein 1
APE1	Apurinic/Apyrimidinic Endonuclease 1
ARDS	Acute respiratory distress syndrome
C57BL/6	C57 black 6 is a common inbred strain of laboratory mouse
CatB	Cathepsin B
CatL	Cathepsin L
CC50	50% Cytotoxic Concentration
ccc DNA	covalently closed circular DNA
CCK-8	Cell Counting Kit-8
CCM –CDs	Curcumin Carbon Dots
CDs	Carbon Dots
CEM-T cells	A line of lymphoblastic cells derived from a child with acute lymphoblastic leukemia
CQDs	Carbon Quantum Dots
CRISPR-Cas9	Clustered Regularly Interspaced Short Palindromic Repeats associated protein 9
DAMP3	Damage Associated Molecular Protein 3
DENV	Dengue Virus
EGFR	Epidermal Growth Factor
dsDNA	Double Stranded Deoxyribonucleic Acid
ED 50	Median Effective Dose
ELISA	Enzyme-Linked Immunosorbent Assay
EMSA	Electrophoretic Mobility Shift Assay
EV71	Enterovirus 71
GEC	Glomerular Endothelial Cells
gp120	Envelope Glycoprotein

H1N1	Hemagglutinin type 1 and Neuraminidases type 1
H6N1	Hemagglutinin type 6 and Neuraminidase type 1
H9N2	Hemagglutinin type 9 and Neuraminidase type2
HA	Haemagglutinin
HBV	Hepatitis B Virus
HBX	Hepatitis B Virus X Protein
HCV	Hepatitis C Virus
HEK 293 T cells	Human Embryonic Kidney 293 cells
HeLa Cells	Henrietta Lacks Cells
HI	Haemagglutination Inhibition
HIV	Human Immunodeficiency Virus
HIV-p24	Human Immunodeficiency Virus protein 24 Capsid Antigen
HMGB1	High-Mobility Group Box 1 Protein
HO-1	Heme Oxygenase-1
HSV-1	Herpes Simplex Virus type 1
HSV-2	Herpes Simplex Virus type 2
IC50	Half-Maximal Inhibitory Concentration
IFN alpha	Type 1 Interferon
IFNs	Interferons
IFV-A	Influenza Virus Type A
IL -1	Interleukin-1
IL- 6- SIL-6R	InterLeukin-6- Soluble InterLeukin-6 Receptor complex
IL-10	Interleukin-10
IL-1β	Interleukin 1 beta
IL-2	Interleukin-2
IL-6	Interleukin 6
IL-8	Interleukin 8
ISGs	Interferon-Stimulated Genes
IκBα	Nuclear Factor of Kappa Light Polypeptide Gene Enhancer in B-cells Inhibitor, alpha
JAK	Janus Kinase
JNK	Jun N-Terminal Kinases
lacZ	Lactose Operon
LTR	Long Terminal Repeat
M1	Matrix Protein
MAPK	Mitogen Activated Protein Kinase
MCP-1	Monocyte Chemoattractant Protein-1

MDCK cells	Madin - Darby Canine Kidney Cells
MIP1α	Macrophage Inflammatory Protein-1α
Mpro	Main protein
mTOR	Mammalian Target Of Rapamycin
MTT assay	(3-(4, 5-dimethylthiazolyl-2)-2, 5-diphenyltetrazolium bromide) Assay
NF-kB	Nuclear Factor Kappa B
NA	Neuraaminidase
NADPH	Nicotinamide Adenine Dinucleotide Phosphate
NLRP3	NLR family Pyrin domain containing 3
NMR	Nuclear Magnetic Resonance
NRF2	Nuclear Factor Erythroid 2–Related Factor 2
NS2B-NS3 protease	A Serine Protease that belongs to chymotrypsin family with a classic serine His-Asp catalytic triadpmbc
NTCP	Sodium Taurocholate Co-transporting Polypeptide
P38	P38 Mitogen Activate Protein Kinases
P53	Tumour Suppressor Gene
P65	Transcription Factor
PAMPs	Pathogen-Associated Molecular Pattern Molecules
PGC-1a	Peroxisome proliferator-activated receptor-Gamma Co-activator
PI3	Phosphatidylinositol 3-kinase
PBMC	Peripheral Blood Mononuclear Cells
RAAS	Renin–Angiotensin–Aldosterone System
RdRp	RNA-dependent RNA polymerase
RT-PCR	Real Time Reverse Transcription Polymerase Chain Reaction
SARS-CoV 2	Severe Acute Respiratory Syndrome Coronavirus 2
STAT3	Signal Transducer and Activator of Transcription 3
Tat	Tyrosine amino transferase
T-cells	T lymphocyte cells
TCID50	Median Tissue Culture Infectious Dose
TGF-β	Transforming Growth Factor Beta
TLR	Toll Like Receptor
TMPRSS2	Transmembrane Protease, Serine 2
TNF-α	Tumor Necrosis Factor
VP-16	Viral Transactivator Protein
Wnt	Wingless-related Integration Site
WST-1	Water Soluble Tetrazolium salt

Introduction to Curcumin

Dried rhizomes of *Curcuma longa* (family: Zingiberaceae), which is well known as Turmeric, (Cooksey, 2017) is commonly used as spice, stabilizer, medicine and as food colour or dye. Curcuminoids, bioactive phenolic compounds which are present in turmeric are curcumin, dimethoxy curcumin and bisdemethoxycurcumin (Amalraj et al., 2017) with relative contents of 70-80%, 10-20%, and 3-6%, respectively (Mukherjee and Kar, 2021). Curcumin is the fundamental curcuminoid found in *Curcuma longa* (Soleimani, Sahebkar and Hosseinzadeh, 2018) which constitutes 2-8% of *Curcuma longa* extract (Giuliani, 2016).

Physicochemical Properties of Curcumin

Curcumin (diferuloylmethane) is a yellow colour pigment (Horev, Ramot and Klapholz, 2015) with chemical name of 1,7-bis-(4-hydroxy-3-methoxy-phenyl)-1,6-heptadiene-3,5-dione]

(Li et al., 2011) with molecular formula of $C_{21}H_{20}O_6$. It has a molecular mass of 368.37 g/mol and melts at 183°C. The structure of curcumin contains two aromatic rings in the form of methylated phenols attached by heptadiene-3,5-diketone responsible for its yellow colour (Itokawa et al., 2008). Curcumin is a very highly lipophilic complex with log P value varying from 2.3 to 2.6 (Heger et al., 2014). Owing to its lipophilicity, curcumin has limited aqueous solubility which does not dissolve in water, however it gets solubilized in solvents such as dimethyl sulphoxide, methanol, alcohol, acetonitrile, ethyl acetate and chloroform (Priyadarsini, 2014). Due to its limited water solubility and low permeability, it is classified in the biopharmaceutics classification system class-IV (Muthu et al., 2019). Its 1% solution exhibits optical density of 1650 absorbance units (Javed et al., 2020). The pka values for the dissociation of two phenolic protons is observed between 7.7–8.5 and 8.5–10.4, respectively while dissociation of enolic protons results in pka value between 9.5–10.7 (Dei Cas and Ghidoni, 2019). Curcumin exhibits keto-enol tautomerism depending on the pH of solution. At acidic and neutral pH, keto form predominates while at alkaline pH, enol form predominates (Lestari and Indrayanto, 2014).

The IR spectrum of curcumin reveals a broad peak near 3500 cm^{-1} confirming the presence of the -OH group. Sharp peaks near 1625 cm^{-1} and

1600 cm^{-1} are observed because of C=O group and C=C aromatic stretching. The presence of C-O and C-O-C is identified by peaks at 1455 cm^{-1} and 1025 cm^{-1}, respectively (Valand, Patel and Menon, 2015; Ismail, et al., 2014). NMR spectrum of curcumin display sharp peak at 7.29 ppm due to aromatic protons, at 3.81 ppm due to -OCH3 group and at 9.62 ppm due to -OH groups (Lestari and Indrayanto, 2014). Mass spectrum of curcumin produces a sharp peak at m/z 368 due to molecular ion peak (Bagchi, et al., 2015) and at m/z 177 due to base peak (Halket et al., 2005; Nurjanah and Saepudin, 2019). Figure 1 depicts various physicochemical properties of curcumin.

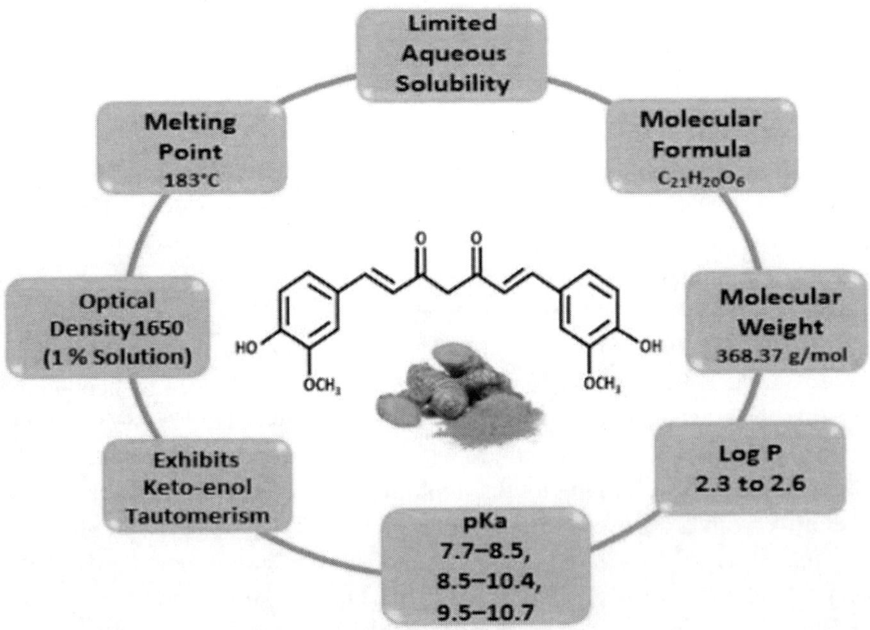

Figure 1. Physicochemical properties of curcumin.

Pharmacology of Curcumin

Curcumin, which is referred to as 'Indian Solid Gold'(Aggarwal et al., 2007), is said to possess numerous health benefits and pharmacological properties (Alok, et al., 2015) owing to its unique structure and functionalities.

Curcumin possesses anti-inflammatory activity by controlling release of inflammatory mediators and by regulating inflammation signaling pathways (Peng, et al., 2021). Reports suggest that the anti-inflammatory effect of curcumin is attributed to its capability to up regulate PPAR-γ (Jacob, et al., 2008). Its anti-inflammatory action is also exhibited by inhibition of various enzymes namely cyclooxygenase 2, lipoxygenase and inducible nitric oxide synthase (Wal, et al., 2019). Reports also reveal the promising wound healing activity of curcumin (Akbik et al., 2014; Tejada et al., 2016). Curcumin has also emerged as a potential anti- cancer molecule for different categories of cancer namely colorectal cancer, renal cancer, hepatic cancer and bone cancer either by arresting the cell cycle cycle, through apoptosis or by autophagy (Ahmad, et al., 2020). Curcumin shows a vital function of inhibiting various processes involved in carcinogenesis and tumor formation (Wilken, et al., 2011). It also inhibits cancer cell multiplication and thus prevents metastasis (Liu and Ho, 2018). Curcumin acts as immunosuppressant by suppressing lymphocyte proliferation and cytokine production (Yadav, et al., 2005).

Apart from above pharmacological activities, the antiviral effect of curcumin is also widely explored. Curcumin hinders the binding of influenza A virus, hepatitis C virus, dengue virus, zika virus, and chikungunya virus to the host cell (Balasubramanian et al., 2019). Figure 2 highlights various viruses against which curcumin shows antiviral activity. This chapter reviews Curcumin's role in preventing various viral infections. Additionally, in depth mechanisms of Curcumin's activity against SARS-CoV-2 are discussed.

Curcumin as Potential Antiviral Agent

Dengue

Dengue virus (DENV) is widespread in more than 100 countries of tropical and subtropical regions of the world (Jing and Wang, 2019). Dengue virus is a species of genus Flavivirus belonging to family Flaviviridae (Ross, 2010), and it comprises of four serotypes : DENV-1, DENV-2, DENV-3, and DENV-4 (Halstead, 2007). All the four serotypes of the virus are transmitted in humans by the bite of *Aedes* mosquitoes, the principal vector being *Aedes aegypti* (Gratz, 2004). The symptoms of the typical dengue fever include abrupt onset of fever, headache, severe myalgia, and arthralgia (Chen and Wilson, 2010).

Curcumin was reported to be effective against different serotypes of DENV virus by inhibition of viral replication in MTT plaque assay when used with 6- gingerol. The CC50 was found to be 108 μM and the IC50 was found to be serotype dependent. (Ardebili et al., 2021; Nugraha Halim et al., 2021). Nano emulsion of curcumin inhibited proliferation of A549 cell in MTT assay by inducing apoptosis. Significant inhibition was observed for DENV type 1 and 2 with CC50 of 52.97 μg/ml. (Nabila et al., 2019). Curcumin with cytotoxicity of 30 μM inhibits the formation of plaque in DENV type 2 infection. It acts on viral membrane envelopes and liposomes and disrupts the cell membrane's integrity. The method used was plaque assay, HI, MTT assay and the IC50 was found to be 4μM (Chen et al., 2013). Curcumin, bisdemethoxycurcumin, acyclic analogue of curcumin, cyclopentanone analogue of curcumin and cyclohexanone analogue of curcumin act on dengue virus to cause inhibition of viral protease which suppresses the infectivity of the virus with CC50 as 49.01 μM, 43.37 μM, 32.34 μM, 87.40 μM, 25.50μM respectively as checked by CCK-8, RT- PCR and Plaque assay (Balasubramanian et al., 2019). Bis demethoxy curcumin acts on type 2 infected cells by suppression of ubiquitin proteasome system which leads to a decrease in viral particles with IC50 of 11.51 μM and CC50 of 29.5 μM, as studied by western blot and MTT methods (Padilla-S et al., 2014). Curcumin also disrupts Dengue NS2B-NS3 Protease's active conformation with IC 50 of 7.18 μM, the binding to protease was studied by NMR (Lim et al., 2020).

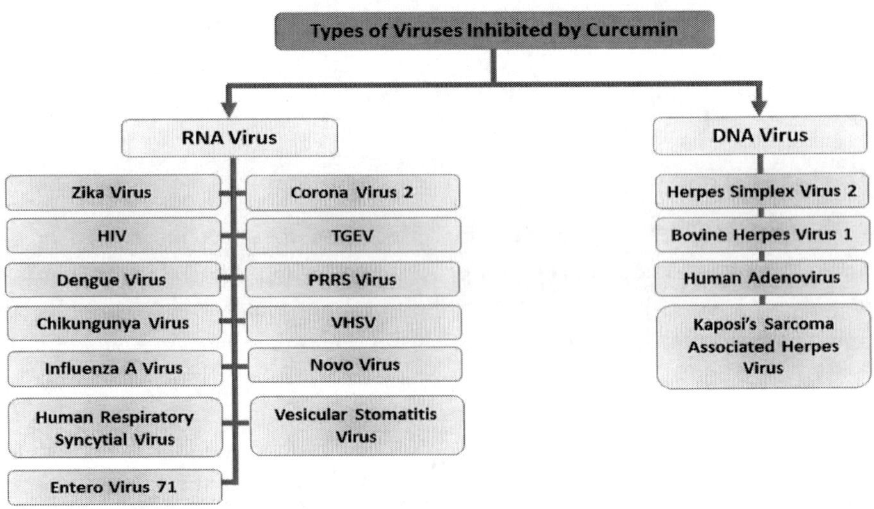

Figure 2. Types of viruses inhibited by curcumin.

A benzenesulfonyl curcumin analogue, (3E, 5E)-3, 5-bis (4-methoxy-benzylidene)-1-(phenylsulfonyl) piperidin-4-one, was found to have activity against DEN2 NS2B/NS3. (Zamri et al., 2019). To study the outcome of curcumin in contradiction of DENV 2, immunocytochemistry technique was used and quasi experimental study was performed with the secure cytotoxic concentration of curcumin of 6.25 ppm (Marbawati et al., 2013).

HIV

HIV belongs to the family of Retroviridae, of the genus Lentivirus, of subfamily Orthoretrovirinae (Seitz, 2016). HIV are of two types— HIV-1 and HIV-2 (Barré-Sinoussi, 1996). Human immunodeficiency virus (HIV) infection in its last stage causes Acquired immunodeficiency syndrome (AIDS) (Weiss, 1993). The majority of cases of AIDS are due to exposure to seminal fluid, blood, or blood products (Conant et al., 1986). AIDS is an incurable chronic illness having many psychosocial implications (Siegel and Lekas, 2002).

Curcumin inhibits HIV-1 protease and HIV-2 protease at IC50 of 100 μM and 250 μM respectively (Prasad and Tyagi, 2015). Curcumin dimer prepared by managing the central keto-enol groups of the two curcumin units to a boron atom enhances anti-HIV activity by more than 10-fold (Sui et al., 1993). Curcumin induces Tat-protein degradation for HIV-1 as proved by a western blotting assay in a dose dependent manner with CC50 between 20 to 120 μM (Ardebili et al., 2021; Ali and Banerjea, 2016). Study revealed that curcumin at concentration of 10 to 100 nM causes 70 to 80% inhibition of Tat transactivation of HIV1-LTR lacZ in HeLa cells (Barthelemy et al., 1998). Additionally, curcumin's anti-inflammatory activity is beneficial for protection of mucosal barrier against HIV-1gp120 (Ferreira et al., 2015). Curcumin also inhibits HIV integrase by acting on the central catalytic domain with IC50 of 40 μM (Mazumder et al., 1995). Docking studies were done to find out potential binding pose of curcumin derivatives to the active site of HIV-1 integrase (Gupta et al., 2011). Curcumin is found to be effective in treatment of HIV associated diarrhea as it acts on TNF-α and inhibits the cytokines (Conteas et al., 2009). Acyclic analog of curcumin was found to have better stability in serum (stable up to 24 hours) as well as serum free media compared to curcumin and was also proven to have retained the activity against HIV-1 in CEM-T and PBMC cells (Kumari et al., 2015). Curcumin targets AMPK or NF-κB factors to inhibit Tat-regulated transcription to inhibit HIV-1 as studied by the MTT method (Zhang et al., 2011). Curcumin stabilized silver nanoparticles act on HIV-1 by inhibiting NF-κB nuclear translocation and by suppressing expression of IL-1β, IL-6 and TNF-α (Sharma et al., 2017). Mesoporous curcumin which are encapsulated by iron-phenanthroline nanoclusters act on type 1 HIV virus and inhibit release of IL-1β, IL-8, TNFα, MCP-1 and MIP1α and decreases HIV-p24 expression by 41% (Sharma et al., 2019).

Chikungunya

Chikungunya virus, an alphavirus, is mosquito-borne that causes joint pains and fever in humans (Petersen and Powers, 2016). The first outbreak of this virus was reported between 1952 and 1953 from the Makonde Plateau (Ross, 1955). The principal vector is *Aedes aegypti* (Coffey et al., 2014).

Pre-incubation of curcumin with lentiviral vectors pseudo typed with the E1 and E2 Chikungunya virus envelope proteins inhibits cell entry or attachment with an IC50 value of 10.79 μM, preventing the infection of HEK 293 T cells without impairing viral reproduction. (Von Rhein et al., 2016). Curcumin with IC50 of 11.6 μM reduces infectivity and disrupts integrity of the viral membrane envelope in a dose dependent manner (Mounce et al., 2017) on the HELa cell line (Kovacikova and van Hemert, 2020). Due to its lipophilicity, dimethoxy curcumin interferes with Chikungunya virus membrane which was found to be more effective than curcumin (Subudhi et al., 2018). Studies revealed that the larvicidal effects of synthetic curcumin, natural turmeric and synthetic curcumin formulated with sucrose against *Aedes aeglypti* larvae is enhanced in presence of sunlight (de Souza et al., 2019). It is in combination with D-mannitol acts on *Aedes aeglypti* and leads to 71.3% mortality after 48 hours (Mezzacappo et al., 2021).

Influenza

Influenza, a viral infection majorly affecting respiratory tract, is caused by different viruses namely *Influenzavirus A*, *Influenzavirus B*, *Influenzavirus C* and *Influenzavirus D* (Krammer et al., 2018). Influenza virus belongs to the Orthomyxoviridae family and is transmitted through sneezing or coughing (Abdullahi et al., 2021).

Monoacetylcurcumin is used for the treatment of influenza infection; it acts by inhibition of PI3K/Akt activation thus lowering its replication in cells. In combination with curcumin, monoacetylcurcumin has synergistic effects

(Richart et al., 2018). Curcumin inhibits Influenzavirus *A* infection and prevents associated pneumonia by reducing oxidative stress, and by inhibiting TLR2/4, NF-κB and p38/JNK MAPK pathways (Dai et al., 2018). It also downregulates cytokines by promoting the IκBα expression which inhibits NF-κB signaling pathway and by preventing translocation of P65 from cytoplasm to nucleus (Xu and Liu, 2017). Anti IFV-A activity of curcumin was studied by plaque assay, Haemagglutination inhibition (HI) test and Western blot analysis with CC50 of 43 μM against MDCK cells. Curcumin hinders synthesis of viral proteins, such as HA, M1 and NA (Chen et al., 2010). Curcumin was found to be more efficacious against *Influenzavirus A* virus than its tetrahydro curcumin. (Aggarwal et al., 2015; Ou et al., 2013). Structural activity relationship studies indicated that the double bonds which are present in the middle seven-carbon chain of curcumin enhanced activity against influenza infection and Petasiphenol, a structural analogue of curcumin, was found to be less effective in comparision to curcumin (Ou et al., 2013). Curcumin also inhibits myocarditis induced by type A virus by inhibiting the signaling of Wnt/β-catenin. (Liu et al., 2013). Influenza A neuraminidase inhibition assays (for types H1N1 and H9N2) were performed to check the inhibitory effect of curcumin by neuraminidases which were studied by Lineweaver-Burk and Dixon plots (Dao et al., 2012).

Hepatitis

Hepatitis, characterized by inflammation of liver tissue, is of 5 types A, B, C, D, and E. (Razavi, 2020), out of which B, C, and D types are chronic. (Burckhardt and Reichen, 2003). Type A spreads by contaminated food, drinks and objects of an infected person whereas type B spreads through blood, and body fluid. Type C spreads through sexual contact and blood. (Center for Disease Control and Prevention, 2017). Dimethoxy curcumin acts on hepatitis C virus by restricting its access into liver cells. It acts on fluidity of viral envelope and prevents cell to cell spread with CC50 of 5-25 μM (Ardebili et al., 2021) as studied by MTT, RT-PCR, TCID50 method however it doesn't affect viral assembly (Anggakusuma et al., 2014). Curcumin has an inhibitory outcome on type B virus through down-regulation of PGC-1a which is the metabolic co-activator of HBV transcription (Mouler Rechtman et al., 2010). Bis demethoxy curcumin is known for dose and time dependent down-regulation of acetylation of ccc DNA-bound histone with CC50 of 5-30 μM (Ardebili et al., 2021) as studied by CCK8 and Western blot analysis experiments (Wei et al., 2017). It inhibits replication of type C virus by suppressing the Akt-SREBP-1 pathway which leads to a decrease HCV gene expression with CC50 of 5-15 μM (Ardebili et al., 2021) and IFN alpha has a synergistic effect when used with curcumin (Kim et al., 2010). Curcumin inhibits type B viral entry by binding with NTCP with CC50 of 30 μM which was checked by performing RT-PCR, MTT, ELISA test (Thongsri et al., 2021). Curcumin enhances the P53 protein accumulation and represses the replication of HBX gene and the process of transcription thus inhibiting hepatitis B virus replication at concentration of 200 mg/l and 500 mg/l as studied by southern blotting, RT-PCR, MTT and western blotting (Kim et al., 2009). It inhibits type C virus by inhibiting replication through induction of expression of HO-1 and inhibition of PI3-Akt signaling pathway at CC50 of 5-25 μM (Ardebili et al., 2021) as studied by MTT, Western blotting and RT-PCR methods (Chen et al., 2012). Curcumin in form of nano-micelles, decreases gene expression of type C virus by suppression of Akt-SREBP-1 pathway, it prevents viral attachment and entry with highest concentration of 0.256 μM and IC50 of 0.1647 mg/ml as studied by MTT, Real time PCR methods. (Naseri et al., 2017). Curcumin strongly interacts with 4EWA proteins involved in multiplication of hepatitis C infection (Wahyuni et al., 2018).

Herpes

Herpes simplex virus (HSV) causes infections of oral and facial mucosal surfaces in HSV-1 type and genital mucosal surfaces in HSV-2 type (Taylor et al., 2002). HSV is a dsDNA virus belonging to the Herpesviridae family (Dadwal and Ito, 2016) and the Alphaherpesviridae subfamily (Roizman and Baines, 1991).

Curcumin has anti-inflammatory effect and decreases replication of HSV type 2 in primary GECs and infected T-cells as assessed by trypan blue method with no type 2 virus detected at 50 μM (Ferreira et al., 2015). Curcumin acts against Kaposi sarcoma associated herpesvirus by APE1 inhibition, which leads to reduction of AP-1 and NF-κB's transcription activity with CC50 of 23.56 μM and IC50 of 8.76 μM as studied by EMSA method (Li et al., 2019). Curcumin at concentrations of 10 to 100 μM act on type 1 and type 2 and prevents entry of virus but does not affect penetration in cultured vero cells and prevents replication of HSV-1 and HSV- 2 at 30 μM as studied by WST-1 assay and plaque assay (Flores et al., 2016). The in-vitro antiviral effect of curcumin and its derivatives- Cu-curcumin and gallium curcumin against HSV-1 with CC50 of 484.2 μg/ml, 326.6 μg/ml and 255.8 μg/ml, respectively studied by TCID50 and trypan blue methods (Zandi et al., 2010).

Curcumin acts on early gene expression of HSV-1 by interfering with RNA polymerase II which is mediated by VP-16 with CC50 of 20 μM (Ardebili et al., 2021) and IC50 of 25 μM as studied by plaque assay, RT-PCR and western blotting (Kutluay et al., 2008). It suppresses the duplication of HSV -2 in-vitro with concentration of 100 mg/ml and ED 50 of 0.32 mg/ml in a plaque reduction assay. The in-vivo studies were done using a mouse model for type 2 genital infection (Bourne et al., 1999). Due to its anti-inflammatory activity, 0.5 mg of the nanoparticle containing curcumin was found to reduce tissue inflammation and severity of HSV-2 in genital epithelial cells of female C57BL/6 mice (Vitali et al., 2020). Hydro-alcoholic extract of curcumin at concentration of 2 mg/ml was evaluated for cytotoxicity on vero cell line by plaque reduction assay, in contrast to acyclovir which reduced plaque by 94.4% at 2.5 mg/ml (Fani et al., 2015).

COVID-19

SARS-CoV-2 responsible for COVID-19 pandemic, is the most novel coronavirus (CoV) to infect humans (Hasöksüz, 2020). A novel beta coronavirus, SARS-CoV-2 has an incubation period between 2 to 14 days (Lauer, 2020), mostly entering human hosts through the respiratory system. This virus is spread by the infected person airborne droplet and fomites (Morawska and Milton, 2020; Xiao et al., 2017).

Various literature revealed about the potential use of curcumin and its derivatives/analoges against SARS-CoV-2. *In vitro* analysis of curcumin against the SARS-CoV in Vero-E6 cells revealed that curcumin at concentrations of 3-10 μM inhibits viral replication (Marín-Palma et al., 2021). Curcumin disrupts the SARS-CoV19 viral envelope and affects the spike protein and also acts on ACE receptor which is present on alveolar type-2 cell, thereby preventing the docking of the S protein of corona to ACE receptor (Chen et al., 2013). S Glycoprotein interacts with the ACE2 receptor to cause interaction between virus host cell and the virus and cause fusion and internalization of the virus (Dieterle et al., 2020). According to a recent study, CRISPR-Cas9 is used in genome wide screening of SARS-CoV-2 infection. HMGB1 acts as a pro-viral host factor (Wei et al., 2021). During infection, HMGB1 can translocate from the nucleus to the extracellular space;

extracellular HMGB1 mediates inflammation (Wang et al., 2004). HMGB1 is a non-histone protein which can bind to DNA as a compositional element inside the cell (Chikhirzhina et al., 2020). Curcumin inhibits enzyme HMGB1 and also prevents the entry of viruses into the cell by repressing the S2 expression (Harris et al., 2012). It also prevents encapsulated viruses from entering host cells such as type 2 pneumocyte epithelial cells (Thimmulappa et al., 2021). Curcumin acts on a positive regulation enzyme called NRF2 and 4-octyl-itaconate, a pharmacological agonist of transcription (Olagnier et al., 2020). Additionally, curcumin mediates immunomodulatory responses by inhibiting cytokines response syndrome and oxidative stress and thus mitigating the progression of pneumonia and ARDS (Wang et al., 2020).

THE Potential Targets of Curcumin in the Entry of Corona Virus and Its Replication

Spike protein of virus binds with ACE receptor, Basigin receptor and a protease enzyme TMPRSS2 which facilitates the entry of virus into the host cell by virus enzymatic mechanism (Wang et al., 2019; Lan et al., 2020; Ragotte et al., 2021). Virus needs endosomal acidification and CatB/L (Cathepsin B/l) enzyme to enter into the cell and replicate, which is inhibited by curcumin. (Khan et al., 2020). RNA dependent RNA polymerase enzyme (RdRp) and Main protein (Mpro), these two enzymes are important for viral duplication. Curcumin has the potential for inhibiting both RdRp and Mpro. Hence after acting on the main protease enzyme, curcumin also prevents the liberation of virus from the infected cell (Pendyala and Petras, 2020).

The three mechanisms by which curcumin inhibits entry of SARS-CoV-2 into the cell and the replication is described in detail below:

Inhibition of the ACE2 Receptor

Angiotensin is released from the liver by the action of RAAS. Angiotensin is converted into the angiotensin-I, angiotensin- I is changed by the action of ACE enzyme to angiotensin- II. Angiotensin- II causes internalization of ACE2 along with SARS-CoV2, so it facilitates the entry of viruses. Angiotensin- II stimulates two types of cell receptors i.e., angiotensin AT1 and Angiotensin AT2 receptor. Activation of Angiotensin-AT1 receptor during covid infection, leads to vasoconstriction, inflammation, fibrosis and cardiac hypertrophy. Curcumin inhibits ACE receptors and declines the formation of angiotensin- II enzymes (Bourgonje et al., 2020; Pang et al.,

2015; Dhar and Bhattacharjee, 2021). Curcumin acts on angiotensin AT1 receptor, and also encourages the angiotensin AT2 receptor and Mas receptor to stimulate the vasorelaxation\ vasodilation, prevents inflammation and fibrosis and also increases the cardiac output (Hoffmann et al., 2020; Vitiello et al., 2020).

Through Cellular Signaling

Angiotensin AT1 receptor combines with Gq enzyme by various molecular mechanisms leading to inhibition of NADPH oxidase, thereby stimulating NF-kB and producing MCP-1. NF-kB and MCP-1 are responsible for inflammation, mayo constriction and hypertrophy (Praditya et al., 2019) Curcumin has potential for inhibiting the NF-kB and MCP-1 cellular signaling pathway. Angiotensin AT1 receptors also have another action, they stimulate

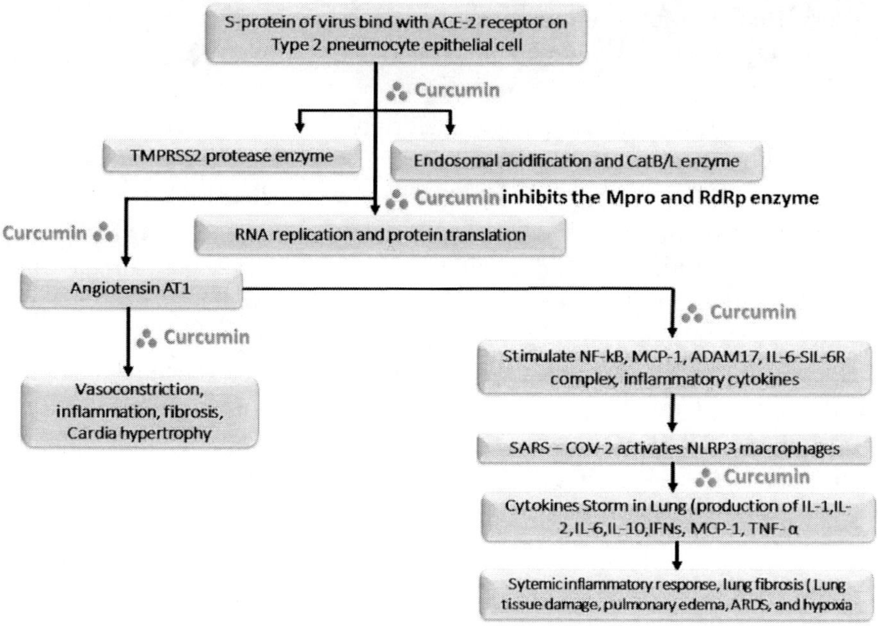

Figure 3. Possible targets of curcumin in COVID-19 infection.

ADAM17 (A disintegrin and metalloprotease 17) protein which helps in the IL-6-SIL-6R complex formation. High levels of IL-6 indicate cytokine storms that occur in COVID patients. The IL-6-SIL-6R complex activates the various mechanisms such as JAK, STAT3, which are responsible for production of inflammatory cytokines (Soni et al., 2020; Eguchi et al., 2020). Curcumin acts on ADAM17 and prevents the IL-6-SIL-6R complex formation enhancing the degradation of EGFR. Curcumin is also found to obstruct mTOR which in turn results in inhibition of STAT3 enzyme and reduces the production of inflammatory cytokines (Jiang et al., 2022; Soni et al., 2020).

Inhibition of Cytokines Storm

Two important mediators namely DAMP 3 and PAMPs are released in infected cells through the exocytosis process. TLR helps in the entry of DAMP3 as well as PAMPs through NF-kB and STAT3, which releases NLRP3 inflammasome. NLRP3 is responsible for high level of inflammatory cytokines IL-1, IL-2, IL-10, TGF-β, IFNs and TNF-α (Nasirzadeh et al., 2021). This results in a cytokine storm and damages multiple organs. Curcumin prevents the cytokine storm by acting on TLR, NF-kB and NLRP3 inflammasome (Murakami, Kamimura and Hirano, 2019; Saeedi-Boroujeni et al., 2021). Figure 3 shows a pictorial presentation of various targets of curcumin in COVID-19 infection.

Recent advancement included formulation of nanoparticle based preparation which could help in enhancement of curcumin's bioavailability and production of a synergistic effect (Ting et al., 2018). Carbon Quantum Dots derived from curcumin (Cur CQDs) are efficient anti-enteroviral drugs (EV71). Applications of Carbon Dots (CDs) against various coronaviruses were examined, along with their potential to fight COVID-19. CDs can alter the penetration and prevent the replication of viruses. CDs alter the detachment and release to combat coronavirus infection. They may be crucial against frontline treatment of COVID-19 or other emerging infectious diseases (Li et al., 2022). CCM-CDs are CDs with application of curcumin which are stable cationic carbon dot forms, they have antiviral qualities and were synthesized by a one-step method. A coronavirus model; PEDV, was used to study CCM-CDs inhibitory effect on viral propagation (Ting et al., 2018). CCM-CDs therapy can alter the structure of surface protein viruses and inhibit the viral entrance. It can prevent the synthesis of a negative-strong form of viral RNA. It aids the synthesis of cytokines that promote inflammation and interferon-stimulated genes (ISGs) to prevent viral replication (Zahedipour et al., 2020).

Conclusion

Curcumin has been studied globally for its various pharmacological activities for decades. This miracle molecule has shown significant antiviral activity against various viruses including SARS-CoV-2. However, the poor water solubility and low bioavailability of curcumin are major limiting factors for its clinical applications. Formulations technologies namely nanosystems and use of bioenhancers such as piperine are found promising to overcome these drawbacks.

References

Abdullahi, H., Elnahas, A., and Konje, J. C. (2021). Seasonal influenza during pregnancy. *European Journal of Obstetrics & Gynecology and Reproductive Biology*, 235–239.

Aggarwal, B. B., Deb, L., and Prasad, S. (2015). Curcumin differs from tetrahydrocurcumin for molecular targets, signaling pathways and cellular responses. *Molecules*, 185–205.

Aggarwal, B. B., Sundaram, C., Malani, N., and Ichikawa, H. (2007). Curcumin: the Indian solid gold. *The molecular targets and therapeutic uses of curcumin in health and disease*, 1-75.

Ahmad, R. S., Hussain, M. B., Sultan, M. T., Arshad, M. S., Waheed, M., Shariati, M. A., Plygun, S., and Hashempur, M. H. (2020). Biochemistry, safety, pharmacological activities, and clinical applications of turmeric: A mechanistic review. *Evidence-based Complementary and Alternative Medicine*, 1-14.

Akbik, D., Ghadiri, M., Chrzanowski, W., and Rohanizadeh, R. (2014). Curcumin as a wound healing agent. *Life sciences*, 1-7.

Ali, A., and Banerjea, A. C. (2016). Curcumin inhibits HIV-1 by promoting Tat protein degradation. *Scientific Reports*, 1–9.

Alok, A., Singh, I. D., Singh, S., Kishore, M., and Jha, P. C. (2015). Curcumin–pharmacological actions and its role in oral submucous fibrosis: A review. *Journal of Clinical and Diagnostic Research,* ZE01–ZE03.

Amalraj, A., Pius, A., Gopi, S., and Gopi, S. (2017). Biological activities of curcuminoids, other biomolecules from turmeric and their derivatives–A review. *Journal of Traditional and Complementary Medicine*, 205-233.

Anggakusuma, Colpitts, C. C., Schang, L. M., Rachmawati, H., Frentzen, A., Pfaender, S., Behrendt, P., Brown, R. J. P., Bankwitz, D., Steinmann, J., Ott, M., Meuleman, P., Rice, C. M., Ploss, A., Pietschmann, T., and Steinmann, E. (2014). Turmeric curcumin inhibits entry of all hepatitis C virus genotypes into human liver cells. *Gut*, 1137–1149.

Ardebili, A., Pouriayevali, M.H., Aleshikh, S., Zahani, M., Ajorloo, M., Izanloo, A., Siyadatpanah, A., Nikoo, H.R., Wilairatana, P., Coutinho, H.D.M. (2021). Antiviral therapeutic potential of curcumin: An update. *Molecules*, 1–23

Bagchi, A., Mukherjee, P., Bhowmick, S. and Raha, A. (2015). Synthesis, characterization and antibacterial activity of a novel curcumin metal complex. *International Journal of Drug Development and Research*, 11-14.

Balasubramanian, A., Pilankatta, R., Teramoto, T., Sajith, A. M., Nwulia, E., Kulkarni, A. and Padmanabhan, R. (2019). Inhibition of dengue virus by curcuminoids. *Antiviral Research*, 71-78.

Barré-Sinoussi, F. (1996). HIV as the cause of AIDS. *Lancet*, 31–35.

Barthelemy, S., Vergnes, L., Moynier, M., Guyot, D., Labidalle, S., and Bahraoui, E. (1998). Curcumin and curcumin derivatives inhibit Tat-mediated transactivation of type 1 human immunodeficiency virus long terminal repeat. *Research in Virology*, 43–52.

Bourgonje, A. R., Abdulle, A. E., Timens, W., Hillebrands, J., Navis, G. J., Gordijn, S. J., Bolling, M. C., Dijkstra, G., Voors, A. A., Osterhaus, A. D. M. E., et al. (2020). Angiotensin-converting enzyme 2 (ACE2), SARS-CoV -2 and the pathophysiology of coronavirus disease (2019) (COVID -19). *J. Pathol.*, 251, 228–248.

Bourne, K. Z., Bourne, N., Reising, S. F., and Stanberry, L. R. (1999). Plant products as topical microbicide candidates: Assessment of *in vitro* and *in vivo* activity against herpes simplex virus type 2. *Antiviral research*, 219–226.

Burckhardt, B., and Reichen, J. (2003). *Therapeutische Umschau* [*Therapeutic Review*]. *Revue therapeutique*, 651–656.

Center for Disease Control and Prevention, (2017). HIV and viral hepatitis factsheets. *South Carolina State Documents Depository*, 22–24.

Chen, D. Y., Shien, J. H., Tiley, L., Chiou, S. S., Wang, S. Y., Chang, T. J., Lee, Y. J., Chan, K. W., and Hsu, W. L. (2010). Curcumin inhibits influenza virus infection and haemagglutination activity. *Food Chemistry*, 1346–1351

Chen, L. H. and Wilson, M. E. (2010). Dengue and chikungunya infections in travelers. *Current Opinion in Infectious Diseases*, 438-444.

Chen, M. H., Lee, M. Y., Chuang, J. J., Li, Y. Z., Ning, S. T., Chen, J. C., and Liu, Y. W. (2012). Curcumin inhibits HCV replication by induction of heme oxygenase-1 and suppression of AKT. *International Journal of Molecular Medicine*, 1021–1028.

Chen, T. Y., Chen, D. Y., Wen, H. W., Ou, J. L., Chiou, S. S., Chen, J. M., Wong, M. L., and Hsu, W. L. (2013). Inhibition of enveloped viruses' infectivity by curcumin. *PloS One*, e62482.

Chikhirzhina, E., Starkova, T., Beljajev, A., Polyanichko, A., and Tomilin, A. (2020). Functional diversity of non-histone chromosomal protein HmgB1. *International Journal of Molecular Sciences*, 7948.

Coffey, L. L., Failloux, A. B., and Weaver, S. C. (2014). Chikungunya virus–vector interactions. *Viruses*, 4628-4663.

Colpitts, C. C., Schang, L. M., Rachmawati, H., Frentzen, A., Pfaender, S., Behrendt, P., Brown, R. J., Bankwitz, D., Steinmann, J., Ott, M., and Meuleman, P. (2014). *Turmeric curcumin inhibits entry of all hepatitis C virus genotypes into human liver cells*. 1137-1149.

Conant, M., Spicer, D., and Levy, J. A. (1986). Condoms prevent transmission of AIDS-associated retrovirus. *JAMA*, 1706

Conteas, C. N., Panossian, A. M., Tran, T. T., and Singh, H. M. (2009). Treatment of HIV-associated diarrhea with curcumin. *Digestive Diseases and Sciences*, 2188–2191.

Cooksey, C. J. (2017). Turmeric: old spice, new spice. *Biotechnic & Histochemistry*, 309-314.

Dadwal, S. S., and Ito, J. I. (2016). Herpes Simplex Virus Infections. *Thomas'. Hematopoietic Cell Transplantation: Stem Cell Transplantation*, 1078–1086.

Dai, J., Gu, L., Su, Y., Wang, Q., Zhao, Y., Chen, X., Deng, H., Li, W., Wang, G., and Li, K. (2018). Inhibition of curcumin on influenza A virus infection and influenzal pneumonia via oxidative stress, TLR2/4, p38/JNK MAPK and NF-κB pathways. *International Immunopharmacology*, 177–187.

Dao, T. T., Nguyen, P. H., Won, H. K., Kim, E. H., Park, J., Won, B. Y., and Oh, W. K. (2012). Curcuminoids from *Curcuma longa* and their inhibitory activities on influenza A neuraminidases. *Food Chemistry*, 21–28.

De Souza, L. M., Inada, N. M., Venturini, F. P., Carmona-Vargas, C. C., Pratavieira, S., de Oliveira, K. T., Kurachi, C., and Bagnato, V. S. (2019). Photolarvicidal effect of curcuminoids from *Curcuma longa* Linn. against *Aedes aegypti* larvae. *Journal of Asia-Pacific Entomology*, 151–158.

Dei Cas, M., and Ghidoni, R. (2019). Dietary curcumin: correlation between bioavailability and health potential. *Nutrients*, 2147.

Dhar, S., and Bhattacharjee, P. (2021). Promising role of curcumin against viral diseases emphasizing COVID-19 management: A review on the mechanistic insights with reference to host-pathogen interaction and immunomodulation. *Journal of Functional Foods*, 104503.

Dieterle, M. E., Haslwanter, D., Bortz III, R. H., Wirchnianski, A. S., Lasso, G., Vergnolle, O., Abbasi, S. A., Fels, J. M., Laudermilch, E., Florez, C., and Mengotto, A. (2020). A replication-competent vesicular stomatitis virus for studies of SARS-CoV-2 spike-mediated cell entry and its inhibition. *Cell Host & Microbe*, 486-496

Eguchi, S., Kawai, T., Scalia, R., and Rizzo, V. (2018). Understanding angiotensin II type 1 receptor signaling in vascular pathophysiology. *Hypertension*, 804-810.

Fani, M. M., Motamedifar, M., and Kordshouli, M. Z. (2015). *In vitro* assessment of the anti-viral effect of Curcumin longa on Herpes Simplex virus type 1. *Journal of Biology and Today's World*, 115-119.

Ferreira, V. H., Nazli, A., Dizzell, S. E., Mueller, K., and Kaushic, C. (2015). The anti-inflammatory activity of curcumin protects the genital mucosal epithelial barrier from disruption and blocks replication of HIV-1 and HSV-2. *PLoS One*, 1–18.

Flores, D. J., Lee, L. H., and Adams, S. D. (2016). Inhibition of Curcumin-Treated Herpes Simplex Virus 1 and 2 in Vero Cells. *Advances in Microbiology*, 276–287.

Giuliani, A. (2016). *Encyclopedia of Food and Health Colors: Properties and Determination of Natural Pigments,* 273–283.

Gratz, N. G. (2004). Critical review of the vector status of *Aedes albopictus*. *Medical and Veterinary Entomology*, 215-227.

Gupta, P., Garg, P., and Roy, N. (2011). Comparative docking and CoMFA analysis of curcumine derivatives as HIV-1 integrase inhibitors. *Molecular Diversity*, 733–750.

Guzman, M. G., and Harris, E. (2015). Dengue. *The Lancet*, 453-465

Halim, J. A. N., Halim, S. N., Denis, D., Haryanto, S., Dharmana, E., Hapsari, R., Sasmono, R. T. and Yohan, B. (2021). Antiviral activities of curcumin and 6-gingerol against infection of four dengue virus serotypes in A549 human cell line in vitro. *Indonesian Journal of Biotechnology*, 41-47.

Halket, J. M., Waterman, D., Przyborowska, A. M., Patel, R. K., Fraser, P. D., and Bramley, P. M. (2005). Chemical derivatization and mass spectral libraries in metabolic profiling by GC/MS and LC/MS/MS. *Journal of Experimental Botany*, 219-243.

Halstead, S. B. (2007). Dengue. *The Lancet*, 1644-1652.

Harris, H. E., Andersson, U., and Pisetsky, D. S. (2012). HMGB1: a multifunctional alarmin driving autoimmune and inflammatory disease. *Nature Reviews Rheumatology*, 195-202.

Hasöksüz, M., Kilic, S., and Saraç, F. (2020). Coronaviruses and sars-cov-2. *Turkish Journal of Medical Sciences*, 549-556.

Heger, M., van Golen, R. F., Broekgaarden, M., and Michel, M. C. (2014). The molecular basis for the pharmacokinetics and pharmacodynamics of curcumin and its metabolites in relation to cancer. *Pharmacological Reviews*, 222-307.

Hoffmann, M., Kleine-Weber, H., Schroeder, S., Krüger, N., Herrler, T., Erichsen, S., Schiergens, T. S., Herrler, G., Wu, N. H., Nitsche, A., and Müller, M. A. (2020). SARS-CoV-2 cell entry depends on ACE2 and TMPRSS2 and is blocked by a clinically proven protease inhibitor. *Cell*, 271-280.

Horev, L., Ramot, Y., and Klapholz, L. (2015). Yellow feet in a patient with breast and thyroid carcinoma, due to oral intake of turmeric. *Drug Safety-Case Reports*, 1-3.

Ismail, E. H., Sabry, D. Y., Mahdy, H., and Khalil, M. M. H. (2014). Synthesis and Characterization of some Ternary Metal Complexes of Curcumin with 1, 10-phenanthroline and their Anticancer Applications. *Journal of Scientific Research*, 509-519.

Itokawa, H., Shi, Q., Akiyama, T., Morris-Natschke, S. L., and Lee, K. H. (2008). Recent advances in the investigation of curcuminoids. *Chinese Medicine*, 1-13.

Jacob, A., Wu, R., Zhou, M. and Wang, P. (2008). Mechanism of the anti-inflammatory effect of curcumin: PPAR-γ activation. *PPAR Research*, 2007.

Javed, A., Shahzad, M., A., Khan, F., Niaze, K (2020). Curcuminoids, *Recent Advances in Natural Product Analysis*, 147-161.

Jiang, Y., Zhao, T., Zhou, X., Xiang, Y., Gutierrez-Castrellon, P., and Ma, X. (2022). Inflammatory pathways in COVID-19: Mechanism and therapeutic interventions. *MedComm*, 1-37.

Jing, Q., and Wang, M. (2019). Dengue epidemiology. *Global Health Journal*, 37-45.

Khan, N., Chen, X., and Geiger, J. D. (2020). Role of endolysosomes in severe acute respiratory syndrome coronavirus-2 infection and coronavirus disease (2019) pathogenesis: implications for potential treatments. *Frontiers in Pharmacology*.

Kim, H. J., Yoo, H. S., Kim, J. C., Park, C. S., Choi, M. S., Kim, M., Choi, H., Min, J. S., Kim, Y. S., Yoon, S. W., and Ahn, J. K. (2009). Antiviral effect of Curcuma longa Linn extract against hepatitis B virus replication. *Journal of Ethnopharmacology*, 189–196.

Kim, K. J., Kim, K. H., Kim, H. Y., Cho, H. K., Sakamoto, N., and Cheong, J. H. (2010). Curcumin inhibits hepatitis C virus replication via suppressing the Akt-SREBP-1 pathway. *FEBS Letters*, 707–712.

Kovacikova, K., and van Hemert, M. J. (2020). Small-Molecule Inhibitors of Chikungunya Virus: Mechanisms of Action and Antiviral Drug Resistance. *Antimicrobial Agents and Chemotherapy*, e01788-20

Krammer, F., Smith, G. J. D., Fouchier, R. A. M., Peiris, M., Kedzierska, K., Doherty, P. C., Palese, P., Shaw, M. L., Treanor, J., Webster, R. G., and García-Sastre, A. (2018). Influenza. *Nature Reviews. Disease Primers*, 1–21.

Kumari, N., Kulkarni, A. A., Lin, X., McLean, C., Ammosova, T., Ivanov, A., Hipolito, M., Nekhai, S., and Nwulia, E. (2015). Inhibition of HIV-1 by curcumin A, a novel curcumin analog. *Drug Design, Development and Therapy*, 5051–5060.

Kutluay, S. B., Doroghazi, J., Roemer, M. E., and Triezenberg, S. J. (2008). Curcumin inhibits herpes simplex virus immediate-early gene expression by a mechanism independent of p300/CBP histone acetyltransferase activity. *Virology*, 239–247.

Lan, J., Ge, J., Yu, J., Shan, S., Zhou, H., Fan, S., Zhang, Q., Shi, X., Wang, Q., Zhang, L., and Wang, X. (2020). Structure of the SARS-CoV-2 spike receptor-binding domain bound to the ACE2 receptor. *Nature*, 215-220.

Lauer, S. A., Grantz, K. H., Bi, Q., Jones, F. K., Zheng, Q., Meredith, H. R., Azman, A. S., Reich, N. G., and Lessler, J. (2020). The incubation period of coronavirus disease 2019 (COVID-19) from publicly reported confirmed cases: *estimation and application. Annals of Internal Medicine*, 577-582.

Lestari, M. L., and Indrayanto, G. (2014). Curcumin. *Profiles of Drug Substances, Excipients and Related Methodology*, 113-204.

Li, H., Zhong, C., Wang, Q., Chen, W., and Yuan, Y. (2019). Curcumin is an APE1 redox inhibitor and exhibits an antiviral activity against KSHV replication and pathogenesis. *Antiviral Research*, 98–103.

Lim, L., Dang, M., Roy, A., Kang, J., Song, J., (2020). Curcumin Allosterically Inhibits the Dengue NS2B-NS3 Protease by Disrupting Its Active Conformation. *ACS Omega*, 25677–25686.

Li, P., Sun, L., Xue, S., Qu, D., An, L., Wang, X., and Sun, Z. (2022). Recent advances of carbon dots as new antimicrobial agents. *SmartMat*, 226-248.

Li, S., Yuan, W., Deng, G., Wang, P., Yang, P., and Aggarwal, B. (2011). Chemical composition and product quality control of turmeric (*Curcuma longa* L.), *Pharmaceutical Crops*, 28-54

Liu, H. T., and Ho, Y. S. (2018). Anticancer effect of curcumin on breast cancer and stem cells. *Food Science and Human Wellness*, 134-137.

Liu, X., Liu, M., Yuan, W., Chang, H., Li, Y., Chen, Z., Deng, Y., Li, R., Wan, Y., Jiang, Z., Fan, X., Wang, Y., Wu, X., and Mo, X. (2013). Anti-viral effects of curcumin on influenza A virus-induced myocarditis via inhibiting Wnt/β-catenin signaling. *Central European Journal of Immunology*, 328–335.

Liu, Z., and Ying, Y. (2020). The inhibitory effect of curcumin on virus-induced cytokine storm and its potential use in the associated severe pneumonia. *Frontiers in cell and Developmental Biology*, 479.

Marbawati, D., Umniyati, S. R., Hudayani, R., Kusnanto, H., Humardewayanti, R., Rana, M. S., Syaket, M., and Shakil, A. (2013). The Effects of Curcumin against Dengue-2 Virus Based on immunocytochemistry technique. *Tropical Medicine Journal*, 95–102.

Marín-Palma, D., Tabares-Guevara, J. H., Zapata-Cardona, M. I., Flórez-Álvarez, L., Yepes, L. M., Rugeles, M. T., Zapata-Builes, W., Hernandez, J. C., and Taborda, N. A. (2021). Curcumin inhibits *in vitro* SARS-CoV-2 infection in vero E6 cells through multiple antiviral mechanisms. *Molecules.* 1-17.

Maurya, V. K., Kumar, S., Prasad, A. K., Bhatt, M. L., and Saxena, S. K. (2020). Structure-based drug designing for potential antiviral activity of selected natural products from Ayurveda against SARS-CoV-2 spike glycoprotein and its cellular receptor. *Virus Disease*, 179-193.

Mazumder, A., Raghavan, K., Weinstein, J., Kohn, K. W., and Pommier, Y. (1995). Inhibition of human immunodeficiency virus type-1 integrase by curcumin. *Biochemical Pharmacology*, 1165–1170.

Mezzacappo, N. F., de Souza, L. M., Inada, N. M., Dias, L. D., Garbuio, M., Venturini, F. P., Corrêa, T. Q., Moura, L., Blanco, K. C., de Oliveira, K. T., and Bagnato, V. S. (2021). Curcumin/d-mannitol as photolarvicide: induced delay in larval development time, changes in sex ratio and reduced longevity of *Aedes aegypti*. *Pest Management Science*, 2530–2538.

Morawska, L., and Milton, D. K. (2020). It is time to address airborne transmission of coronavirus disease 2019 (COVID-19). *Clinical Infectious Diseases*, 2311-2313.

Mouler Rechtman, M., Har-Noy, O., Bar-Yishay, I., Fishman, S., Adamovich, Y., Shaul, Y., Halpern, Z., and Shlomai, A. (2010). Curcumin inhibits hepatitis B virus via down-regulation of the metabolic coactivator PGC-1α. *FEBS Letters*, 2485–2490.

Mounce, B. C., Cesaro, T., Carrau, L., Vallet, T. and Vignuzzi, M. (2017). Curcumin inhibits Zika and chikungunya virus infection by inhibiting cell binding. *Antiviral Research*, 148-157.

Mukherjee, S., and Kar, S. K. (2021). Curcuminoids: The novel molecules of nature. In *Herbs and Spices-New Processing Technologies*. IntechOpen.

Murakami, M., Kamimura, D., and Hirano, T. (2019). Pleiotropy and specificity: insights from the interleukin 6 family of cytokines. *Immunity*, 812-831.

Muthu, M. J., Kavitha, K., Chitra, K. S., and Nandhineeswari, S. (2019). Soluble curcumin prepared by solid dispersion using four different carriers: Phase solubility, molecular modelling and physicochemical characterization. *Tropical Journal of Pharmaceutical Research*, 1581-1588.

Nabila, N., Suada, N. K., Denis, D., Yohan, B., Adi, A. C., Veterini, A. S., Anindya, A. L., Sasmono, R. T., and Rachmawati, H. (2020). Antiviral action of curcumin encapsulated in nanoemulsion against four serotypes of dengue virus. *Pharmaceutical Nanotechnology*, 54-62.

Naseri, S., Darroudi, M., Aryan, E., Gholoobi, A., Rahimi, H. R., Ketabi, Movaqar A., Abdoli, M., Gouklani, H., and Teimourpou, R., M. Z. (2017). The Antiviral Effects of Curcumin Nanomicelles on the Attachment and Entry of Hepatitis C Virus. *Iranian Journal of Virology*, 29-35.

Nasirzadeh, A., Bazeli, J., Hajavi, J., Yavarmanesh, N., Zahedi, M., Abounoori, M., Razavi, A., Maddah, M. M., Mortazavi, P., Moradi, M., and Heidarzadeh, S. (2021). Inhibiting IL-6 during Cytokine Storm in COVID-19: Potential Role of Natural Products, *Preprints*, 2021060131.

Nurjanah, N., and Saepudin, E. (2019). November. Curcumin isolation, synthesis and characterization of curcumin isoxazole derivative compound. In *AIP Conference Proceedings*, 020065.

Olagnier, D., Farahani, E., Thyrsted, J., Blay-Cadanet, J., Herengt, A., Idorn, M., Hait, A., Hernaez, B., Knudsen, A., Iversen, M. B., and Schilling, M. (2020). SARS-CoV2-mediated suppression of NRF2-signaling reveals potent antiviral and anti-inflammatory activity of 4-octyl-itaconate and dimethyl fumarate. *Nature Communications*, 1-12.

Ou, J. L., Mizushina, Y., Wang, S. Y., Chuang, D. Y., Nadar, M., and Hsu, W. L. (2013). Structure-activity relationship analysis of curcumin analogues on anti-influenza virus activity. *The FEBS Journal*, 5829–5840.

Padilla-s, L., Rodríguez, A., Gonzales, M. M., Gallego-g, J. C., and Castaño-o, J. C. (2014). Inhibitory effects of curcumin on dengue virus type 2-infected cells *in vitro*. *Archives of virology*, 573-579.

Pak, J. E., Sharon, C., Satkunarajah, M., Auperin, T. C., Cameron, C. M., Kelvin, D. J., Seetharaman, J., Cochrane, A., Plummer, F. A., Berry, J. D., and Rini, J. M. (2009). Structural insights into immune recognition of the severe acute respiratory syndrome coronavirus S protein receptor binding domain. *Journal of Molecular Biology*, 815-823.

Pang, X. F., Zhang, L. H., Bai, F., Wang, N. P., Garner, R. E., McKallip, R. J., and Zhao, Z. Q. (2015). Attenuation of myocardial fibrosis with curcumin is mediated by modulating expression of angiotensin II AT1/AT2 receptors and ACE2 in rats. *Drug Design, Development and Therapy*, 6043-6054.

Pendyala, B., and Patras, A. (2020). In silico screening of food bioactive compounds to predict potential inhibitors of COVID-19 main protease (Mpro) and RNA-dependent RNA polymerase (RdRp). *Agriculture and Food Chemistry*, 1-11.

Peng, Y., Ao, M., Dong, B., Jiang, Y., Yu, L., Chen, Z., Hu, C., and Xu, R. (2021). Anti-inflammatory effects of curcumin in the inflammatory diseases: Status, limitations and countermeasures. *Drug design, Development and Therapy*, 4503.

Petersen, L. R., and Powers, A. M. (2016). Chikungunya: epidemiology. *F1000Research*, 5.

Praditya, D., Kirchhoff, L., Brüning, J., Rachmawati, H., Steinmann, J., and Steinmann, E. (2019). Anti-infective properties of the golden spice curcumin. *Frontiers in Microbiology*, 912.

Prasad, S., and Tyagi, A. K. (2015). Curcumin and its analogues: a potential natural compound against HIV infection and AIDS. *Food & Function*, 3412–3419.

Priyadarsini, K. I. (2014). The chemistry of curcumin: from extraction to therapeutic agent. *Molecules*, 20091-20112.

Ragotte, R. J., Pulido, D., Donnellan, F. R., Hill, M. L., Gorini, G., Davies, H., Brun, J., McHugh, K., King, L. D., Skinner, K., and Miura, K. (2021). Human basigin (CD147) does not directly interact with SARS-CoV-2 spike glycoprotein. *Msphere*, e0064721.

Razavi, H. (2020). Global Epidemiology of Viral Hepatitis. *Gastroenterology Clinics*, 179–189.

Richart, S. M., Li, Y. L., Mizushina, Y., Chang, Y. Y., Chung, T. Y., Chen, G. H., Tzen, J. T. C., Shia, K. S., and Hsu, W. L. (2018). Synergic effect of curcumin and its structural analogue (Monoacetylcurcumin) on anti- influenza virus infection. *Journal of Food and Drug Analysis*, 1015–1023.

Roizman, B., and Baines, J. (1991). The diversity and unity of herpesviridae. *Comparative Immunology, Microbiology and Infectious Diseases*, 63–79.

Ross, R. W. (1955). The Newala epidemic: III. The virus: isolation, pathogenic properties and relationship to the epidemic. *Epidemiology & Infection*, 177-191.

Ross, T. M. (2010). Dengue virus. *Clinics in laboratory medicine*, 149-160.

Saeedi-Boroujeni, A., Mahmoudian-Sani, M. R., Bahadoram, M., and Alghasi, A. (2021). COVID-19: A Case for Inhibiting NLRP3 Inflammasome, Suppression of Inflammation with Curcumin? *Basic & Clinical Pharmacology & Toxicology*, 37-45.

Seitz, R. (2016). Human Immunodeficiency Virus (HIV). *Transfusion Medicine and Hemotherapy*, 203–222.

Sharma, A., Yadav, A., Gupta, N., Sharma, S., Kakkar, R., Cwiklinski, K., Quaye, E., Mahajan, S. D., Schwartz, S. A., and Kumar Sharma, R. (2019). Multifunctional mesoporous curcumin encapsulated iron- phenanthroline nanocluster: A new Anti-HIV agent. *Colloids and Surfaces B: Biointerfaces*, 289–297.

Sharma, R. K., Cwiklinski, K., Aalinkeel, R., Reynolds, J. L., Sykes, D. E., Quaye, E., Oh, J., Mahajan, S. D., and Schwartz, S. A. (2017). Immunomodulatory activities of curcumin-stabilized silver nanoparticles: Efficacy as an antiretroviral therapeutic. *Immunological Investigations*, 833–846.

Siegel, K., and Lekas, H. M. (2002). AIDS as a chronic illness: psychosocial implications. *Aids*, S69-S76.

Soleimani, V., Sahebkar, A., and Hosseinzadeh, H. (2018). Turmeric (*Curcuma longa*) and its major constituent (curcumin) as nontoxic and safe substances. *Phytotherapy Research*, 985-995.

Soni, V. K., Mehta, A., Ratre, Y. K., Tiwari, A. K., Amit, A., Singh, R. P., Sonkar, S. C., Chaturvedi, N., Shukla, D., and Vishvakarma, N. K. (2020). Curcumin, a traditional spice component, can hold the promise against COVID-19? *European Journal of Pharmacology*, 173551.

Subudhi, B. B., Chattopadhyay, S., Mishra, P., and Kumar, A. (2018). Current strategies for inhibition of chikungunya infection. *Viruses*, 235.

Sui, Z., Salto, R., Li, J., Craik, C., and Ortiz de Montellano, P. R. (1993). Inhibition of the HIV-1 and HIV-2 proteases by curcumin and curcumin boron complexes. *Bioorganic & Medicinal Chemistry*, 415–422.

Taylor, T. J., Brockman, M. A., Mcnamee, E. E., and Knipe, D. M. (2002). Herpes Simplex Virus. *Frontiers in Bioscience-Landmark*, 752–764.

Tejada, S., Manayi, A., Daglia, M., F Nabavi, S., Sureda, A., Hajheydari, Z., Gortzi, O., Pazoki-Toroudi, H. and M Nabavi, S., (2016). Wound healing effects of curcumin: A short review. *Current Pharmaceutical Biotechnology*, 1002-1007.

Thimmulappa, R. K., Mudnakudu-Nagaraju, K. K., Shivamallu, C., Subramaniam, K. T., Radhakrishnan, A., Bhojraj, S., and Kuppusamy, G. (2021). Antiviral and immunomodulatory activity of curcumin: A case for prophylactic therapy for COVID-19. *Heliyon*, 06350.

Thongsri, P., Pewkliang, Y., Borwornpinyo, S., Wongkajornsilp, A., Hongeng, S., and Sangiamsuntorn, K. (2021). Curcumin inhibited hepatitis B viral entry through NTCP binding. *Scientific Reports*, 1–12.

Ting, D., Dong, N., Fang, L., Lu, J., Bi, J., Xiao, S., and Han, H. (2018). Multisite inhibitors for enteric coronavirus: antiviral cationic carbon dots based on curcumin. *ACS Applied Nano Materials*, 5451-5459.

Valand, N. N., Patel, M. B., and Menon, S. K. (2015). Curcumin-p-sulfonatocalix [4] resorcinarene (p-SC [4] R) interaction: thermo-physico chemistry, stability and biological evaluation. *RSC Advances*, 8739-8752.

Vitali, D., Bagri, P., Wessels, J. M., Arora, M., Ganugula, R., Parikh, A., Mandur, T., Felker, A., Garg, S., Kumar, M. N. V. R., and Kaushic, C. (2020). Curcumin can decrease tissue inflammation and the severity of HSV-2 infection in the female reproductive mucosa. *International Journal of Molecular Sciences,* 337.

Vitiello, A., and Ferrara, F. (2020). Correlation between renin-angiotensin system and Severe Acute Respiratory Syndrome Coronavirus 2 infection: What do we know? *European Journal of Pharmacology*, 173373.

Von Rhein, C., Weidner, T., Henß, L., Martin, J., Weber, C., Sliva, K. and Schnierle, B. S. (2016). Curcumin and *Boswellia serrata* gum resin extract inhibit chikungunya and vesicular stomatitis virus infections *in vitro*. *Antiviral Research*, 51-57.

Wahyuni, T. S., Permatasari, A. A., Widiandani, T., Fuad, A., Widyawaruyanti, A., Aoki-Utsubo, C., and Hotta, H. (2018). Antiviral activities of curcuma genus against hepatitis C virus. *Natural Product Communications*, 1579–1582.

Wal, P., Saraswat, N., Pal, R. S., Wal, A., and Chaubey, M. (2019). A detailed insight of the anti-inflammatory effects of curcumin with the assessment of parameters, sources of ROS and associated mechanisms. *Open Medicine Journal*, 64-76.

Wang, H., Yang, H., and Tracey, K. J. (2004). Extracellular role of HMGB1 in inflammation and sepsis. *Journal of Internal Medicine*, 320-331.

Wang, K., Chen, W., Zhou, Y. S., Lian, J. Q., Zhang, Z., Du, P., Gong, L., Zhang, Y., Cui, H. Y., Geng, J. J., and Wang, B. (2020). SARS-CoV-2 invades host cells via a novel route: CD147-spike protein. *biorxiv*, 1-10

Wei, J., Alfajaro, M. M., DeWeirdt, P. C., Hanna, R. E., Lu-Culligan, W. J., Cai, W. L., Strine, M. S., Zhang, S. M., Graziano, V. R., Schmitz, C. O., and Chen, J. S. (2021). Genome-wide CRISPR screens reveal host factors critical for SARS-CoV-2 infection. *Cell*, 76-91.

Wei, Z. Q., Zhang, Y. H., Ke, C. Z., Chen, H. X., Ren, P., He, Y. L., Hu, P., Ma, D. Q., Luo, J., and Meng, Z. J. (2017). Curcumin inhibits hepatitis B virus infection by down-regulating cccDNA-bound histone acetylation. *World Journal of Gastroenterology*, 6252–6260.

Weiss, R. A. (1993). How does HIV cause AIDS? *Science*, 1273-1279.

Wilken, R., Veena, M. S., Wang, M. B., and Srivatsan, E. S. (2011). Curcumin: A review of anti-cancer properties and therapeutic activity in head and neck squamous cell carcinoma. *Molecular Cancer*, 1-19.

Xiao, S., Li, Y., Wong, T. W., and Hui, D. S. (2017). Role of fomites in SARS transmission during the largest hospital outbreak in Hong Kong. *PloS One,* e0181558.

Xu, Y., and Liu, L. (2017). Curcumin alleviates macrophage activation and lung inflammation induced by influenza virus infection through inhibiting the NF-κB signaling pathway. *Influenza and Other Respiratory Viruses*, 457–463.

Yadav, V. S., Mishra, K. P., Singh, D. P., Mehrotra, S., and Singh, V. K. (2005). Immunomodulatory effects of curcumin. *Immunopharmacology and Immunotoxicology*, 485-497.

Zahedipour, F., Hosseini, S. A., Sathyapalan, T., Majeed, M., Jamialahmadi, T., Al-Rasadi, K., Banach, M., and Sahebkar, A. (2020). Potential effects of curcumin in the treatment of COVID-19 infection. *Phytotherapy Research*, 2911-2920

Zamri, A., Teruna, H. Y., Rahmawati, E. N., Frimayanti, N., and Ikhtiarudin, I. (2019). Synthesis and in silico studies of a benzenesulfonyl curcumin analogue as a new anti-dengue virus type 2 (DEN2) NS2B/NS3. *Indonesian Journal of Pharmacy*, 84–90.

Zandi, K., Ramedani, E., Khosro, M., Tajbakhsh, S., Dailami, I., Rastian, Z., Fouladvand, M., Yousefi, F., and Farshadpour, F. (2010). Evaluation of antiviral activities of curcumin derivatives against HSV-1 in Vero cell line. *Natural Product Communications*, 8–11.

Zhang, H. S., Ruan, Z., and Sang, W. W. (2011). HDAC1/NFκB pathway is involved in curcumin inhibiting of Tat-mediated long terminal repeat transactivation. *Journal of Cellular Physiology*, 3385–3391.

Chapter 5

Curcumin: Green Extraction Techniques, Synthetic Approaches and Its Anti-Inflammatory, Antioxidant and Anti-Neoplastic Effects

Lucas D. Dias[1,*]
Adrieli Oliveira Raminelli[2]
Bruno Lemes Marques[3]
and Ricardo C. Parreira[1]

[1]Centro Universitário de Mineiros, Campus Trindade, Trindade, GO, Brazil
[2]Laboratório de Psicofarmacologia, Departamento de Neurociências e Ciências do Comportamento da Faculdade de Medicina de Ribeirão Preto, Hospital das Clínicas da Faculdade de Medicina de Ribeirão Preto, Universidade de São Paulo, Ribeirão Preto, SP, Brazil
[3] Departamento de Farmacologia, Instituto de Ciências Biológicas, Universidade Federal de Goiás, Goiânia, GO, Brazil

Abstract

Curcumin is a useful natural product applied in Medicine including treatment and diagnosis. In this regard, it has been used for treatment of neurodegenerative diseases and as anti-inflammatory and anticancer agents. This natural product can be obtained by extraction from a natural source (turmeric powder) or via synthetic approaches (batch and/or flow chemistry). Herein, we describe general green extraction methods using alternative media and synthetic procedures for curcumin through

* Corresponding Author's Email: lucasdanillodias@gmail.com.

In: Curcumin and Its Role in Health and Disease
Editor: Kathryn Woltjer
ISBN: 979-8-88697-491-1

continuous flow chemistry as well as its production in up-scale, high purity, and low cost for medical use. Moreover, some recent advances on pharmacological effects of curcumin as anti-inflammatory, antioxidant and anti-neoplastic agents are reported and discussed. In this chapter, we did not produce a systematic review; instead, we highlighted selected green extraction methods (using alternative solvents) and synthetic procedure (combining batch and flow chemistry) for curcumin and its possibilities and limitations as a medicine.

Keywords: curcumin, green extraction, green synthesis, anti-inflammatory, antioxidant, anti-neoplastic

Introduction

Over the years, pharmaceutical industries and researchers have searched and developed new medicines to treat different diseases (Hussein, Meihua et al. 2013) (Conn and Roth 2008) (Atanasov, Zotchev et al. 2021). In this regard, natural products have been widely used as medicine and/or as precursors for synthetic modulation (Newman and Cragg 2020) aiming to develop active and low toxic drugs. Among them, curcumin (a traditional food additive) is considered an useful natural product for biomedical applications (Hatcher, Planalp et al. 2008) which have been described as antibacterial (Adamczak, Ozarowski et al. 2020), antioxidant (Menon and Sudheer 2007), anticancer (Ojo, Adeyemo et al. 2022) agents and also for biophotonics applications (e.g.: as a photosensitizer for antimicrobial photodynamic therapy) (Dias, Blanco et al. 2020).

Regarding its production, curcumin can be obtained by synthetic approaches (Singh, Pandey et al. 2021) (Priyadarsini 2014) and extraction methodologies from the turmeric (*Curcuma longa*) rhizome (Zielinska, Alves et al. 2020). However, due to the demand to develop drugs on a large scale, low cost and high purity, synthetic methodologies following the 12 Principles of Green Chemistry have been selected and applied (Li and Trost 2008). In this chapter, we reported an overview about green extraction approaches and synthetic methodologies for curcumin and also its application as antioxidant, anti-inflammatory, and anti-neoplastic agents. Moreover, we presented some possibilities and limitations on use of curcumin for treatment of diseases (Figure 1).

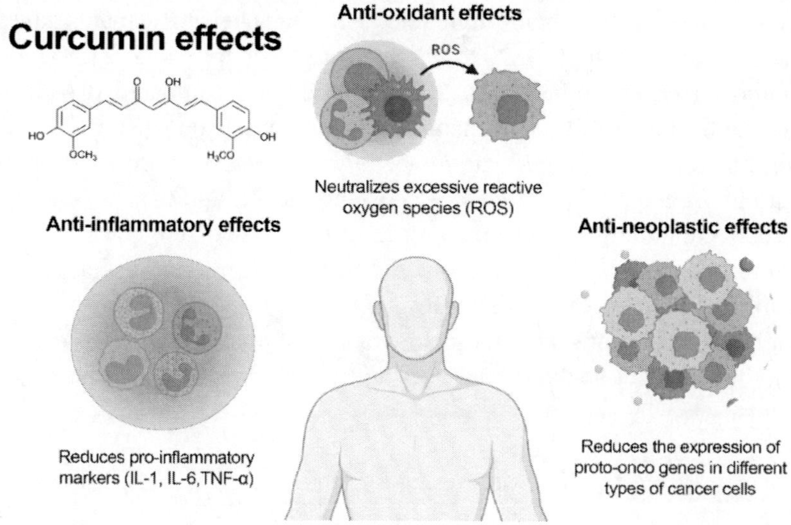

Figure 1. Schematic illustration of curcumin biomedical applications reported in this chapter.

Extraction of Curcumin Using Alternative Media

As previously mentioned, curcumin is largely used in culinary, food industry and as medicine (Fuloria, Mehta et al. 2022) (Raduly, Raditoiu et al. 2021). Its extraction and separation from natural source (turmeric powder) have been reported using different methodologies such as organic solvents (e.g.: ethanol, ethyl acetate, and acetone) and chromatographic techniques for separation/ purification (Tripathy, Verma et al. 2021) (Yadav, Sharma et al. 2017) (Jiang, Ghosh et al. 2021). However, the curcumin extracted from *Curcuma longa L* (turmeric) represents a group of curcuminoids namely curcumin (majority molecular structure), demethoxycurcumin and bis-demethoxycurcumin (Figure 2) but their chemical profile (proportion of curcuminoids) depend on origin and the climatic and soil conditions (Nelson, Dahlin et al. 2017). According to literature, these curcuminoids have been already extracted, separated using analytical techniques, and characterized by a set of spectroscopic tools (Zhu, Chen et al. 2022) (Hoang, Fauster et al. 2022).

Among the extraction methods for curcumin reported so far, we highlighted the ones that are according to the Green Chemistry philosophy aiming to use non-toxic reagents, reduce waste (mostly toxic organic solvents), and also to obtain high selectivity and yield (Chemat, Vian et al. 2012) (Chemat, Vian et al. 2020). As selected example, in 2021, Degot and co-authors (Degot, Huber et al. 2021) applied and compared two different green and bio-based surfactant-free microemulsion (SFME) namely water/ethanol/triacetin and water/diacetin/triacetin as extraction solvents for curcumin from *Curcuma longa.* According to the authors, the mixture of solvents containing water/ethanol/triacetin showed the best yield for curcuminoids (~18% more than water/diacetin/triacetin and ~53% more than ethanol/water mixture). Furthermore, comparing this method with a Soxhlet apparatus, the last shows higher yields for curcuminoids but it consumes more energy (permanent heating), and uses a large number of hazardous and toxic solvents.

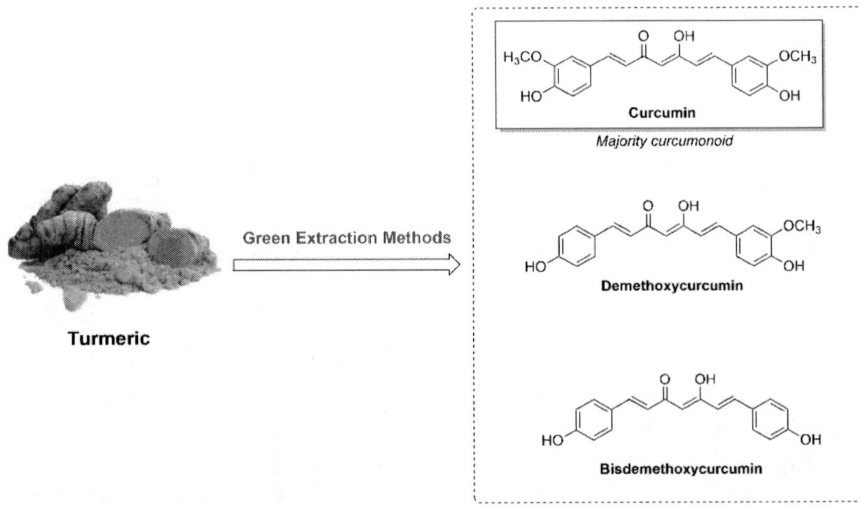

Figure 2. Chemical composition of curcumin powder from *Curcuma longa L* (turmeric).

In this regard, in 2020, Gokdemir and co-authors investigated 1-butyl-3-methylimidazolium bis (trifluoromethylsulfonyl) imide ([BMIM][Tf$_2$N]) as an alternative extraction system instead of toxic classical organic solvents for curcumin from turmeric. In this study, the authors applied response surface methodology (RSM) to evaluate the influence of different parameters such as the time (10 to 60 min), temperature (25 to 55°C), and volume of solvent (10 to 30 mL) (Gokdemir, Baylan et al. 2020). From the analysis of results, the authors observed that the yield was influenced by the extraction time, temperature and volume of solvent. Additionally, the authors obtained the best yield (2.94%) using the following extraction conditions: extraction time of 60 min, temperature of 55ºC and solvent volume of 30 mL. Overall, these examples using green conditions and chemicals/solvents represent good sustainable methods for curcumin extraction from turmeric. These should be chosen in order to produce less waste, using non-toxic reagents and high activity extraction systems.

Synthetic Method for Curcumin by Flow Chemistry

Due to the need to use curcumin on a large scale with low cost and high purity, synthetic methodologies have been developed and described in the literature (Yixuan, Qaria et al. 2021). On the other hand, these methods mostly used a large number of toxic reagents/solvents and high energy consumption. In order to meet some principles of Green Chemistry and decrease the cost of curcumin, Oliveira and co-authors developed a synthetic method for curcumin combining batch and continuous flow chemistry (Carmona-Vargas, Alves et al. 2017). The flow chemistry technology presents some advantages regarding a chemical engineering view when compared to the methods described so far (Burange, Osman et al. 2022). In this study, the authors divided the synthesis of curcumin in 3 steps. Initially, boron complex **1** was synthesized by reaction of acetylacetone and B_2O_3/B(O-n-Bu)$_3$ followed by its reaction with vanillin (*via* aldol condensation) yielding the intermediate boron complex **2**. Then, the decomplexation of the boron complex was performed using HCl yielding curcumin with high purity, as described in Figure 3.

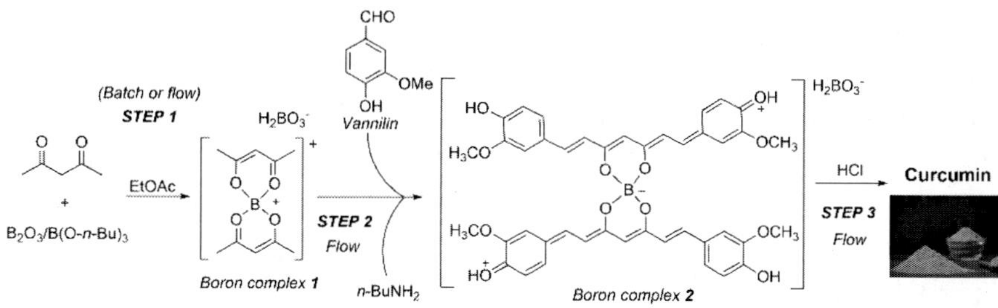

Figure 3. Synthesis of curcumin by combining batch and continuous flow chemistry.

Biomedical Applications of Curcumin

Experimental and pharmacological trials have demonstrated efficacy of curcumin in various diseases. Regarding literature, some authors have pointed out that this plant exerts actions such as anti-inflammatory, anti-neoplastic and antioxidant, among others (Jakubczyk, Druzga et al. 2020, Peng, Ao et al. 2021). In this chapter we will discuss these three curcumin effects on some pathologies.

Anti-Inflammatory Effects of Curcumin

Inflammation is a normal and adaptive reaction to damaging stimuli, and it may be evident in diseases like infections and tissue damage. Inflammation is a complicated physiological and pathological process that aids in the preservation of bodily homeostasis. Various cell types, including neutrophils, macrophages, mast cells and lymphocytes participate in the inflammatory response. The inflammatory process is viewed as the body's defense response to an aggressive agent. Defense reactions are typically advantageous to the organism, operating to reduce invading pathogen survival and proliferation while encouraging tissue survival, repair, and recovery (Ammon, Safayhi et al. 1993).

Inflammation is characterized by five symptoms, redness, heat, pain, swelling and reduced function. Heat and redness are consequences of vasodilation, which increases blood circulation and concentration in the inflamed area (hyperemia), increasing the temperature. Swelling is a consequence of the increase in vascular permeability that allows the leakage of vascular fluids and, therefore, the formation of edema. Such edema can compress the nerve endings, causing pain, while the body releases chemical substances (cytokines, chemokines, and prostaglandins) in response to tissue injury. The loss of function happens especially in joints and tissues or limbs, limiting the individual's movements (Ammon, Safayhi et al. 1993).

An important aspect of inflammation is that it can be divided into acute and chronic. If left untreated, it can be considered highly harmful to the body. Vasoactive amines, arachidonic acid metabolites, leukotrienes, thromboxanes, platelet activating factor (PAF), chemokines, tumor necrosis factor (TNF), and other cytokines (interleukins (IL) IL-1, IL-6, and IL-18) are the mediators implicated in acute inflammation. The body's complicated physiological reaction is to neutralize, inactivate, and remove the inflammatory agent while also replacing tissues destroyed by fibrosis, culminating in tissue healing and inhibiting the inflammatory response. However, chronic inflammation is characterized by the simultaneous occurrence of inflammatory activation and tissue destruction. The chronic inflammatory process evolves gradually, depending on the duration of injury, permanence of the aggressor and the body's difficulty in eliminating tissue or cell damage. It can also entail complicated interactions between various cells and the mediators they release, such as the cytokines IL-17, IL-12, and IL-23. Inflammation aggravates illnesses, which increase inflammation, producing a vicious cycle that makes therapy difficult. As a result, we must emphasize the importance of inflammation in the onset and progression of illnesses, and therapeutic medications must have anti-inflammatory properties (Calder 2015).

Some medicinal plants have been evaluated for anti-inflammatory properties in prior research. Curcumin has piqued the curiosity of many researchers due to its activity, and it is regarded as one of the natural substances with the highest promise for illness therapy. Curcumin has antioxidant, immunomodulatory, and anti-inflammatory properties. The final one works by modulating signaling pathways and reducing mediator synthesis, and numerous preclinical and clinical studies have been conducted to investigate its influence on inflammatory disorders such as arthritis, psoriasis, depression, atherosclerosis, and COVID-19 (Cole, Teter et al. 2007, Thimmulappa, Mudnakudu-Nagaraju et al. 2021).

Many *in vitro* and animal studies demonstrated that Curcumin acts on various levels of the arachidonic acid inflammatory cascade and on various enzymes and cytokines. The development of chronic diseases such as autoimmune, cardiovascular, endocrine, neurodegenerative, and neoplastic disorders are intrinsically connected with inflammation. Interestingly, curcumin binds to toll-like receptors (TLRs) and controls its different intracellular signaling pathways (nuclear factor kappa-B (NF-B), mitogen-activated protein kinases (MAPK), activator protein 1 (AP-1)). Hence, it can control inflammatory mediators and could possibly be used in inflammatory disorders. It inhibits NF-B by acting on the peroxisome proliferator-activated receptor gamma (PPAR). It can also have anti-inflammatory effects via modulating the inflammatory signaling pathway janus kinase/signal transducer and activator of transcription (JAK/STAT) (Peng, Ao et al. 2021).

Curcumin has been demonstrated to promote reduced levels of pro-inflammatory mediators in several different in vivo studies (Meng, Yan et al. 2013, Chowdhury, Banerjee et al. 2019). Furthermore, curcumin administration demonstrated statistically significant improvements in plasma levels of C-reactive protein (CRP) and TNF in a randomized, double-blind, placebo-controlled clinical experiment (Singh, Passsari et al. 2016).

Curcumin appears to be efficient at lowering inflammatory mediator levels, and its anti-inflammatory characteristics may benefit disorders such as osteoarthritis, the most prevalent joint condition associated with inflammation. Apparently, curcumin has the ability to lessen joint inflammation and pain symptoms due to its anti-inflammatory and cartilaginous protecting properties (Peng, Ao et al. 2021).

Psoriasis is a chronic inflammatory skin disease with an inflammatory pathogenesis. Dendritic cells are recognized to be involved in the early stages of psoriasis. Myeloid dendritic cell secretion of pro-inflammatory markers results in the production of inflammatory cytokines such as IL-17, IFN-, Interferon-gamma (TNF), and IL-22, which initiates the psoriasis-associated tissue-damage cascade. This results in the development of psoriasis, which is characterized by keratinocyte proliferation, erythema caused by skin thickness, and local tissue infiltration. (Glitzner, Korosec et al. 2014, Barnes, Kumar et al. 2016). Hence, this compound is a great possibility of insertion as an adjuvant in the treatment of health problems. As demonstrated, Curcumin can aid in lighter and more severe cases of inflammation.

The role of oxidative stress and inflammation in the etiology of metabolic syndrome has also been explored. Subjects with metabolic syndrome were randomly assigned to receive Curcuminoids or a placebo for eight weeks in this randomized, double-blind, placebo-controlled experiment. To boost oral bioavailability, curcuminoids were supplied at a daily dosage of 1g and supplemented with piperine (10mg/day). At the beginning and conclusion of the trial, serum superoxide dismutase activity, malondialdehyde, and C-reactive protein (CRP) concentrations were examined. In comparison to placebo, supplementation with the Curcuminoid-piperine combination increased serum superoxide dismutase activity and decreased malondial-dehyde and CRP concentrations (Panahi, Hosseini et al. 2015).

Curcumin's anti-inflammatory impact was also detected in a randomized, double-blind, placebo-controlled study of type 2 diabetic nephropathy. Curcumin treatment was observed to lower blood levels of TGF- and IL-8 in this investigation. Curcumin, as previously said, is a natural anti-inflammatory agent, and multiple experimental and pharmacological investigations have confirmed its efficacy in the treatment of various illnesses. Curcumin, in addition to its anti-inflammatory properties, has been found in recent study to aid in the treatment of cancer (Bansal, Kausar et al. 2011, Mohan, Narayanan et al. 2013).

Anti-Neoplastic Effects of Curcumin

Cancer is the second most lethal illness and one of the world's most serious public health issues. Cancer diagnoses and deaths are predicted to rise dramatically as people grow old and adopt cancer-risking lifestyle choices. This is especially significant in low- and middle-income countries when they go through economic transitions such as increased automation of transportation and labor, cultural transformations in women's roles, and more exposure and access to foreign markets. As a result, many of the lifestyle risk factors that are currently prominent in high-income countries, such as tobacco smoking, physical inactivity, excess body weight, and reproductive patterns, are also becoming more frequent (Mattiuzzi and Lippi 2019).

Cancer disease starts when a group of cells breaks free from normal growth restraints and rapidly promotes uncontrolled cell division and spreads through distinct sites. Although the term "cancer" refers to more than 100 forms of the disease, all of them share some basic pathological development stages that unites them around this term. Interestingly, almost every tissue in the body can be host to a form of cancer, although some can bear more than one type. These differences arise from a multifactorial system that promote changes in the cell microenvironment, which therefore triggers responses that further increase the uncontrolled cell growth (Cullen and Breen 2016).

While normal cells reproduce only when there is a physiological change in the environment, generally caused by secretion of several growth-inducer factors by nearby cells, tumoral cells undergo uncontrolled cell proliferation even when the environment is not changed by the surrounding cells. Additionally, neoplastic cells can also migrate from their primary site and invade nearby tissues, where they can form tumoral masses that can disrupt tissue and organ functionality (Cullen and Breen 2016).

We now know that the malignant transformation of a cell derives from the accumulation of mutations in specific classes of genes. Essentially, there are two gene classes that plays major roles in the cancer development: proto-oncogenes and tumor suppressor genes, where the first one is responsible for the promotion of cell growth and the later inhibit it (Turnbull, Sud et al. 2018, Kontomanolis, Koutras et al. 2020).

Mutations that occur in proto-oncogenes further drive them to become carcinogenic oncogenes that stimulate excessive cell growth. Usually, these mutations can increase the production of different growth-stimulatory proteins or enhance the activity of several growth-inducing signaling pathways. In contrast, the mutations that occur in tumor suppressor genes usually disrupts their ability to inhibit cell proliferation by inactivation of their expression. The resulting imbalance between the stimulation of oncogenes and inhibition of tumor suppressor genes is sufficient to trigger the development of a tumoral cell, and therefore cancer disease itself (Turnbull, Sud et al. 2018, Kontomanolis, Koutras et al. 2020).

Several different processes can cause significant genetic mutation that leads to the development of cancer. For instance, exposure to ionizing radiation, alkylating chemical agents, some infectious agents, and even chemotherapeutic drugs can further increase the susceptibility of cancer development. Moreover, chronical illnesses that disrupts the activity of the immune system can also significantly increase the arise of tumoral cells. This is mainly due to the imbalance between an overstimulated inflammatory response, that ultimately leads to cell and DNA damage, and a suppressed antitumoral activity from specific immune cells (Spranger and Gajewski 2018).

Interestingly, the production of reactive oxygen species (ROS) and inflammatory cytokines plays major roles in the development of tumoral masses. Briefly, as discussed in the chapters above, chronic inflammatory process evolves gradually through signaling pathways related to the arachidonic acid cascade, which in turn activate cellular responses that inhibits antioxidant cell defenses and increases the production of ROS. This “vicious cycle” enhances the susceptibility of tumorigenesis by markedly increasing cellular damage, thus promoting the activation of proto-oncogenes that sustains the uncontrolled cell growth (Perillo, Di Donato et al. 2020).

While the actual pharmacological treatment for most cancers relies mostly on the impairment of the cell cycle, and thus prevention of enhanced tumorigenesis, recent research is focusing on different antioxidant and anti-inflammatory compounds that can stop the creation of a pro-tumorigenic microenvironment(Saluja, Arciero et al. 2018).

Indeed, Curcumin is one of the promising compounds that is being tested for its anti-neoplastic activity. One important feature of Curcumin anticancer effect is related to with its ability to exert immunomodulatory effects. Several in-vitro and in-vivo studies have shown that Curcumin can inhibit the activity of NF-κB, a pro-inflammatory transcription factor associated with tumorigenesis and cancer progression (Giordano and Tommonaro 2019, Wang, Jiang et al. 2019). Furthermore, Curcumin treatment significantly reduces the expression of the transcriptional factor AP-1 (Activator Protein-1), which is known to be involved in the regulation of pro-apoptotic, mitogenic, and pro-angiogenic genes. Finally, in addition to modulating the expression of these transcription factors, this substance influences the activity of various immune cells, including macrophages, dendritic cells, and both T and B lymphocytes (Giordano and Tommonaro 2019, Wang, Jiang et al. 2019).

Curcumin is being tested in different types of cancer and is showing promising results in in-vitro and in-vivo studies among many of them. For instance, administration of Curcumin in breast cancer cells inhibited cell growth and tumorigenesis. Breast cancer is a widespread malignant tumor present in the female population, being the leading cause of death by means of cancer in women. The activity of Curcumin in this cancer is mainly due to the interaction with the human epidermal growth factor receptor 2 (HER2), a tyrosine kinase receptor directly correlated with the development of breast cancer. Moreover, this interaction results in the downregulation of intracellular pathways related with cell survival and growth, such as the PI3K/Akt signaling (Liu and Ho 2018, Saxena, Ilic et al. 2020, Meiyanto, Husnaa et al. 2021).

Lung cancer also appears to benefit from the administration of Curcumin. Lung cancer is also a widespread tumoral diseases that causes most of the cancer-related death in men worldwide. Curcumin demonstrated its therapeutic efficacy in lung cancer therapy by downregulating NF-κB in human lung cancer cell lines A549 and by suppressing JAK2 activity via the JAK2/STAT3 signaling pathway. Moreover, evidence suggest that curcumin inhibits MMP-2 and MMP-9 expression levels in the human large cell lung cancer 801D cell line through reducing the Rac1/PAK1 signaling pathway, which eventually affects cell migration and invasion (Liu, Gao et al. 2018, Zhang, Chen et al. 2018, Ashrafizadeh, Rafiei et al. 2020).

A growing number of studies have shown that taking Curcumin can help cure glioblastoma. Glioblastoma multiforme is the most prevalent and aggressive brain tumor in adults, yet research has shown that solo or combination therapy with various microRNAs and Curcumin has diverse effects on glioma cell behaviors such as proliferation, migration, and apoptosis. Curcumin inhibited GSC proliferation, sphere formation, and colony formation in a controlled study on Glio3 and Glio9 (non-adherent and adherent glioma stem cells, respectively). Another study discovered that

Curcumin had powerful anti-apoptotic effects on GSCs (Walker and Mittal 2020, Wang, Liu et al. 2020, Wong, Kamarudin et al. 2021).

Curcumin's clinical application is still being researched, both as a monotherapy and in combination with other medications. Curcumin was utilized alone as an oral formulation in 15 colorectal cancer patients in a phase I clinical study. After two months of Curcumin treatment, the authors observed no toxicity, the development of considerable diarrhea in two patients, and two patients with stable illness (Greil, Greil-Ressler et al. 2018, Pricci, Girardi et al. 2020).

However, there are some clinical trials that failed to demonstrate significant effect with the administration of Curcumin. Indeed, a multicenter, randomized phase II trial comparing docetaxel (a common anti-neoplastic) with Curcumin to docetaxel alone in the first-line therapy of metastatic castration-resistant prostate cancer clearly showed that adding Curcumin to the treatment strategy was not efficacious(Passildas-Jahanmohan, Eymard et al. 2021). Moreover, a randomized, double-blind, placebo-controlled study was conducted on prostate cancer patients who underwent intermittent androgen deprivation (IAD) to assess the anticancer activity of oral Curcumin. The authors showed that Six months of oral Curcumin supplementation had no effect on the total off-treatment duration of IAD. During the Curcumin treatment phase, however, Curcumin consumption inhibited PSA rise (Choi, Han et al. 2019).

Truthfully, there is still limited clinical trials evaluating the potential benefits of Curcumin treatment in a broad range of cancers. Either by analyzing the monotherapy with Curcumin or combined therapy with other anti-neoplastic agents, it is crucial to develop new trials to further enlighten the clinical usefulness of this compound in cancer therapy.

Antioxidant Effects of Curcumin

In recent years, there has been a considerable increase in the number of studies on oxidative stress and free radicals (ROS). ROS and oxidative stress are linked to cell damage, which exacerbates several diseases. Researchers are looking at ways to lessen the damaging effects of reactive oxygen species (ROS) and, as a result, boost the body's antioxidant capacity. The consumption of oxygen during cell development results in the production of several ROS. They are created continually by the body's routine utilization of oxygen, such as breathing and some cell-mediated immunological processes. (Sokmen and Khan 2016).

ROS comprise both free radicals like superoxide anion radicals ($O_2^{\cdot-}$) and hydroxyl radicals ($OH^{\cdot}$) as well as non-free radicals such hydrogen peroxide (H_2O_2) and singlet oxygen ($^1O_2$). ROS are continually created during normal physiological processes and can readily trigger membrane lipid peroxidation, resulting in the buildup of lipid peroxides. ROS are also capable of causing DNA damage, which may lead to mutations, and of destroying critical biomolecules such as nucleic acids, lipids, proteins, and carbohydrates. If ROS are not efficiently scavenged, they can cause sickness (Ak and Gulcin 2008).

There are some nutrients and food components that have become the target of research due to their antioxidant activity. These nutrients can transform and/or reduce the oxidation action of free radicals, preventing such action from causing damage to the body. Oxidative stress occurs when there is an imbalance between the generation of free radicals and their elimination by antioxidant defenses. By damaging membranes, nucleic acids, proteins, and polysaccharides, oxidative stress can induce cellular damage, leading to functional alterations and the development of various illnesses (Ak and Gulcin 2008).

Curcumin is known to have a variety of pharmacological activities and therapeutic properties, in addition to having strong antioxidant action in relation to food and biological systems (Sokmen and Khan 2016). The antioxidant structure of Curcuminoids is due to their chemical structure. Cell damage that occurs in chronic diseases such as diabetes, cancer, cardiovascular disease is associated with ROS, these are formed during normal cellular aerobic respiration. Neutrophils, which are extremely complex cells that aggressively seek out, swallow, and eliminate harmful bacteria, also produce reactive oxygen species. Neutrophils employ their antimicrobial activity to cause host defense, which involves the usage of ROS as oxidants. Antioxidants are critical in neutralizing ROS and protecting cells from oxidative damage. Curcumin, a fat-soluble herb, works as an antioxidant because the ROS produced by curcumin and curcuminoids are linked to apoptotic activity in tumor cells (Mishra, Kapoor et al. 2005, Sokmen and Khan 2016)

Curcumin's chemical structure and the presence of hydroxyl and methoxy groups have been linked to a variety of activities, including antioxidant, antibacterial, anti-inflammatory, anti-angiogenic, and antimutagenic effects (Kocaadam and Sanlier 2017, Jakubczyk, Druzga et al. 2020). Curcumin is a potentially beneficial supplement for the treatment of irritable bowel syndrome (IBS) due to its unique activity, including antioxidant and anti-inflammatory properties, as well as the capacity to alter the intestinal microbiota (Appleton and Day 2019).

Furthermore, the antioxidant capabilities of Curcumin have been linked to the protection of the reproductive system. Curcumin has been demonstrated in studies to maintain the structural integrity and functional activity of sperm, especially when oxidative damage to germ cells is significant, due to its phenol group, which protects oxidative cell damage. Curcumin has been shown in studies with mice treated with Metronidazole, an antibiotic having antibacterial effect, to increase the antioxidant state and function of reproductive cells and tissues. Curcumin therapy lowered indicators linked with oxidative stress in another investigation done on mice subjected to prolonged stress (Galano, Alvarez-Diduk et al. 2009, Daverey and Agrawal 2016).

Researchers have also investigated the possible antioxidant effect of Curcumin on astrocytes, and this has been shown to protect them from oxidative stress, which is associated with most neurodegenerative diseases. In an *in vitro* study, it was found that Curcumin inhibited oxidative stress and its adverse effects as well as protected astrocytes because it showed antioxidant activity through the improvement of astrogliosis markers (GFAP and Vimentin) and suppression of the upregulation of Prdx6 induced by oxidative stress. And finally, Curcumin also promoted the recovery of mitochondria damaged by oxidative stress (Daverey and Agrawal 2016). In another *in vitro* study, it was observed that after treatment with Curcumin, protein expression and enzymatic activity of thioredoxin in rat brain cortical neurons were increased, which gave them protection against cell injury (Wu, Zhang et al. 2015).

The antioxidant activity of several dosages of powdered *Curcuma longa* L. root was tested in a pilot randomized, double-blind, crossover study in healthy males. Nine healthy males were given a low dosage, a moderate dose, and a high dose of C. longa. Plasma Curcumin levels rose in all groups after 20 and 90 minutes of C. longa consumption. The postprandial incremental area under the antioxidant capacity curve was smaller at the high dosage than in the low or moderate dose. The researchers hypothesized that a low dose of C. longa increased antioxidant capacity in healthy males while large doses of C. longa decreased antioxidant capacity in healthy men. Despite these studies demonstrated the Curcumin efficacy the own authors recommended that new research to happen to strengthen previous scientific results (Wu, Zhang et al. 2015).

The hazards connected with Curcumin have been shown to be modest, and like with other supplements and drugs, the tolerance and acceptability of Curcumin diminishes with increasing dose. Side effects (dosage dependent) include included gastrointestinal distress, reflux, bloating, and stomach pain (Fadus et al. 2017). For hundreds of years, Curcumin has been used as a therapeutic plant product, with its most current advances allowing it to possibly be used as therapy. Such idea is exciting and challenging, with laboratory and clinical trials still necessary to prove its effectiveness and safety for future treatments.

Futures Perspectives

Initially, Curcumin was widely used in cooking and cosmetics. However, its medicinal use as teas and ointments was only recognized in the 19th century, when its active principle was isolated, purified and described (Tsuda 2018, Kotha and Luthria 2019). The growing increase in experimental and clinical research involving the anti-inflammatory, chemoprophylactic and antioxidant properties of curcumin has been quite evident in the last decade. Some authors have suggested that further research is needed to study how to improve the bioavailability of curcumin. Several researchers are investigating the efficacy, safety, and pharmacokinetics of curcumin since the literature on these topics is limited and the understanding of the long-term adverse effects of curcumin is necessary due to its therapeutic use.

It is of the utmost importance that additional studies take place to validate and reinforce the results on the clinical efficacy of curcumin in various diseases, including cancer and neurodegenerative diseases. It was also suggested that further research is taking place with the aim of identifying the appropriate formulation and delivery system for each biomedical application. It is imperative that researchers identify the molecular targets of curcumin, in addition to its mechanisms of action against various diseases, as this will serve as a basis for the development of more specific structural molecules that can exert a more exact therapeutic action against the target disease of the study (Tsuda 2018, Sohn, Priya et al. 2021).

The biological effects of Curcumin in health promotion and disease prevention have become increasingly noticed (Sharifi-Rad, El Rayess et al. 2020). In addition to the three effects of Curcumin mentioned above, the literature has pointed out that this phytochemical also has hepatoprotective, pulmonoprotective, immunoregulatory, neuroprotective, cardioprotective, anti-thrombotic, cognition-enhancin, pain-relieving, lipid-modifying and anti-depressant properties (Zangui, Atkin et al. 2019). However, new clinical trials still need to be performed to confirm these beneficial effects of Curcumin in different clinical conditions (Sharifi-Rad, El Rayess et al. 2020). Natural products are becoming the target of research, and an example of this is Curcumin itself (Yusuf, Sadiya et al. 2022). Nanoformulations that contain curcuminoids, either alone or associated with another product, are currently widely studied in pharmaceutical industries with the objective of improving the bioavailability of Curcumin, the greatest therapeutic limitation of this plant nowadays (Salehi, Calina et al. 2020).

Acknowledgments

L. D. Dias and R. C. Parreira thank Centro Universitário de Mineiros (UNIFIMES) for support.

References

Adamczak, A., M. Ozarowski and T. M. Karpinski (2020). "Curcumin, a Natural Antimicrobial Agent with Strain-Specific Activity." *Pharmaceuticals* **13**(7): 153.

Ak, T. and I. Gulcin (2008). "Antioxidant and radical scavenging properties of curcumin." *Chemico-Biological Interactions* **174**(1): 27-37.

Ammon, H. P. T., H. Safayhi, T. Mack and J. Sabieraj (1993). "Mechanism of Antiinflammatory Actions of Curcumine and Boswellic Acids." *Journal of Ethnopharmacology* **38**(2-3): 113-119.

Appleton, L. and A. S. Day (2019). "Re: A Meta-Analysis of the Clinical Use of Curcumin for Irritable Bowel Syndrome." *Journal of Clinical Medicine* **8**(11): 1885.

Ashrafizadeh, M., H. Rafiei, R. Mohammadinejad, E. G. Afshar, T. Farkhondeh and S. Samarghandian (2020). "Potential therapeutic effects of curcumin mediated by JAK/STAT signaling pathway: a review." *Phytotherapy Research* **34**(8): 1745-1760.

Atanasov, A. G., S. B. Zotchev, V. M. Dirsch, C. T. Supuran and T. Int Nat Prod Sci (2021). "Natural products in drug discovery: advances and opportunities." *Nature Reviews Drug Discovery* **20**(3): 200-216.

Bansal, S. S., H. Kausar, F. Aqil, J. Jeyabalan, M. V. Vadhanam, R. C. Gupta and S. Ravoori (2011). "Curcumin implants for continuous systemic delivery: safety and biocompatibility." *Drug Delivery and Translational Research* **1**(4): 332-341.

Barnes, E. C., R. Kumar and R. A. Davis (2016). "The use of isolated natural products as scaffolds for the generation of chemically diverse screening libraries for drug discovery." *Natural Product Reports* **33**(3): 372-381.

Burange, A. S., S. M. Osman and R. Luque (2022). "Understanding flow chemistry for the production of active pharmaceutical ingredients." *Iscience* **25**(3): 103892.

Calder, P. C. (2015). "Marine omega-3 fatty acids and inflammatory processes: Effects, mechanisms and clinical relevance." *Biochimica Et Biophysica Acta-Molecular and Cell Biology of Lipids* **1851**(4): 469-484.

Carmona-Vargas, C. C., L. D. Alves, T. J. Brocksom and K. T. de Oliveira (2017). "Combining batch and continuous flow setups in the end-to-end synthesis of naturally occurring curcuminoids." *Reaction Chemistry & Engineering* **2**(3): 366-374.

Chemat, F., M. A. Vian and G. Cravotto (2012). "Green Extraction of Natural Products: Concept and Principles." *International Journal of Molecular Sciences* **13**(7): 8615-8627.

Chemat, F., M. A. Vian, A. S. Fabiano-Tixier, M. Nutrizio, A. R. Jambrak, P. E. S. Munekata, J. M. Lorenzo, F. J. Barba, A. Binello and G. Cravotto (2020). "A review of sustainable and intensified techniques for extraction of food and natural products." *Green Chemistry* **22**(8): 2325-2353.

Choi, Y. H., D. H. Han, S. W. Kim, M. J. Kim, H. H. Sung, H. G. Jeon, B. C. Jeong, S. I. Seo, S. S. Jeon and H. M. Lee (2019). "A randomized, double-blind, placebo-controlled trial to evaluate the role of curcumin in prostate cancer patients with intermittent androgen deprivation." *The Prostate* **79**(6): 614-621.

Chowdhury, I., S. Banerjee, A. Driss, W. Xu, S. Mehrabi, C. Nezhat, N. Sidell, R. N. Taylor and W. E. Thompson (2019). "Curcumin attenuates proangiogenic and proinflammatory factors in human eutopic endometrial stromal cells through the NF-kappa B signaling pathway." *Journal of Cellular Physiology* **234**(5): 6298-6312.

Cole, G. M., B. Teter and S. A. Frautschy (2007). Neuroprotective effects of curcumin. *Molecular Targets and Therapeutic Uses of Curcumin in Health and Disease.* B. B. Aggarwal, Y. J. Surh and S. Shishodia. **595:** 197-212.

Conn, P. J. and B. L. Roth (2008). "Opportunities and challenges of psychiatric drug discovery: Roles for scientists in academic, industry, and government settings." *Neuropsychopharmacology* **33**(9): 2048-2060.

Cullen, J. M. and M. Breen (2016). "An overview of molecular cancer pathogenesis, prognosis, and diagnosis." *Tumors in domestic animals*: 1-26.

Daverey, A. and S. K. Agrawal (2016). "Curcumin alleviates oxidative stress and mitochondrial dysfunction in astrocytes." *Neuroscience* **333**: 92-103.

Degot, P., V. Huber, E. Hofmann, M. Hahn, D. Touraud and W. Kunz (2021). "Solubilization and extraction of curcumin from *Curcuma longa* using green, sustainable, and food-approved surfactant-free microemulsions." *Food Chemistry* **336**: 127660.

Dias, L. D., K. C. Blanco, I. S. Mfouo-Tynga, N. M. Inada and V. S. Bagnato (2020). "Curcumin as a photosensitizer: From molecular structure to recent advances in antimicrobial photodynamic therapy." *Journal of Photochemistry and Photobiology C-Photochemistry Reviews* **45**: 100384.

Fuloria, S., J. Mehta, A. Chandel, M. Sekar, N. Rani, M. Y. Begum, V. Subramaniyan, K. Chidambaram, L. Thangavelu, R. Nordin, Y. S. Wu, K. V. Sathasivam, P. T. Lum, D. U. Meenakshi, V. Kumarasamy, A. Azad and N. K. Fuloria (2022). "A Comprehensive

Review on the Therapeutic Potential of *Curcuma longa* Linn. in Relation to its Major Active Constituent Curcumin." *Frontiers in Pharmacology* **13**: 820806.

Galano, A., R. Alvarez-Diduk, M. T. Ramirez-Silva, G. Alarcon-Angeles and A. Rojas-Hernandez (2009). "Role of the reacting free radicals on the antioxidant mechanism of curcumin." *Chemical Physics* **363**(1-3): 13-23.

Giordano, A. and G. Tommonaro (2019). "Curcumin and cancer." *Nutrients* **11**(10): 2376.

Glitzner, E., A. Korosec, P. M. Brunner, B. Drobits, N. Amberg, H. B. Schonthaler, T. Kopp, E. F. Wagner, G. Stingl, M. Holcmann and M. Sibilia (2014). "Specific roles for dendritic cell subsets during initiation and progression of psoriasis." *Embo Molecular Medicine* **6**(10): 1312-1327.

Gokdemir, B., N. Baylan and S. Cehreli (2020). "Application of a Novel Ionic Liquid as an Alternative Green Solvent for the Extraction of Curcumin from Turmeric with Response Surface Methodology: Determination and Optimization Study." *Analytical Letters* **53**(13): 2111-2121.

Greil, R., S. Greil-Ressler, L. Weiss, C. Schönlieb, T. Magnes, B. Radl, G. T. Bolger, B. Vcelar and P. P. Sordillo (2018). "A phase 1 dose-escalation study on the safety, tolerability and activity of liposomal curcumin (Lipocurc™) in patients with locally advanced or metastatic cancer." *Cancer chemotherapy and pharmacology* **82**(4): 695-706.

Hatcher, H., R. Planalp, J. Cho, F. M. Tortia and S. V. Torti (2008). "Curcumin: From ancient medicine to current clinical trials." *Cellular and Molecular Life Sciences* **65**(11): 1631-1652.

Hoang, L. T., T. Fauster, K. Haas and H. Jaeger (2022). "Aqueous Extraction of Curcuminoids from *Curcuma longa*: Effect of Cell Disintegration Pre-treatment and Extraction Condition." *Food and Bioprocess Technology* **15**(6): 1359-1373.

Hussein, M. Z., J. T. Meihua, S. Fakurazi and H. Ithnin (2013). "The evolutionary development in drug discovery and delivery." *Journal of Drug Delivery Science and Technology* **23**(3): 195-205.

Jakubczyk, K., A. Druzga, J. Katarzyna and K. Skonieczna-Zydecka (2020). "Antioxidant Potential of Curcumin-A Meta-Analysis of Randomized Clinical Trials." *Antioxidants* **9**(11): 1092.

Jiang, T., R. Ghosh and C. Charcosset (2021). "Extraction, purification and applications of curcumin from plant materials-A comprehensive review." *Trends in Food Science & Technology* **112**: 419-430.

Kocaadam, B. and N. Sanlier (2017). "Curcumin, an active component of turmeric (*Curcuma longa*), and its effects on health." *Critical Reviews in Food Science and Nutrition* **57**(13): 2889-2895.

Kontomanolis, E. N., A. Koutras, A. Syllaios, D. Schizas, A. Mastoraki, N. Garmpis, M. Diakosavvas, K. Angelou, G. Tsatsaris and A. Pagkalos (2020). "Role of oncogenes and tumor-suppressor genes in carcinogenesis: a review." *Anticancer research* **40**(11): 6009-6015.

Kotha, R. R. and D. L. Luthria (2019). "Curcumin: Biological, Pharmaceutical, Nutraceutical, and Analytical Aspects." *Molecules* **24**(16): 2930.

Li, C. J. and B. M. Trost (2008). "Green chemistry for chemical synthesis." *Proceedings of the National Academy of Sciences of the United States of America* **105**(36): 13197-13202.

Liu, F., S. Gao, Y. Yang, X. Zhao, Y. Fan, W. Ma, D. Yang, A. Yang and Y. Yu (2018). "Antitumor activity of curcumin by modulation of apoptosis and autophagy in human lung cancer A549 cells through inhibiting PI3K/Akt/mTOR pathway." *Oncology reports* **39**(3): 1523-1531.

Liu, H. T. and Y. S. Ho (2018). "Anticancer effect of curcumin on breast cancer and stem cells." *Food science and human wellness* **7**(2): 134-137.

Mattiuzzi, C. and G. Lippi (2019). "Current Cancer Epidemiology." *J Epidemiol Glob Health* **9**(4): 217-222.

Meiyanto, E., U. Husnaa, R. F. Kastian, H. Putri, Y. A. Larasati, A. Khumaira, D. D. P. Pamungkas, R. I. Jenie, M. Kawaichi and B. Lestari (2021). "The target differences of anti-tumorigenesis potential of curcumin and its analogues against HER-2 positive and triple-negative breast cancer cells." *Advanced Pharmaceutical Bulletin* **11**(1): 188.

Meng, Z., C. Yan, Q. Deng, D. F. Gao and X. L. Niu (2013). "Curcumin inhibits LPS-induced inflammation in rat vascular smooth muscle cells *in vitro* via ROS-relative TLR4-MAPK/NF-kappa B pathways." *Acta Pharmacologica Sinica* **34**(7): 901-911.

Menon, V. P. and A. R. Sudheer (2007). Antioxidant and anti-inflammatory properties of curcumin. *Molecular Targets and Therapeutic Uses of Curcumin in Health and Disease*. B. B. Aggarwal, Y. J. Surh and S. Shishodia. **595:** 105-125.

Mishra, S., N. Kapoor, A. M. Ali, B. V. V. Pardhasaradhi, A. L. Kumari, A. Khar and K. Misra (2005). "Differential apoptotic and redox regulatory activities of curcumin and its derivatives." *Free Radical Biology and Medicine* **38**(10): 1353-1360.

Mohan, A., S. Narayanan, S. Sethuraman and U. M. Krishnan (2013). "Combinations of Plant Polyphenols & Anti-Cancer Molecules: A Novel Treatment Strategy for Cancer Chemotherapy." *Anti-Cancer Agents in Medicinal Chemistry* **13**(2): 281-295.

Nelson, K. M., J. L. Dahlin, J. Bisson, J. Graham, G. F. Pauli and M. A. Walters (2017). "The Essential Medicinal Chemistry of Curcumin." *Journal of Medicinal Chemistry* **60**(5): 1620-1637.

Newman, D. J. and G. M. Cragg (2020). "Natural Products as Sources of New Drugs over the Nearly Four Decades from 01/1981 to 09/2019." *Journal of Natural Products* **83**(3): 770-803.

Ojo, O. A., T. R. Adeyemo, D. Rotimi, G. E. Batiha, G. Mostafa-Hedeab, M. E. Iyobhebhe, T. C. Elebiyo, B. Atunwa, A. B. Ojo, C. M. G. Lima and C. A. Conte-Junior (2022). "Anticancer Properties of Curcumin Against Colorectal Cancer: A Review." *Frontiers in Oncology* **12**: 881641.

Panahi, Y., M. S. Hosseini, N. Khalili, E. Naimi, M. Majeed and A. Sahebkar (2015). "Antioxidant and anti-inflammatory effects of curcuminoid-piperine combination in subjects with metabolic syndrome: A randomized controlled trial and an updated meta-analysis." *Clinical Nutrition* **34**(6): 1101-1108.

Panahi, Y., A. R. Rahimnia, M. Sharafi, G. Alishiri, A. Saburi and A. Sahebkar (2014). "Curcuminoid Treatment for Knee Osteoarthritis: A Randomized Double-Blind Placebo-Controlled Trial." *Phytotherapy Research* **28**(11): 1625-1631.

Passildas-Jahanmohan, J., J. C. Eymard, M. Pouget, F. Kwiatkowski, I. Van Praagh, L. Savareux, M. Atger, X. Durando, C. Abrial and D. Richard (2021). "Multicenter randomized phase II study comparing docetaxel plus curcumin versus docetaxel plus placebo in first-line treatment of metastatic castration-resistant prostate cancer." *Cancer Medicine* **10**(7): 2332-2340.

Peng, Y., M. Y. Ao, B. H. Dong, Y. X. Jiang, L. Y. Yu, Z. M. Chen, C. J. Hu and R. C. Xu (2021). "Anti-Inflammatory Effects of Curcumin in the Inflammatory Diseases: Status, Limitations and Countermeasures." *Drug Design Development and Therapy* **15**: 4503-4525.

Perillo, B., M. Di Donato, A. Pezone, E. Di Zazzo, P. Giovannelli, G. Galasso, G. Castoria and A. Migliaccio (2020). "ROS in cancer therapy: The bright side of the moon." *Experimental & Molecular Medicine* **52**(2): 192-203.

Pricci, M., B. Girardi, F. Giorgio, G. Losurdo, E. Ierardi and A. Di Leo (2020). "Curcumin and colorectal cancer: from basic to clinical evidences." *International Journal of Molecular Sciences* **21**(7): 2364.

Priyadarsini, K. I. (2014). "The Chemistry of Curcumin: From Extraction to Therapeutic Agent." *Molecules* **19**(12): 20091-20112.

Raduly, F. M., V. Raditoiu, A. Raditoiu and V. Purcar (2021). "Curcumin: Modern Applications for a Versatile Additive." *Coatings* **11**(5): 519.

Rodrigues, H. C. N., T. F. P. Martins, N. Santana, C. C. Braga, M. A. C. Silva, L. C. da Cunha, C. S. D. Sugizaki, A. Freitas, N. A. Costa and M. D. G. Peixoto (2021). "Antioxidant and anti-inflammatory response to curcumin supplementation in hemodialysis patients: A randomized, double-blind, placebo-controlled clinical trial." *Clinical Nutrition Espen* **44**: 136-142.

Salehi, B., D. Calina, A. O. Docea, N. Koirala, S. Aryal, D. Lombardo, L. Pasqua, Y. Taheri, C. M. S. Castillo, M. Martorell, N. Martins, M. Iriti, H. A. R. Suleria and J. Sharifi-Rad (2020). "Curcumin's Nanomedicine Formulations for Therapeutic Application in Neurological Diseases." *Journal of Clinical Medicine* **9**(2): 430.

Saluja, R., V. S. Arciero, S. Cheng, E. McDonald, W. W. L. Wong, M. C. Cheung and K. K. W. Chan (2018). "Examining trends in cost and clinical benefit of novel anticancer drugs over time." *Journal of Oncology Practice* **14**(5): e280-e294.

Saxena, A. R., Z. Ilic, V. Sripada and D. R. Crawford (2020). "Lower concentrations of curcumin inhibit Her2-Akt pathway components in human breast cancer cells, and other dietary botanicals potentiate this and lapatinib inhibition." *Nutrition Research* **78**: 93-104.

Sharifi-Rad, J., Y. El Rayess, A. A. Rizk, C. Sadaka, R. Zgheib, W. Zam, S. Sestito, S. Rapposelli, K. Neffe-Skocinska, D. Zielinska, B. Salehi, W. N. Setzer, N. S. Dosoky, Y. Taheri, M. El Beyrouthy, M. Martorell, E. A. Ostrander, H. A. R. Suleria, W. C. Cho, A. Maroyi and N. Martins (2020). "Turmeric and Its Major Compound Curcumin on Health: Bioactive Effects and Safety Profiles for Food, Pharmaceutical, Biotechnological and Medicinal Applications." *Frontiers in Pharmacology* **11**: 01021.

Singh, G., A. K. Passsari, V. V. Leo, V. K. Mishra, S. Subbarayan, B. P. Singh, B. Kumar, S. Kumar, V. K. Gupta, H. Lalhlenmawia and S. K. Nachimuthu (2016). "Evaluation of Phenolic Content Variability along with Antioxidant, Antimicrobial, and Cytotoxic

Potential of Selected Traditional Medicinal Plants from India." *Frontiers in Plant Science* **7**.

Singh, S., P. Pandey, M. Q. Akhtar, A. S. Negi and S. Banerjee (2021). "A new synthetic biology approach for the production of curcumin and its glucoside in Atropa belladonna hairy roots." *Journal of Biotechnology* **328**: 23-33.

Sohn, S. I., A. Priya, B. Balasubramaniam, P. Muthuramalingam, C. Sivasankar, A. Selvaraj, A. Valliammai, R. Jothi and S. Pandian (2021). "Biomedical Applications and Bioavailability of Curcumin-An Updated Overview." *Pharmaceutics* **13**(12): 2102.

Sokmen, M. and M. A. Khan (2016). "The antioxidant activity of some curcuminoids and chalcones." *Inflammopharmacology* **24**(2-3): 81-86.

Spranger, S. and T. F. Gajewski (2018). "Impact of oncogenic pathways on evasion of antitumour immune responses." *Nature Reviews Cancer* **18**(3): 139-147.

Thimmulappa, R. K., K. K. Mudnakudu-Nagaraju, C. Shivamallu, K. J. T. Subramaniam, A. Radhakrishnan, S. Bhojraj and G. Kuppusamy (2021). "Antiviral and immunomodulatory activity of curcumin: A case for prophylactic therapy for COVID-19." *Heliyon* **7**(2): e06350.

Tripathy, S., D. K. Verma, M. Thakur, A. R. Patel, P. P. Srivastav, S. Singh, A. K. Gupta, M. L. Chavez-Gonzalez, C. N. Aguilar, N. Chakravorty, H. K. Verma and G. L. Utama (2021). "Curcumin Extraction, Isolation, Quantification and Its Application in Functional Foods: A Review With a Focus on Immune Enhancement Activities and COVID-19." *Frontiers in Nutrition* **8**.

Tsuda, T. (2018). "Curcumin as a functional food-derived factor: degradation products, metabolites, bioactivity, and future perspectives." *Food & Function* **9**(2): 705-714.

Turnbull, C., A. Sud and R. S. Houlston (2018). "Cancer genetics, precision prevention and a call to action." *Nature genetics* **50**(9): 1212-1218.

Walker, B. C. and S. Mittal (2020). "Antitumor activity of curcumin in glioblastoma." *International Journal of Molecular Sciences* **21**(24): 9435.

Wang, M., S. Jiang, L. Zhou, F. Yu, H. Ding, P. Li, M. Zhou and K. Wang (2019). "Potential mechanisms of action of curcumin for cancer prevention: focus on cellular signaling pathways and miRNAs." *International Journal of Biological Sciences* **15**(6): 1200.

Wang, Z., F. Liu, W. Liao, L. Yu, Z. Hu, M. Li and H. Xia (2020). "Curcumin suppresses glioblastoma cell proliferation by p-AKT/mTOR pathway and increases the PTEN expression." *Archives of Biochemistry and Biophysics* **689**: 108412.

Wong, S. C., M. N. A. Kamarudin and R. Naidu (2021). "Anticancer mechanism of curcumin on human glioblastoma." *Nutrients* **13**(3): 950.

Wu, J. X., L. Y. Zhang, Y. L. Chen, S. S. Yu, Y. Zhao and J. Zhao (2015). "Curcumin pretreatment and post-treatment both improve the antioxidative ability of neurons with oxygen-glucose deprivation." *Neural Regeneration Research* **10**(3): 481-489.

Yadav, D. K., K. Sharma, A. Dutta, A. Kundu, A. Awasthi, A. Goon, K. Banerjee and S. Saha (2017). "Purity Evaluation of Curcuminoids in the Turmeric Extract Obtained by Accelerated Solvent Extraction." *Journal of Aoac International* **100**(3): 586-591.

Yixuan, L., M. A. Qaria, S. Sivasamy, S. Jianzhong and Z. Daochen (2021). "Curcumin production and bioavailability: A comprehensive review of curcumin extraction, synthesis, biotransformation and delivery systems." *Industrial Crops and Products* **172**: 114050.

Yusuf, M., Sadiya, B. Ahmed and M. Gulfishan (2022). "Modern Perspectives of Curcumin and its Derivatives as Promising Bioactive and Pharmaceutical Agents." *Biointerface Research in Applied Chemistry* **12**(6): 7177-7204.

Zangui, M., S. L. Atkin, M. Majeed and A. Sahebkar (2019). "Current evidence and future perspectives for curcumin and its analogues as promising adjuncts to oxaliplatin: state-of-the-art." *Pharmacological Research* **141**: 343-356.

Zhang, T., Y. Chen, Y. Ge, Y. Hu, M. Li and Y. Jin (2018). "Inhalation treatment of primary lung cancer using liposomal curcumin dry powder inhalers." *Acta Pharmaceutica Sinica B* **8**(3): 440-448.

Zhu, Z. P., J. Chen, Y. Chen, Y. T. Ma, Q. S. Yang, Y. Q. Fan, C. M. Fu, B. Limsila, R. Li and W. Liao (2022). "Extraction, structural characterization and antioxidant activity of turmeric polysaccharides." *Lwt-Food Science and Technology* **154**: 112805.

Zielinska, A., H. Alves, V. Marques, A. Durazzo, M. Lucarini, T. F. Alves, M. Morsink, N. Willemen, P. Eder, M. V. Chaud, P. Severino, A. Santini and E. B. Souto (2020). "Properties, Extraction Methods, and Delivery Systems for Curcumin as a Natural Source of Beneficial Health Effects." *Medicina-Lithuania* **56**(7): 336.

Chapter 6

Preventive Combined Effects of Exercise Training and Curcumin Supplementation in Chronic Disease: Possible Effects of Immune Responses

M. Molanouri Shamsi[1,*], PhD
and S. Amani-Shalamzari[2], PhD
[1]Department of Physical Education & Sport Sciences,
Faculty of Humanities, Tarbiat Modares University, Tehran, Iran
[2]Department of Exercise Physiology,
Faculty of Physical Education & Sport Sciences,
Kharazmi University, Tehran, Iran

Abstract

Numerous studies have confirmed curcumin's anti-inflammatory and antioxidant effects due to its biological activities. Also, the positive effects of curcumin on various immune system indices have been established in multiple studies. Acute and chronic responses to physical exercise can be effective in physiological responses and, at the same time, innate and adaptive immune responses. It has been suggested that regular physical exercise can effectively prevent several diseases, including cancer, cardiovascular disease, neuromuscular disorders, and diabetes. Adipose tissue is considered the leading risk factor for chronic diseases. The possible effects of curcumin on adipose tissue and the proven positive effects of exercise training on weight control can be effective in modulating immune system responses in adipose tissue and preventing

[*] Corresponding Author's Email: molanouri@modares.ac.ir.

In: Curcumin and Its Role in Health and Disease
Editor: Kathryn Woltjer
ISBN: 979-8-88697-491-1

weight gain. In addition, according to new studies, higher intensities of physical exercise are effective in preventing some chronic diseases. However, this exercise is associated with further muscle damage and inflammation. It has been suggested that curcumin can modulate the inflammatory responses created following intensive physical exercise. The synergistic effects of exercise training and curcumin supplementation modulate immune responses effectively. The physiological and metabolic effects of exercise training combined with curcumin supplementation can probably be effective in preventing chronic disease by improving immune responses.

Keywords: physical exercise, curcumin supplementation, chronic disease, immune system

Abbreviations

AMPK	AMP-activated protein kinase
CRP	C-reactive protein
CVD	Cardiovascular disease
FFA	Free-fatty acid
HOMA-IR	Homeostatic model assessment for insulin resistance
LPS	Lipopolysaccharide
NAFLD	Non-alcoholic fatty liver disease
NF-kB	Nuclear factor kappa-light-chain-enhancer of activated B cells
NK	Natural killer
QUICKI	Quantitative insulin sensitivity check index
ROS	Reactive oxygen stress
TLRs	Toll-like receptors
WAT	White adipose tissue

Introduction

Overweight and obesity are considered global problems, playing a role in chronic diseases such as cardiovascular disease, diabetes, cancers, nervous system disorders, and mortality (Ogden et al., 2007, Ogden et al., 2006). Recent evidence supports the effects of some dietary components such as spices on preventing and treating obesity and related metabolic disorders.

Among these spices, turmeric and its active ingredient curcumin have been considered in recent years. Various in vivo and in vitro evidence confirm its anti-inflammatory, anti-tumour, and antioxidant effects and its involvement in the hypolipidemic process (Kempaiah and Srinivasan 2004, Kochhar 2008).

In addition to the effects on the fatty tissue of curcumin, possible effects on modulating immune function can probably be effective in preventing chronic diseases (He et al., 2015). However, despite extensive studies on curcumin, more studies are needed on the doses used and its long-term effects, especially in obese and overweight populations. Recommended doses for this supplement have been considered without toxicity. However, some studies suggested that consuming curcumin in higher doses can probably show modulatory effects on metabolic responses (Aggarwal 2010, Aggarwal and Harikumar 2009).

Regular physical exercise along with nutritional interventions has always been considered for controlling obesity, improving immune system responses, and preventing chronic diseases (Shao et al., 2021, Shamsi et al., 2022). Like curcumin, regular exercise training can show antioxidant and anti-inflammatory effects (Gomez-Cabrera, Domenech, and Viña 2008). Some studies suggested that curcumin may show pro-oxidant side effects when it is taken at the same time as exercise training (Hewlings and Kalman 2017). Using some supplements such as curcumin and physical exercise and their combined effects on the modulating immune responses are also debatable. In recent years, more intense and interval physical exercise has been considered due to the positive physiological and metabolic effects (De Nardi et al., 2018). However, these physical activities can be associated with muscle damage and inflammatory and oxidative responses (MacInnis and Gibala 2017). In the present chapter, we will highlight the effects of regular physical exercise and curcumin supplementation on immune system responses, especially in obesity and related metabolic disorders. Also, the combined effects of physical exercise and curcumin supplementation on immune function will be discussed.

Exercise Training, Preventive Effects on Chronic Disease and Immune System

Physical exercise is the movement of the body by skeletal muscles that leads to increased energy expenditure. Training refers to regular exercises performed purposefully to improve physical fitness and the functioning of the body's organs, especially the immune system. In recent years, new areas related to exercise training have emerged that exercise is considered to have prophylactic effects and is an effective therapy for many disorders and diseases (Barker and Eickmeyer 2020). In this regard, it was shown that regular physical exercise could alleviate the symptoms of many metabolic disorders. Hence, according to studies and meta-analyses, the risk of cardiovascular disease- (CVD) related and cancer-related mortality in athletes compared with non-athletes is reduced by 40–70% and 30–50%, respectively (Liu et al., 2019, Runacres, Mackintosh, and McNarry 2021). Additionally, running-based exercise training has protective effects on neurological health and reduces the risk of dementia diseases such as Alzheimer's and Parkinson's (Church et al., 2004).

It is approved that regular physical exercise reduces the risk of chronic metabolic and cardiorespiratory diseases, mainly because of the anti-inflammatory effects of exercise. The anti-inflammatory effects of exercise have been mediated via three possible mechanisms: the reduction in visceral fat mass, an increase in production and release of anti-inflammatory cytokines from contracting skeletal muscle, and a reduced expression of Toll-like receptors (TLRs) on monocytes and macrophages(Gleeson et al., 2011, Rezaei et al., 2017). Regular physical exercise can reduce abdominal and visceral fat and waist circumference, which are related to all causes of mortality. Also, white adipose tissue (WAT) is an active tissue with metabolic and immunologic responses. Excessive WAT produces pro-inflammatory cytokines that can adversely affect other tissues in the body and cause a chronic low-grade systemic inflammatory state (Gleeson et al., 2011, Kershaw and Flier 2004, Molanouri Shamsi et al., 2016). Exercise training also increases adiponectin levels, which is accompanied by improving metabolic status. Researchers confirm that physical exercise has anti-inflammatory effects, and long-term exercise can protect against the development of chronic diseases (Pedersen and Saltin 2006, Naderi et al., 2022).

Also, skeletal muscle during exercise produces some myokines, which act in autocrine and paracrine manners. Myokines play a significant role in the cross-talk between muscle-liver, muscle-adipose, and muscle-brain. Moreover, myokines exert beneficial effects on energy metabolism (glucose uptake and transport, fat oxidation, lipolysis), angiogenesis (proliferation of endothelial cells), myogenesis (regulation of myoblast growth cycle), regulation of blood vessels, and prevention and treatment of metabolic and inflammatory diseases (Pedersen 2011, So et al., 2014, Shamsi, Chekachak, et al., 2017).

Moreover, it is approved that acute and chronic exercise training profoundly affects the normal functioning of both components of both arms of the innate and the acquired immune system. The response depends on the intensity, duration, and mode of physical exercise and changes in body temperature, blood flow, and hydration status. Growing evidence demonstrates that regular and moderate physical exercise could promote innate and adaptive immune functions (Simpson et al., 2015, Scheffer and Latini 2020, Lancaster and Febbraio 2014). In this regard, improved function of T-cells (proliferation and migration) and neutrophils (degranulation, oxidative burst) and increased numbers and activation of NK cells with long-term, moderate exercise has been reported in most communities from obese to old populations (Simpson et al., 2015).

In addition, in the context of the elderly, there are two new words: inflammaging and inflamminactivity. Inflammaging is influenced by immunosenescence, which is the combination of "inflammation + aging." It shows that chronic, low-grade inflammation is related to the aging process (Franceschi et al., 2000). Inflamminactivity means that a sedentary lifestyle is more important than aging to induce inflammation and highlights physical exercise is an essential component in the inflammation model (Flynn, Markofski, and Carrillo 2019). However, physical exercise and an active lifestyle can counteract this situation. Moderate-intensity exercise training will help boost the immune system at any age. In the elderly population, clinical and exercise professionals are gradually applying physical exercise as a therapy to neutralize age-associated dysregulation of immune function. Also, physical exercise can promote apoptosis of aging T lymphocytes and stimulates the synthesis of new, fully functional immune cells, thereby improving immune function (Malaguarnera et al., 2008).

Aging leads to a decline in the normal functioning of the immune system, which is called the term "immunosenescence." This situation is associated with poorer vaccine responses and the enhanced incidence of infection and chronic diseases in the elderly. Moderate-exercise training enhances vaccination responses, T-cell proliferative capacity, neutrophil phagocytic activity, and NK-cell cytotoxic activity. It lowers the numbers of senescent T-cells, circulatory levels of inflammatory cytokines, and inflammatory response in aging humans (Simpson et al., 2012, Shamsi, Najedi, et al., 2017). Therefore, regular physical exercise could modulate the immune system and delay the onset of immunosenescence. Figure 1 summarizes the effects of acute or chronic physical exercise on immune responses.

Sports scientists have recently highlighted the benefits of high-intensity exercise in most populations, from children to the elderly. However, intense exercise causes more inflammation and muscle damage. It is generally accepted that regular moderate-intensity training is immuno-enhancing, while prolonged high-intensity workouts can depress immunity (Simpson et al., 2015). Heavy exercise may impair T-cell, NK-cell, and neutrophil function, change the cytokine balance, and eventually suppress the immune function (Smith et al., 1996). Therefore, using nutraceuticals that can mitigate the harmful effects of intense and prolonged exercise is a proper solution.

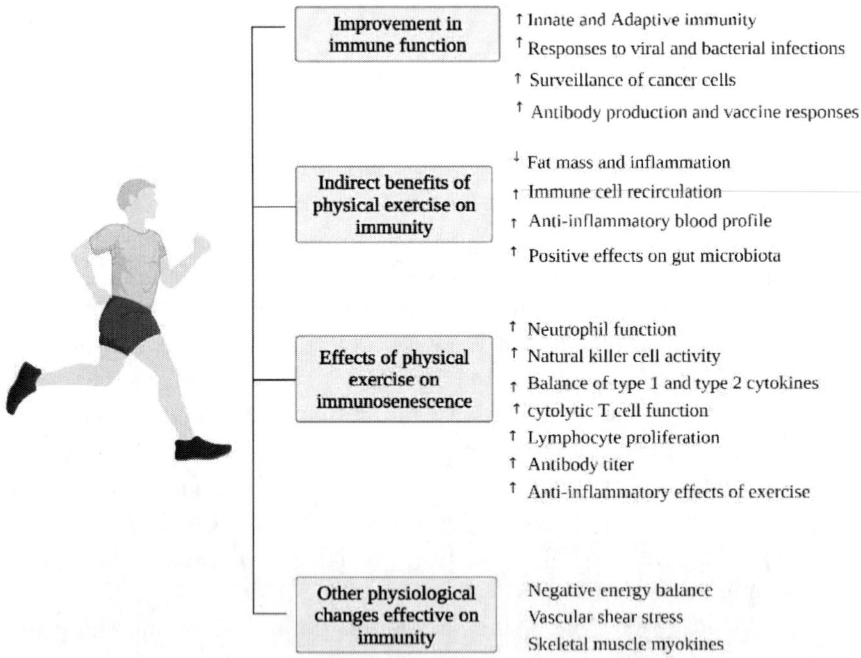

Figure 1. Effects of acute or chronic physical exercise on immune responses. Physical exercise improves immune function with a direct impact on innate and adaptive immune responses and indirect effects of exercise training on the immune system. Regular physical exercise effectively affects immune responses in older adults and delays the onset of immunosenescence. Physiological responses induced by physical exercise can act as a possible mechanism in the modulatory effects of exercise on immune responses.

Curcumin, Preventive Effects on Chronic Disease and Immune System

Being overweight and obese is a serious global health problem now. According to data obtained in 2016, about 39% of adults worldwide are overweight and obese; by 2030, this number will reach about 60% of adults. Obesity has been identified as a risk factor in the etiopathology of several chronic diseases such as cardiovascular disease, hyperlipidemia, diabetes mellitus, some cancers, and some gastrointestinal tract diseases (Tanabe et al., 2015, Tanabe et al., 2019).

Possible effects of curcumin due to its natural effects on cellular biochemical and physiological responses have been introduced as suggested pathways in the prevention and control of obesity. Curcumin can be effective in some metabolic mechanisms, including inhibiting adipogenesis, regulating lipid metabolism, and stimulating energy expenditure in obesity and obesity-related diseases. Several studies have shown the regulation of inflammatory responses associated with immune-related responses following curcumin supplementation (Saraf-Bank et al., 2019, He et al., 2015, Peng et al., 2021). Also, various molecular mechanisms such as transcription factors, cellular receptors, growth factors, enzymes, cytokines, and chemokines are proposed as possible mechanisms in the modulation of inflammation with curcumin administration (Shehzad et al., 2011, Shimizu et al., 2019).

In curcumin supplementation studies, modulating circulatory inflammatory markers in obesity and some related diseases appear. Taking curcumin capsules/day for three months at a dose of two 40 mg capsules/day has reduced serum inflammatory markers in obese patients with non-alcoholic fatty liver disease (NAFLD) (Jazayeri-Tehrani et al., 2019). Also, consuming one g/day of curcumin for eight weeks effectively reduces serum inflammatory and chemotaxis indices in people with metabolic syndrome (Panahi et al., 2016). Concomitant use of 500 mg daily curcumin with a weight loss diet has effectively reduced serum inflammatory markers in adolescent girls (Saraf-Bank et al., 2019). However, taking 1 gram per day of curcumin for four weeks did not affect some inflammatory markers in obese people (Ganjali et al., 2014). Decreased levels of free-fatty acid (FFA) as a factor for inducing the production of inflammatory factors have also been observed in patients with type 2 diabetes following three months of supplementation with 300 mg/day of curcumin (Na et al., 2013, Glass and Olefsky 2012).

Some components of the immune system, such as eosinophils, neutrophils, monocytes, and macrophages, are involved in the production of reactive oxygen species that are effective in activation of nuclear factor kappa-light-chain-enhancer of activated B cells (NF-κB), overproduction of cytokines, and stimulation of inflammatory processes (Coelho, Oliveira, and Fernandes 2013, Castro, Macedo-de la Concha, and Pantoja-Meléndez 2017). Reactive oxygen species are also involved in the high regulation of TLR-2 and TLR-4, which are pathways involved in the inflammatory processes of vascular dysfunction and insulin resistance (Meneses et al., 2019, Böni-Schnetzler et al., 2009). It has been shown that polyphenols, one of curcumin's natural compounds, affect oxidative stress and inflammatory status (Kasprzak-Drozd et al., 2022).

Also, as we know, intestinal microbiota-related disorders can affect the distribution of proper structures and function of intestinal barriers, which can lead to penetration of microorganisms or their fragments such as lipopolysaccharide (LPS) and induction of chronic inflammation (Khan et al., 2016). A process that also occurs during obesity and causes chronic inflammation and activated pro-inflammatory responses and metabolic dysfunction in WAT (Hersoug, Møller, and Loft 2016). The protective effects of curcumin against a high-fat diet have been observed in animal specimens through the reduction of adiposity and inflammatory responses in white adipose tissue that may be due to alterations in gut microbiota composition (Neyrinck et al., 2013).

Adipose tissue beyond adipocytes also has resident immune cells that interactions created by these cells with other tissues can be effective in the aetiology and progression of various diseases, including type 2 diabetes, cardiovascular disease, liver disease, and cancers (Varì et al., 2021). Activation of immune cells in adipose tissue and their profile depends on the condition of adipocytes and adipokines secreted from them (Kershaw and Flier 2004, Weisberg et al., 2003). It has been shown that using curcumin, especially in higher doses, can be effective in modulating the inflammatory responses of adipokines and increasing anti-inflammatory adipokines (Chuengsamarn et al., 2014, Navekar et al., 2017). Using 1500 mg/d for six months in diabetic people decreased leptin levels as a pro-inflammatory adipokine and increased adiponectin as an anti-inflammatory indicator released from adipose tissue (Chuengsamarn et al., 2014). In another study, 12 weeks of supplementation with 3,000 mg /d for 12 weeks effectively reduced serum leptin levels in people with NAFLD (Navekar et al., 2017).

In addition to the direct effects of curcumin on the signalling pathways involved in stimulating the inflammatory status of adipocytes (Varì et al., 2021), several studies have shown the therapeutic effects of curcumin in reducing the invasion of macrophages into adipose tissue in obese mouse models (Zhao et al., 2017, Meydani and Hasan 2010). Curcumin is probably involved in the interactions between adipose tissue and immune system cells to control the inflammatory status.

In addition to the effects on adipose tissue, curcumin has anti-inflammatory and antioxidant effects, which prevent some chronic diseases. Direct effects of curcumin on various tissues, especially in vitro and animal models, for the prevention of related conditions have been shown. It is suggested that curcumin can effectively suppress cancer cells with effects on molecular mechanisms such as survival signal reduction, proapoptotic promotion, anti-inflammatory actions, and reactive oxygen stress (ROS) scavenging to different degrees in the tumour environment (Park et al., 2013). In addition to the regulatory effects of curcumin on molecular markers, various cellular components of the immune system, such as macrophages, dendritic cells, and B and T lymphocytes, are also affected by curcumin, which can be effective in preventing cancer (Momtazi-Borojeni et al., 2018). Curcumin is also effective in cell-mediated immunity in cancer. It is shown that curcumin can prevent the loss of T cells, is influential in the development of T cell populations, reverses the type 2 immune bias, and reduces the tumour-induced inhibition of T-cell proliferation in tumour-bearing hosts as mechanisms for cell-dependent tumour eradication (Filipowicz, Bhattacharyya, and Sonenberg 2008). Curcumin has also been shown to be effective in inhibiting immunosuppressive cytokines and increasing the activity of CD8+ T cells to enhance host immunity against tumours (Luo et al., 2011).

The supportive effects of curcumin have also been observed in preventing cardiovascular disease. It has been suggested that curcumin can prevent isoproterenol-induced cardiac hypertrophy, oxidative stress, inflammatory bowel disease, necrosis, and neutrophil infiltration into chromocytes and protect them from cellular injury (Nirmala and Puvanakrishnan 1996, Izem-Meziane et al., 2012). Some studies have also supported the protective effects of curcumin in hypertension (Hlavačková et al., 2011, Nakmareong et al., 2011).

Moreover, considering neuroinflammation is a crucial factor in the process of neurodegenerative diseases. A decrease in the expression of inflammatory cytokines in lipopolysaccharide-stimulated microglia following administration of curcumin in a dose-dependent pattern has been observed

(Cho, Lee, and Kim 2007). It has been suggested that curcumin may effectively stimulate microglial phagocytosis, eliminate beta-amyloid, and promote heat stress responses (Yilmaz et al., 2020).

Also, the process of aging and senescent cells is associated with aging-related diseases, especially neurodegenerative diseases (Naylor, Baker, and van Deursen 2013). Aging is associated with inflammation caused by aging, which can be involved in people suffering from various diseases at this age. Polyphenol compounds can effectively control the inflammation caused by aging with their anti-inflammatory and antioxidant effects. However, there is some evidence for preventing aging-related diseases by considering curcumin's anti-inflammatory and antioxidant effects (Shimizu et al., 2019, Peng et al., 2021). However, whether curcumin compounds can effectively prevent cellular senescence has not been confirmed ce. Some studies seem to confirm the modulatory effects of curcumin on the cellular aging process through a possible impact on mechanisms such as sirtuins and AMP-activated protein kinase (AMPK) that have anti-senescent properties in the cell (Bielak-Zmijewska et al., 2019, Naylor, Baker, and van Deursen 2013). However, cytostatic doses can play a role in inhibiting sirtuins and AMPK, thus increasing cellular senescence. Figure 2 summarizes the possible effects of curcumin on the prevention of chronic diseases.

Despite the positive effects of curcumin on some metabolic and immunological aspects, especially in some metabolic diseases and cancer, the role of curcumin in the disease prevention process is not clear until now. The concentration and cell formulation may be involved in absorption and positive curcumin effects. In addition, side effects such as nausea, diarrhoea, headache, and yellow stool are observed following curcumin supplementation, which may be due to low absorption, rapid metabolism, and systemic absorption. Another point about the use of curcumin is its cytostatic, cytotoxic, and genotoxic agent effects at higher doses (Bielak-Zmijewska et al., 2019). Some studies have suggested the role of curcumin in regulating metabolic pathways related to exercise activities. Also, the using curcumin as a supplement for preventing inflammatory responses and muscle damage caused by strenuous exercise has been mentioned. In the following, we will examine the possible effects of a combination of exercise training and curcumin supplementation on the prevention of chronic diseases by considering the immune system responses.

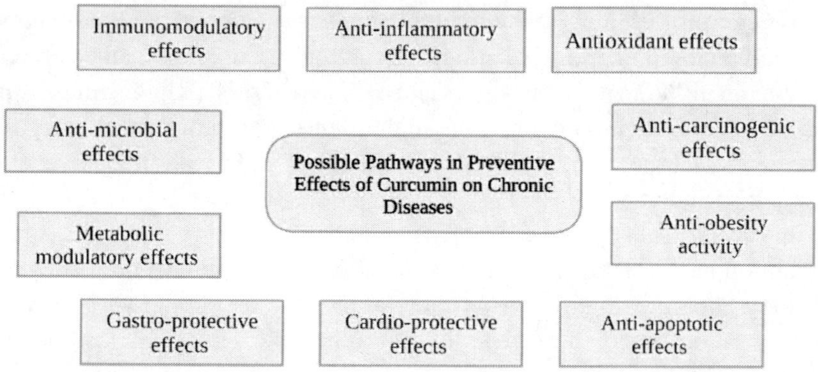

Figure 2. Potential effects of curcumin on prevention of chronic diseases.

Exercise Training and Curcumin, Preventive Effects on Chronic Disease and Immune System

In recent years, nutritional and physical activity interventions have been considered two main parts of lifestyle changes in preventing chronic diseases. According to studies, exercise training can prevent chronic diseases with specific effects on immune system-related indicators. At the same time, the results of curcumin and exercise training on metabolic indicators and fat tissue have been confirmed in various studies that can effectively prevent diseases associated with fat mass. The synergistic effects of moderate regular physical exercise and curcumin supplementation can be effective in creating anti-inflammatory and antioxidant impact; and improving some indicators of the immune system in preventing chronic diseases, especially in people with obesity and metabolic complications. However, limited studies have been performed on the combination of exercise training and curcumin supplementation and their effects on indicators related to the immune system and adipose tissue.

Dolati et al., (2019) showed that although curcumin did not affect waist circumference, hip circumferences, Waist-to-hip ratio, serum insulin, the homeostatic model assessment for insulin resistance (HOMA-IR), or quantitative insulin sensitivity check index (QUICKI), it caused significant changes in C-reactive protein (CRP) levels (Dolati et al., 2020). Combined moderate exercise training and curcumin supplementation induced substantial changes in CRP levels and improved lipid profile, insulin resistance, and body composition in overweight women (Biswas et al., 2017). The combination of intense exercise training and curcumin supplementation in athletes has been considered due to the positive effects of curcumin. Curcumin can be effective in reducing inflammatory responses and oxidative stress, reducing muscle pain and damage, better recovery and higher muscle performance, improving gastrointestinal function, and better physiological and psychological reactions in athletes (Suhett et al., 2021).

In recent years, the role of intensive exercise training in chronic disease prevention has been considered. The meta-analysis of studies performed with the intervention of high-intensity interval training on people with metabolic syndrome confirmed the effects of this type of exercise on fasting blood glucose, systolic and diastolic blood pressure, and waist circumference (Serrablo-Torrejon et al., 2020). At the same time, studies on the effect of curcumin supplementation in patients with metabolic syndrome have improved indicators related to hyperlipidemia and fasting blood glucose. Still, no change in systolic and waist blood pressure indicators has been observed (Azhdari, Karandish, and Mansoori 2019). The complementary role of high-intensity exercise training and curcumin supplementation can probably be associated with improving metabolic indicators in people with metabolic syndrome. However, high-intensity exercise can be associated with increased inflammatory markers and oxidative stress, and inactive and non-athletic people may experience a further increase in these indicators, resulting in muscle soreness and fatigue (Cerqueira et al., 2020). Various human and animal studies have confirmed the effects of curcumin as anherbal supplement in reducing inflammatory responses and muscle pain following intensive exercise (Peng et al., 2021, Shimizu et al., 2019, Tanabe et al., 2015).

Also, muscle mass loss and sarcopenia can lead to weakened immune systems and some diseases in the aging process. The process of sarcopenia seems multifaceted, and the chronic inflammation created in the aging process plays an essential role in its development (Kalinkovich and Livshits 2015). Physical activity, a proper diet, and using nutritional compounds have been considered effective ways to prevent this process (Landi et al., 2018). Physical exercise models such as strenuous exercise and resistance training can play a role in muscle adaptation and controlling the sarcopenic process. The combined effects of curcumin supplementation with exercise training, especially higher-intensity exercise, have been suggested to improve muscle strength in aging. Lee et al., (2021) showed that curcumin, especially at higher doses, can be used in exercise-based therapy and muscle sarcopenia with anti-apoptotic, anti-inflammatory, and antioxidant effects (Lee et al., 2021). Curcumin can also modulate gene expressions related to muscle degradation and protein synthesis and accelerate mitochondrial biogenesis in skeletal muscle following exercise training (Lee et al., 2021, Ray Hamidie et al., 2015).

However, it should be noted that exercise training is associated with improved antioxidant and anti-inflammatory responses in the body, and the use of other foods that contain antioxidants and anti-inflammatory agents should be considered. Using higher amounts of curcumin in these conditions may not only be ineffective in producing antioxidant responses but may also lead to oxidative responses in the body. It should be noted that to create the desired adaptations, especially in people with obesity or related disorders, the use of appropriate doses of curcumin according to the type, intensity, and duration of physical exercise should be considered (Campbell, Carlini, and Fleenor 2021).

Reports from various human studies and related institutions approved an acceptable daily intake of curcumin at 0.1-3.0 mg/kg body weight. However, higher doses of curcumin showed positive effects, especially in the case of metabolic and hormonal indicators in obesity and metabolic syndrome. Some studies report adverse effects such as diarrhoea, vomiting, discolored stool, headache, and rash at higher doses in some people ((Sharma et al., 2004, Lao et al., 2006). Also, animal studies that have examined the toxicity of curcumin at different doses and for long periods have not observed clinical toxicity(Tsai et al., 2021, Soleimani, Sahebkar, and Hosseinzadeh 2018). However, changes in stained fur, discolored feces, discolored urine, and increased liver weight were observed following the administration of turmeric oleoresin in higher doses (Additives et al., 2020). Some studies proposed that curcumin in higher doses may have pro-oxidant effects and damage some tissues (Aggarwal, Vijayalekshmi, and Sung 2009, Lao et al., 2006, Peng et al., 2021).

Studies conducted on the combined effects of physical exercise and supplements at higher doses have confirmed the protective effects of exercise training against tissue damage or complications caused by high doses of supplementation (Naderi et al., 2022, Shamsi, Chekachak, et al., 2017). The metabolic and immunological regulatory effects observed by acute or chronic physical exercise can be effective in preventing possible destructive effects on different tissues. Also, the release of indicators related to the immune system's responses such as myokines and the creation of cross-talk between some tissues, can be effective in creating protective effects against possible cytostatic, cytotoxic, and genotoxic curcumin at higher doses.

Evaluation of the effects of curcumin at different doses in exercise recovery periods has not shown any side effects in humans. A study by our group confirmed improvement in the symptoms of gastric problems in animal specimens following prolonged strenuous exercise and curcumin supplementation (Gorzi et al., 2021). Simultaneous use of curcumin with exercise has probably been able to neutralize the side effects of higher doses of various supplements, especially in diseases and metabolic and immunological disorders.

Conclusion

Obesity and overweight are considered to be significant risk factors for chronic diseases. The simultaneous effects of exercise training and intake of curcumin as supplements have been assessed in the current study. According to some studies, the complementary effects of exercise training and curcumin supplementation can be considered, especially on metabolic and immunological responses. However, more studies should be considered, especially in obese and overweight people and metabolic syndrome, and the study of different doses of curcumin and different intensities and duration of physical exercise to varying ages on metabolic and immunological responses.

Acknowledgments

We wish to thank the Research Center of Tarbiat Modares University (TMU).

Conflict of Interest

All authors declare they have no conflict of interest.

Ethical Approval for Studies Involving Humans

This article does not contain any studies with human participants performed by any authors.

Ethical Approval for Studies Invoving Animals

This article does not contain any studies with animals performed by any of the authors.

References

Additives, Efsa Panel on, Feed Products or Substances used in Animal, Vasileios Bampidis, Giovanna Azimonti, Maria de Lourdes Bastos, Henrik Christensen, Mojca Kos Durjava, Maryline Kouba, Marta López-Alonso, Secundino López Puente, Francesca Marcon, Baltasar Mayo, Alena Pechová, Mariana Petkova, Fernando Ramos, Yolanda Sanz, Roberto Edoardo Villa, Ruud Woutersen, Paul Brantom, Andrew Chesson, Johannes Westendorf, Lucilla Gregoretti, Paola Manini, and Birgit Dusemund. 2020. "Safety and efficacy of turmeric extract, turmeric oil, turmeric oleoresin and turmeric tincture from *Curcuma longa* L. rhizome when used as sensory additives in feed for all animal species." *EFSA journal. European Food Safety Authority* 18 (6):e06146-e06146. doi: 10.2903/j.efsa.2020.6146.

Aggarwal, B. B., and K. B. Harikumar. 2009. "Potential therapeutic effects of curcumin, the anti-inflammatory agent, against neurodegenerative, cardiovascular, pulmonary, metabolic, autoimmune and neoplastic diseases." *Int. J. Biochem. Cell Biol.* 41 (1):40-59. doi: 10.1016/j.biocel.2008.06.010.

Aggarwal, Bharat B, RV Vijayalekshmi, and Bokyung Sung. 2009. "Targeting inflammatory pathways for prevention and therapy of cancer: short-term friend, long-term foe." *Clinical Cancer Research* 15 (2):425-430.

Aggarwal, Bharat B. 2010. "Targeting inflammation-induced obesity and metabolic diseases by curcumin and other nutraceuticals." *Annual review of nutrition* 30:173-199. doi: 10.1146/annurev.nutr.012809.104755.

Azhdari, M., M. Karandish, and A. Mansoori. 2019. "Metabolic benefits of curcumin supplementation in patients with metabolic syndrome: A systematic review and meta-analysis of randomized controlled trials." *Phytother. Res.* 33 (5):1289-1301. doi: 10.1002/ptr.6323.

Barker, K., and S. Eickmeyer. 2020. "Therapeutic Exercise." *Med. Clin. North Am.* 104 (2):189-198. doi: 10.1016/j.mcna.2019.10.003.

Bielak-Zmijewska, A., W. Grabowska, A. Ciolko, A. Bojko, G. Mosieniak, Ł Bijoch, and E. Sikora. 2019. "The Role of Curcumin in the Modulation of Ageing." *Int. J. Mol. Sci.* 20 (5). doi: 10.3390/ijms20051239.

Biswas, T., M. J. Uddin, A. A. Mamun, S. Pervin, and P. Garnett S. 2017. "Increasing prevalence of overweight and obesity in Bangladeshi women of reproductive age: Findings from 2004 to 2014." *PLoS One* 12 (7):e0181080. doi: 10.1371/journal.pone.0181080.

Böni-Schnetzler, M., S. Boller, S. Debray, K. Bouzakri, D. T. Meier, R. Prazak, J. Kerr-Conte, F. Pattou, J. A. Ehses, F. C. Schuit, and M. Y. Donath. 2009. "Free fatty acids induce a proinflammatory response in islets via the abundantly expressed interleukin-1 receptor I." *Endocrinology* 150 (12):5218-29. doi: 10.1210/en.2009-0543.

Campbell, M. S., N. A. Carlini, and B. S. Fleenor. 2021. "Influence of curcumin on performance and post-exercise recovery." *Crit. Rev. Food Sci. Nutr.* 61 (7):1152-1162. doi: 10.1080/10408398.2020.1754754.

Castro, A. M., L. E. Macedo-de la Concha, and C. A. Pantoja-Meléndez. 2017. "Low-grade inflammation and its relation to obesity and chronic degenerative diseases." *Revista Médica del Hospital General de México* 80 (2):101-105. doi: https://doi.org/10.1016/j.hgmx.2016.06.011.

Cerqueira, Érica, Daniel A. Marinho, Henrique P. Neiva, and Olga Lourenço. 2020. "Inflammatory Effects of High and Moderate Intensity Exercise-A Systematic Review." *Frontiers in physiology* 10:1550-1550. doi: 10.3389/fphys.2019.01550.

Cho, J. W., K. S. Lee, and C. W. Kim. 2007. "Curcumin attenuates the expression of IL-1beta, IL-6, and TNF-alpha as well as cyclin E in TNF-alpha-treated HaCaT cells; NF-kappaB and MAPKs as potential upstream targets." *Int. J. Mol. Med.* 19 (3):469-74.

Chuengsamarn, S., S. Rattanamongkolgul, B. Phonrat, R. Tungtrongchitr, and S. Jirawatnotai. 2014. "Reduction of atherogenic risk in patients with type 2 diabetes by curcuminoid extract: a randomized controlled trial." *J. Nutr. Biochem.* 25 (2):144-50. doi: 10.1016/j.jnutbio.2013.09.013.

Church, T. S., Y. J. Cheng, C. P. Earnest, C. E. Barlow, L. W. Gibbons, E. L. Priest, and S. N. Blair. 2004. "Exercise capacity and body composition as predictors of mortality among men with diabetes." *Diabetes Care* 27 (1):83-8. doi: 10.2337/diacare.27.1.83.

Coelho, Marisa, Teresa Oliveira, and Ruben Fernandes. 2013. "Biochemistry of adipose tissue: an endocrine organ." *Archives of medical science : AMS* 9 (2):191-200. doi: 10.5114/aoms.2013.33181.

De Nardi, A. T., T. Tolves, T. L. Lenzi, L. U. Signori, and Amvd Silva. 2018. "High-intensity interval training versus continuous training on physiological and metabolic variables in prediabetes and type 2 diabetes: A meta-analysis." *Diabetes Res. Clin. Pract.* 137:149-159. doi: 10.1016/j.diabres.2017.12.017.

Dolati, S., K. Namiranian, R. Amerian, S. Mansouri, S. Arshadi, and M. A. Azarbayjani. 2020. "The Effect of Curcumin Supplementation and Aerobic Training on Anthropometric Indices, Serum Lipid Profiles, C-Reactive Protein and Insulin Resistance in Overweight Women: A Randomized, Double-Blind, Placebo-Controlled Trial." *J. Obes. Metab. Syndr.* 29 (1):47-57. doi: 10.7570/jomes19055.

Filipowicz, Witold, Suvendra N Bhattacharyya, and Nahum Sonenberg. 2008. "Mechanisms of post-transcriptional regulation by microRNAs: are the answers in sight?" *Nature Reviews Genetics* 9 (2):102-114.

Flynn, M. G., M. M. Markofski, and A. E. Carrillo. 2019. "Elevated Inflammatory Status and Increased Risk of Chronic Disease in Chronological Aging: Inflamm-aging or Inflamm-inactivity?" *Aging Dis.* 10 (1):147-156. doi: 10.14336/ad.2018.0326.

Franceschi, C., M. Bonafè, S. Valensin, F. Olivieri, M. De Luca, E. Ottaviani, and G. De Benedictis. 2000. "Inflamm-aging. An evolutionary perspective on immuno-senescence." *Ann. N. Y. Acad. Sci.* 908:244-54. doi: 10.1111/j.1749-6632. 2000.tb06651.x.

Ganjali, S., A. Sahebkar, E. Mahdipour, K. Jamialahmadi, S. Torabi, S. Akhlaghi, G. Ferns, S. M. Parizadeh, and M. Ghayour-Mobarhan. 2014. "Investigation of the effects of curcumin on serum cytokines in obese individuals: a randomized controlled trial." *Scientific World Journal* 2014:898361. doi: 10.1155/2014/898361.

Glass, C. K., and J. M. Olefsky. 2012. "Inflammation and lipid signaling in the etiology of insulin resistance." *Cell Metab.* 15 (5):635-45. doi: 10.1016/j.cmet.2012.04.001.

Gleeson, M., N. C. Bishop, D. J. Stensel, M. R. Lindley, S. S. Mastana, and M. A. Nimmo. 2011. "The anti-inflammatory effects of exercise: mechanisms and implications for the prevention and treatment of disease." *Nat. Rev. Immunol.* 11 (9):607-15. doi: 10.1038/nri3041.

Gomez-Cabrera, Mari-Carmen, Elena Domenech, and Jose Viña. 2008. "Moderate exercise is an antioxidant: upregulation of antioxidant genes by training." *Free Radical Biology and Medicine* 44 (2):126-131.

Gorzi, A, M Asadi, FA Voltarelli, and M Molanouri Shamsi. 2021. "Effects of curcumin on antioxidant capacity and gastric mucosal injury following strenuous endurance training in rats." *Comparative Exercise Physiology* 17 (1):17-24.

He, Y., Y. Yue, X. Zheng, K. Zhang, S. Chen, and Z. Du. 2015. "Curcumin, inflammation, and chronic diseases: how are they linked?" *Molecules* 20 (5):9183-213. doi: 10.3390/molecules20059183.

Hersoug, L. G., P. Møller, and S. Loft. 2016. "Gut microbiota-derived lipopolysaccharide uptake and trafficking to adipose tissue: implications for inflammation and obesity." *Obes. Rev.* 17 (4):297-312. doi: 10.1111/obr.12370.

Hewlings, Susan J., and Douglas S. Kalman. 2017. "Curcumin: A Review of Its Effects on Human Health." *Foods (Basel, Switzerland)* 6 (10):92. doi: 10.3390/foods6100092.

Hlavačková, L., A. Janegová, O. Uličná, P. Janega, A. Cerná, and P. Babál. 2011. "Spice up the hypertension diet - curcumin and piperine prevent remodeling of aorta in experimental L-NAME induced hypertension." *Nutr. Metab. (Lond)* 8:72. doi: 10.1186/1743-7075-8-72.

Izem-Meziane, M., B. Djerdjouri, S. Rimbaud, F. Caffin, D. Fortin, A. Garnier, V. Veksler, F. Joubert, and R. Ventura-Clapier. 2012. "Catecholamine-induced cardiac mitochondrial dysfunction and mPTP opening: protective effect of curcumin." *Am. J. Physiol. Heart Circ. Physiol.* 302 (3):H665-74. doi: 10.1152/ajpheart.00467.2011.

Jazayeri-Tehrani, S. A., S. M. Rezayat, S. Mansouri, M. Qorbani, S. M. Alavian, M. Daneshi-Maskooni, and M. J. Hosseinzadeh-Attar. 2019. "Nano-curcumin improves glucose indices, lipids, inflammation, and Nesfatin in overweight and obese patients with non-alcoholic fatty liver disease (NAFLD): a double-blind randomized placebo-controlled clinical trial." *Nutr. Metab. (Lond)* 16:8. doi: 10.1186/s12986-019-0331-1.

Kalinkovich, A., and G. Livshits. 2015. "Sarcopenia--The search for emerging biomarkers." *Ageing Res. Rev.* 22:58-71. doi: 10.1016/j.arr.2015.05.001.

Kasprzak-Drozd, K., T. Oniszczuk, M. Gancarz, A. Kondracka, R. Rusinek, and A. Oniszczuk. 2022. "Curcumin and Weight Loss: Does It Work?" *Int. J. Mol. Sci.* 23 (2). doi: 10.3390/ijms23020639.

Kempaiah, R. K., and K. Srinivasan. 2004. "Influence of dietary curcumin, capsaicin and garlic on the antioxidant status of red blood cells and the liver in high-fat-fed rats." *Ann. Nutr. Metab.* 48 (5):314-20. doi: 10.1159/000081198.

Kershaw, E. E., and J. S. Flier. 2004. "Adipose tissue as an endocrine organ." *J. Clin. Endocrinol. Metab.* 89 (6):2548-56. doi: 10.1210/jc.2004-0395.

Khan, M. J., K. Gerasimidis, C. A. Edwards, and M. G. Shaikh. 2016. "Role of Gut Microbiota in the Aetiology of Obesity: Proposed Mechanisms and Review of the Literature." *J. Obes.* 2016:7353642. doi: 10.1155/2016/7353642.

Kochhar, K. P. 2008. "Dietary spices in health and diseases (II)." *Indian J. Physiol. Pharmacol.* 52 (4):327-54.

Lancaster, G. I., and M. A. Febbraio. 2014. "The immunomodulating role of exercise in metabolic disease." *Trends Immunol.* 35 (6):262-9. doi: 10.1016/j.it.2014.02.008.

Landi, F., R. Calvani, M. Cesari, M. Tosato, A. M. Martone, E. Ortolani, G. Savera, S. Salini, A. Sisto, A. Picca, and E. Marzetti. 2018. "Sarcopenia: An Overview on Current Definitions, Diagnosis and Treatment." *Curr. Protein Pept. Sci.* 19 (7):633-638. doi: 10.2174/1389203718666170607113459.

Lao, C. D., M. T. th Ruffin, D. Normolle, D. D. Heath, S. I. Murray, J. M. Bailey, M. E. Boggs, J. Crowell, C. L. Rock, and D. E. Brenner. 2006. "Dose escalation of a curcuminoid formulation." *BMC Complement Altern. Med.* 6:10. doi: 10.1186/1472-6882-6-10.

Lee, D. Y., Y. S. Chun, J. K. Kim, J. O. Lee, S. K. Ku, and S. M. Shim. 2021. "Curcumin Attenuates Sarcopenia in Chronic Forced Exercise Executed Aged Mice by Regulating Muscle Degradation and Protein Synthesis with Antioxidant and Anti-inflammatory Effects." *J. Agric. Food Chem.* 69 (22):6214-6228. doi: 10.1021/acs.jafc.1c00699.

Liu, Y., D. C. Lee, Y. Li, W. Zhu, R. Zhang, X. Sui, C. J. Lavie, and S. N. Blair. 2019. "Associations of Resistance Exercise with Cardiovascular Disease Morbidity and Mortality." *Med. Sci. Sports Exerc.* 51 (3):499-508. doi: 10.1249/mss.0000000000001822.

Luo, F., X. Song, Y. Zhang, and Y. Chu. 2011. "Low-dose curcumin leads to the inhibition of tumor growth via enhancing CTL-mediated antitumor immunity." *Int. Immunopharmacol.* 11 (9):1234-40. doi: 10.1016/j.intimp.2011.04.002.

MacInnis, Martin J., and Martin J. Gibala. 2017. "Physiological adaptations to interval training and the role of exercise intensity." *The Journal of physiology* 595 (9):2915-2930. doi: 10.1113/JP273196.

Malaguarnera, Lucia, Erika Cristaldi, Maria Vinci, and Mariano Malaguarnera. 2008. "The role of exercise on the innate immunity of the elderly." *European Review of Aging and Physical Activity* 5 (1):43-49. doi: 10.1007/s11556-007-0028-8.

Meneses, M. J., R. Silvestre, I. Sousa-Lima, and M. P. Macedo. 2019. "Paraoxonase-1 as a Regulator of Glucose and Lipid Homeostasis: Impact on the Onset and Progression of Metabolic Disorders." *Int. J. Mol. Sci.* 20 (16). doi: 10.3390/ijms20164049.

Meydani, Mohsen, and Syeda T. Hasan. 2010. "Dietary polyphenols and obesity." *Nutrients* 2 (7):737-751. doi: 10.3390/nu2070737.

Molanouri Shamsi, M, M Mahdavi, LS Quinn, R Gharakhanlou, and A Isanegad. 2016. "Effect of resistance exercise training on expression of Hsp70 and inflammatory cytokines in skeletal muscle and adipose tissue of STZ-induced diabetic rats." *Cell stress and chaperones* 21 (5):783-791.

Momtazi-Borojeni, A. A., S. M. Haftcheshmeh, S. A. Esmaeili, T. P. Johnston, E. Abdollahi, and A. Sahebkar. 2018. "Curcumin: A natural modulator of immune cells in systemic lupus erythematosus." *Autoimmun. Rev.* 17 (2):125-135. doi: 10.1016/j.autrev.2017.11.016.

Na, L. X., Y. Li, H. Z. Pan, X. L. Zhou, D. J. Sun, M. Meng, X. X. Li, and C. H. Sun. 2013. "Curcuminoids exert glucose-lowering effect in type 2 diabetes by decreasing serum free fatty acids: a double-blind, placebo-controlled trial." *Mol. Nutr. Food Res.* 57 (9):1569-77. doi: 10.1002/mnfr.201200131.

Naderi, Mahdi, Hajar Kordestani, Zahra Sahebi, Vahid Khedmati Zare, Sadegh Amani-Shalamzari, Mojtaba Kaviani, Joachim Wiskemann, and Mahdieh Molanouri Shamsi. 2022. "Serum and gene expression profile of cytokines following combination of yoga training and vitamin D supplementation in breast cancer survivors: a randomized controlled trial." *BMC Women's Health* 22 (1):1-11.

Nakmareong, S., U. Kukongviriyapan, P. Pakdeechote, W. Donpunha, V. Kukongviriyapan, B. Kongyingyoes, K. Sompamit, and C. Phisalaphong. 2011. "Antioxidant and vascular protective effects of curcumin and tetrahydrocurcumin in rats with L-NAME-induced hypertension." *Naunyn Schmiedebergs Arch. Pharmacol.* 383 (5):519-29. doi: 10.1007/s00210-011-0624-z.

Navekar, R., M. Rafraf, A. Ghaffari, M. Asghari-Jafarabadi, and M. Khoshbaten. 2017. "Turmeric Supplementation Improves Serum Glucose Indices and Leptin Levels in Patients with Nonalcoholic Fatty Liver Diseases." *J. Am. Coll. Nutr.* 36 (4):261-267. doi: 10.1080/07315724.2016.1267597.

Naylor, R. M., D. J. Baker, and J. M. van Deursen. 2013. "Senescent cells: a novel therapeutic target for aging and age-related diseases." *Clin. Pharmacol. Ther.* 93 (1):105-16. doi: 10.1038/clpt.2012.193.

Neyrinck, A. M., M. Alligier, P. B. Memvanga, E. Névraumont, Y. Larondelle, V. Préat, P. D. Cani, and N. M. Delzenne. 2013. "*Curcuma longa* extract associated with white pepper lessens high fat diet-induced inflammation in subcutaneous adipose tissue." *PLoS One* 8 (11):e81252. doi: 10.1371/journal.pone.0081252.

Nirmala, C., and R. Puvanakrishnan. 1996. "Protective role of curcumin against isoproterenol induced myocardial infarction in rats." *Mol. Cell Biochem.* 159 (2):85-93. doi: 10.1007/bf00420910.

Ogden, C. L., M. D. Carroll, L. R. Curtin, M. A. McDowell, C. J. Tabak, and K. M. Flegal. 2006. "Prevalence of overweight and obesity in the United States, 1999-2004." *JAMA* 295 (13):1549-55. doi: 10.1001/jama.295.13.1549.

Ogden, C. L., M. D. Carroll, M. A. McDowell, and K. M. Flegal. 2007. "Obesity among adults in the United States--no statistically significant change since 2003-2004." *NCHS Data Brief* (1):1-8.

Panahi, Y., M. S. Hosseini, N. Khalili, E. Naimi, L. E. Simental-Mendía, M. Majeed, and A. Sahebkar. 2016. "Effects of curcumin on serum cytokine concentrations in subjects with metabolic syndrome: A post-hoc analysis of a randomized controlled trial." *Biomed. Pharmacother.* 82:578-82. doi: 10.1016/j.biopha.2016.05.037.

Park, W., A. R. Amin, Z. G. Chen, and D. M. Shin. 2013. "New perspectives of curcumin in cancer prevention." *Cancer Prev. Res. (Phila)* 6 (5):387-400. doi: 10.1158/1940-6207.capr-12-0410.

Pedersen, B. K., and B. Saltin. 2006. "Evidence for prescribing exercise as therapy in chronic disease." *Scand. J. Med. Sci. Sports* 16 Suppl 1:3-63. doi: 10.1111/j.1600-0838.2006.00520.x.

Pedersen, Bente Klarlund. 2011. "Muscles and their myokines." *The Journal of experimental biology* 214 (2):337-346.

Peng, Ying, Mingyue Ao, Baohua Dong, Yunxiu Jiang, Lingying Yu, Zhimin Chen, Changjiang Hu, and Runchun Xu. 2021. "Anti-Inflammatory Effects of Curcumin in the Inflammatory Diseases: Status, Limitations and Countermeasures." *Drug design, development and therapy* 15:4503-4525. doi: 10.2147/DDDT.S327378.

Ray Hamidie, R. D., T. Yamada, R. Ishizawa, Y. Saito, and K. Masuda. 2015. "Curcumin treatment enhances the effect of exercise on mitochondrial biogenesis in skeletal muscle by increasing cAMP levels." *Metabolism* 64 (10):1334-47. doi: 10.1016/j.metabol.2015.07.010.

Rezaei, Sajjad, Mahdieh Molanouri Shamsi, Mehdi Mahdavi, Azadeh Jamali, Jonato Prestes, Ramires Alsamir Tibana, James Wilfred Navalta, and Fabrício Azevedo Voltarelli. 2017. "Endurance exercise training decreased serum levels of surfactant protein D and improved aerobic fitness of obese women with type-2 diabetes." *Diabetology & metabolic syndrome* 9 (1):1-8.

Runacres, Adam, Kelly A. Mackintosh, and Melitta A. McNarry. 2021. "Health Consequences of an Elite Sporting Career: Long-Term Detriment or Long-Term Gain? A Meta-Analysis of 165,000 Former Athletes." *Sports medicine (Auckland, N.Z.)* 51 (2):289-301. doi: 10.1007/s40279-020-01379-5.

Saraf-Bank, S., A. Ahmadi, Z. Paknahad, M. Maracy, and M. Nourian. 2019. "Effects of curcumin supplementation on markers of inflammation and oxidative stress among healthy overweight and obese girl adolescents: A randomized placebo-controlled clinical trial." *Phytother. Res.* 33 (8):2015-2022. doi: 10.1002/ptr.6370.

Scheffer, D. D. L., and A. Latini. 2020. "Exercise-induced immune system response: Anti-inflammatory status on peripheral and central organs." *Biochim. Biophys. Acta Mol. Basis Dis.* 1866 (10):165823. doi: 10.1016/j.bbadis.2020.165823.

Serrablo-Torrejon, I., A. Lopez-Valenciano, M. Ayuso, E. Horton, X. Mayo, G. Medina-Gomez, G. Liguori, and A. Jimenez. 2020. "High intensity interval training exercise-induced physiological changes and their potential influence on metabolic syndrome clinical biomarkers: a meta-analysis." *BMC Endocr. Disord.* 20 (1):167. doi: 10.1186/s12902-020-00640-2.

Shamsi, M Molanouri, Soodabeh Chekachak, Sara Soudi, LS Quinn, K Ranjbar, J Chenari, MH Yazdi, and M Mahdavi. 2017. "Combined effect of aerobic interval training and selenium nanoparticles on expression of IL-15 and IL-10/TNF-α ratio in skeletal muscle of 4T1 breast cancer mice with cachexia." *Cytokine* 90:100-108.

Shamsi, M Molanouri, Sh Najedi, ZM Hassan, A Isanejad, and M Mahdavi. 2017. "Short term exercise training enhances cell-mediated responses to HSV-1 vaccine in mice." *Microbial pathogenesis* 110:457-463.

Shamsi, Mahdieh Molanouri, Alieh Vahed, AmirHossin Ahmadi Hekmatikar, and Katsuhiko Suzuki. 2022. "Combined Effects of Exercise Training and Nutritional Supplementation in Cancer Patients in the Context of the COVID-19: A Perspective Study." *Frontiers in Nutrition* 9.

Shao, Tianyi, Henu Kumar Verma, Babita Pande, Vincenzo Costanzo, Weibing Ye, Yuyan Cai, and L. V. K. S. Bhaskar. 2021. "Physical Activity and Nutritional Influence on Immune Function: An Important Strategy to Improve Immunity and Health Status." *Frontiers in physiology* 12:751374-751374. doi: 10.3389/fphys.2021.751374.

Sharma, R. A., S. A. Euden, S. L. Platton, D. N. Cooke, A. Shafayat, H. R. Hewitt, T. H. Marczylo, B. Morgan, D. Hemingway, S. M. Plummer, M. Pirmohamed, A. J. Gescher, and W. P. Steward. 2004. "Phase I clinical trial of oral curcumin: biomarkers of systemic activity and compliance." *Clin. Cancer Res.* 10 (20):6847-54. doi: 10.1158/1078-0432.ccr-04-0744.

Shehzad, A., T. Ha, F. Subhan, and Y. S. Lee. 2011. "New mechanisms and the anti-inflammatory role of curcumin in obesity and obesity-related metabolic diseases." *Eur. J. Nutr.* 50 (3):151-61. doi: 10.1007/s00394-011-0188-1.

Shimizu, K., M. Funamoto, Y. Sunagawa, S. Shimizu, Y. Katanasaka, Y. Miyazaki, H. Wada, K. Hasegawa, and T. Morimoto. 2019. "Anti-inflammatory Action of Curcumin and Its Use in the Treatment of Lifestyle-related Diseases." *Eur. Cardiol.* 14 (2):117-122. doi: 10.15420/ecr.2019.17.2.

Simpson, R. J., H. Kunz, N. Agha, and R. Graff. 2015. "Exercise and the Regulation of Immune Functions." *Prog. Mol. Biol. Transl. Sci.* 135:355-80. doi: 10.1016/bs.pmbts.2015.08.001.

Simpson, Richard J, Thomas W Lowder, Guillaume Spielmann, Austin B Bigley, Emily C LaVoy, and Hawley Kunz. 2012. "Exercise and the aging immune system." *Ageing research reviews* 11 (3):404-420.

Smith, J. A., A. B. Gray, D. B. Pyne, M. S. Baker, R. D. Telford, and M. J. Weidemann. 1996. "Moderate exercise triggers both priming and activation of neutrophil subpopulations." *Am. J. Physiol.* 270 (4 Pt 2):R838-45. doi: 10.1152/ajpregu.1996.270.4.R838.

So, Byunghun, Hee-Jae Kim, Jinsoo Kim, and Wook Song. 2014. "Exercise-induced myokines in health and metabolic diseases." *Integrative Medicine Research* 3 (4):172-179. doi: https://doi.org/10.1016/j.imr.2014.09.007.

Soleimani, V., A. Sahebkar, and H. Hosseinzadeh. 2018. "Turmeric (*Curcuma longa*) and its major constituent (curcumin) as nontoxic and safe substances: Review." *Phytother. Res.* 32 (6):985-995. doi: 10.1002/ptr.6054.

Suhett, L. G., R. de Miranda Monteiro Santos, B. K. S. Silveira, A. C. G. Leal, A. D. M. de Brito, J. F. de Novaes, and C. M. D. Lucia. 2021. "Effects of curcumin supplementation on sport and physical exercise: a systematic review." *Crit. Rev. Food Sci. Nutr.* 61 (6):946-958. doi: 10.1080/10408398.2020.1749025.

Tanabe, Y., K. Chino, T. Ohnishi, H. Ozawa, H. Sagayama, S. Maeda, and H. Takahashi. 2019. "Effects of oral curcumin ingested before or after eccentric exercise on markers of muscle damage and inflammation." *Scand. J. Med. Sci. Sports* 29 (4):524-534. doi: 10.1111/sms.13373.

Tanabe, Y., S. Maeda, N. Akazawa, A. Zempo-Miyaki, Y. Choi, S. G. Ra, A. Imaizumi, Y. Otsuka, and K. Nosaka. 2015. "Attenuation of indirect markers of eccentric exercise-induced muscle damage by curcumin." *Eur. J. Appl. Physiol.* 115 (9):1949-57. doi: 10.1007/s00421-015-3170-4.

Tsai, I. C., C. W. Hsu, C. H. Chang, P. T. Tseng, and K. V. Chang. 2021. "The Effect of Curcumin Differs on Individual Cognitive Domains across Different Patient Populations: A Systematic Review and Meta-Analysis." *Pharmaceuticals (Basel)* 14 (12). doi: 10.3390/ph14121235.

Varì, R., B. Scazzocchio, A. Silenzi, C. Giovannini, and R. Masella. 2021. "Obesity-Associated Inflammation: Does Curcumin Exert a Beneficial Role?" *Nutrients* 13 (3). doi: 10.3390/nu13031021.

Weisberg, S. P., D. McCann, M. Desai, M. Rosenbaum, R. L. Leibel, and A. W. Ferrante, Jr. 2003. "Obesity is associated with macrophage accumulation in adipose tissue." *J. Clin. Invest.* 112 (12):1796-808. doi: 10.1172/jci19246.

Yilmaz, E. N., S. Bay, G. Ozturk, and M. H. Ucisik. 2020. "Neuroprotective Effects of Curcumin-Loaded Emulsomes in a Laser Axotomy-Induced CNS Injury Model." *Int. J. Nanomedicine* 15:9211-9229. doi: 10.2147/ijn.s272931.

Zhao, Y., B. Chen, J. Shen, L. Wan, Y. Zhu, T. Yi, and Z. Xiao. 2017. "The Beneficial Effects of Quercetin, Curcumin, and Resveratrol in Obesity." *Oxid. Med. Cell Longev.* 2017:1459497. doi: 10.1155/2017/1459497.

Chapter 7

The Essential Therapeutic Effects of Curcumin: A Mini Review

Soumitra Shome and Anupam Das Talukdar*
Ethnobotany and Medicinal Plants Research Laboratory,
Department of Life Science and Bioinformatics, Assam University,
Silchar, Assam, India

Abstract

Curcumin is the essential bioactive constituent of *Curcuma longa* that has diverse disease healing effects that majorly includes antibacterial, anticancer, antidiabetic and anti-inflammatory. Curcumin has the potential to exhibit broad-spectrum antibacterial efficacy by a mechanism that includes ROS generation, membrane damage and cell death. The anticancer effectiveness of curcumin has been rigorously investigated, and it is chiefly mediated by inhibition of cyclin D1, preventing NF-ĸB activation and increasing reduced glutathione levels (GSH) in cancerous cells. Curcumin can show good antidiabetic activity using principles that involve enhancing uptake of glucose by increasing GLUT2, GLUT3 and GLUT4 gene expressions, decreasing glucose levels in hepatic cells, increasing release of insulin from pancreatic cells, decreasing resistance to insulin. The anti-inflammatory role of curcumin is largely due to the downregulation of key pathways that include lipooxygenase and cyclooxygenase pathways, thereby inhibiting the generation of important inflammation regulators, such as pro-inflammatory leukotrienes and prostaglandins. However, the aforesaid healing potency of curcumin is limited up to a definite scale due to its

* Corresponding Author's Email: anupam@bioinfoaus.ac.in.

In: Curcumin and Its Role in Health and Disease
Editor: Kathryn Woltjer
ISBN: 979-8-88697-491-1

large size of particle, retarded aqueous dissolution, limited stability that results in decreased bioavailability and cellular uptake. All these shortcomings linked to curcumin can be addressed by synthesizing nanocurcumin as well as conjugating/loading nanocurcumin to another therapeutically bioactive nanoparticle to develop nanoconjugates/ nanocomposites of curcumin having reduced size of particle, improved dissolution in water, enhanced stability and bioavailability thereby resulting in increased level of therapeutic efficacy. Moreover, such curcumin based nanoconjugates/nanocomposites, due to improved properties, can also exhibit multi-targeting therapeutic efficacy.

Keywords: curcumin, nanocurcumin, antibacterial, anticancer, anti-inflammatory, antidiabetic

Introduction

Curcumin can be considered as the non-water soluble, biologically active constituent extracted from the root tissue of a perennial herbaceous plant called *Curcuma longa* L. that is a member of the ginger family (Zingiberaceae) having broad utilization as food and medicine. According to the IUPAC system the nomenclature of curcumin is (1E, 6E)-1, 7-bis (4-hydroxy-3-methoxyphenyl)-1, 6-heptadiene-3,5-dione having molar mass and chemical formula as 368.38 g/mol and $C_{21}H_{20}O_6$ respectively (Figure 1). Curcumin's chemical structure suggested the presence of two aromatic ring arrangements consisting of o-methoxy phenolic groups that is joined with a seven carbon linker. Absorption bands of curcumin fall in both the ultraviolet and visible range of the spectrum, having peak absorption at 265 nm and 410-430 nm, respectively. Curcumin dissolved in methanol can exhibit molar extinction coefficient of about 55,000 dm3/mol per cm at 425 nm. Curcumin acts as an excellent antioxidant and therapeutic drug that is mainly due to its remarkable ability to scavenge reactive oxygen species. Besides the well-established therapeutic role of curcumin, it finds diverse applicability as food also and is popularly used for improving the colour and flavour of food items. Turmeric powder that mostly contains curcumin is widely used for marinating vegetables, fish, meat and is also a key ingredient of several vegetarian and non-vegetarian dishes.

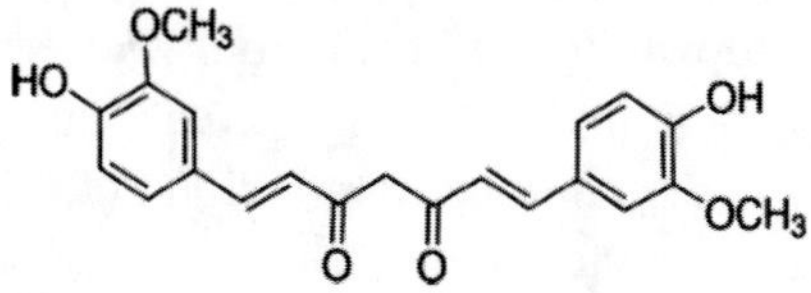

Figure 1. Structure of curcumin.

Literature survey suggested that curcumin has wide-ranging therapeutic and pharmacological activity and this chapter reviews some of its essential therapeutic role that includes antibacterial, anticancer, anti-inflammatory and antidiabetic. Acute multidrug-resistant bacterial epidemic infections can be a clinical emergency and require effective scientific answer to overcome such predictable plight. Globally, about 70,000 patients die because of infections due to multidrug resistant bacteria that is much greater than global demise because of measles, tetanus and cholera taken collectively. In context of this, curcumin and its various nanoformulations seems very capable to handle such crisis as they exhibit efficient antibacterial activity using remarkable and unique mechanism of action against several multi-drug resistant bacteria. Curcumin/nanocurcumin molecule can bind efficiently to the bacterial membrane and mediate elevated ROS generation, bacterial membrane disruption, leakage of cellular contents and cell death. High deaths because of cancer is a matter of global concern and is a serious impediment to improving life span in several countries around the world. As per the reports of World Health Organization (WHO) in the year 2019, many individuals before attaining the age of 70 develop cancer disease and is the first or second principal factor of death in a group of 112 countries while in another group of 23 countries, cancer is the third or fourth reason of death mortality. Curcumin and its essential nanoformulations has the potential to effectively block the process of cancer progression in pancreas, liver, nasopharyngeal tract, stomach and breast by mechanism that includes regulation of ROS synthesis, inhibiting excessive angiogenesis, inducing apoptosis, down-regulating hepatocellular XIAP and survivin and inhibiting *H. pylori* growth in gastric cells etc. Long-term inflammatory ailments is considered being the largest significant factor of mortality worldwide, with nearly 50% of total deaths occur due to various inflammatory diseases like cardiac illness, autoimmune ailment, long-term renal illness, fatty liver ailment, diabetes mellitus and neurodegenerative illness (Furman et al. 2019). In connection to this, several investigations confirm the superior anti-inflammatory and antioxidant efficacy of curcumin/nanocurcumin against severe chronic diseases using processes that majorly includes downregulation of lipoxygenase and cyclooxygenase pathway, inhibiting synthesis of pro-inflammatory leukotrienes and prostaglandins and downregulation of expression of COX-2 and iNOS mRNA, thereby, applying brakes on the acceleration of inflammatory disease. Reports indicated that the frequency of diabetes in the year 2000 was about 2.8% and it was estimated that by the year 2030 cases of diabetes may rise to 4.4%. Several investigations that has been performed by researchers world-wide confirm the antidiabetic effectiveness of curcumin and its various nanoformulations by mechanisms that consists of reduction of oxidative stress, downregulation of ROS generation, enhancing antioxidant enzyme activity, increasing insulin secretion and decreasing blood glucose level etc. Despite the fact that curcumin has multiple pharmacological and therapeutic efficiency and applicability, but due to its big size of particle, retarded bioavailability, decreased aqueous solubility, decreased uptake by cells, and decreased stability, the efficacy of aforementioned therapeutic properties of curcumin gets significantly retarded and is a major drawback associated with curcumin. To defeat this disadvantage of curcumin, nanotechnology/nanobiotechnology based advanced techniques can be used to synthesize nanocurcumin as well as its various nanocomposites/nanoconjugates having improved water solubility and bioavailability.

Nanotechnology is a prospering field of science that finds diverse applicability from medicine (Stephen et al. 2020), agriculture (Majumdar and Keller 2021), dentistry (Handa et al. 2021), food processing/packaging (Singh et al. 2017), disease diagnosis (Nagraik et al. 2021), nanocosmetics (Raj et al. 2012) to semiconductors (Varudkar et al. 2020), sensors (Nagraik et al. 2021), solar cells (Wong et al. 2014) and textiles (Yetisen et al. 2016). Nanotechnology can be defined as the scientific discipline that deal with micro to nano scale objects and is specifically concerned with the synthesis, modelling and characterizing ultra-small particles (nanoparticles) having enhanced characteristics and finds wide applicability in medicine, pharmaceutical and chemical sciences. Nanoparticles can be described as extremely minute nanomaterial that has unique and special characteristics and proportion between 1-100 nm and can demonstrate remarkable wide-ranging pharmacological and therapeutic activity using advanced mechanisms. By employing suitable and efficient nanoparticle synthesis procedure such as green synthesis, coprecipitation, sol gel method, and microemulsion method, the large sized particles of crude curcumin having low bioavailability, decreased dissolution in water and stability can be sliced to generate particles with extremely small dimensions (nanocurcumin) having improved solubility and bioavailability. Further, such synthesized nanocurcumin may be conjugated/ligated to another bioactive and therapeutically efficient nanoparticle, such as metal oxide/metal nanoparticle to develop novel nanoconjugates/nanocomposites having unique and multitargeting therapeutic and pharmacologic mechanisms. In the present review, the well investigated antibacterial, anticancer, anti-inflammatory and antidiabetic effects of curcumin and some of its essential nanoformulations were compiled in a lucid manner to highlight the versatility of curcumin/nanocurcumin.

Curcumin as a Natural Food Additive

Curcumin, along with its multiple disease healing effects, is also an essential food additive and is widely used to enhance food color and flavor. Curcumin, as turmeric powder, is a part of Indian Culture and is used for preparation of various vegetarian and non-vegetarian dishes in India and other Southeast Asia countries. Food items like vegetables, fish and meat are preferably marinated with curcumin (turmeric powder) before cooking which help in disinfecting any germs leaving behind an appetizing colour, aroma and flavour ("US7273630B2 - Process for cleaning and disinfecting food products - Google Patents" n.d.). Besides this curcumin (turmeric) because of its established and popular health benefits like boosting immune system, antioxidant potential, anti-inflammatory effects, aid digestion and liver detoxification activity etc. is also consumed as pickles, turmeric tea and turmeric milk ("You Must Eat Fresh Turmeric Pickle Daily, Read Its Amazing Benefits" n.d.). Nanocurcumin derived from curcumin has also been marketed in the form of capsules (500mg) as food supplements that has improved therapeutic properties like good intestinal absorption, long lasting in blood stream, enhanced antioxidant, anti-inflammatory effects and superior blood-brain barrier penetrability.

Antibacterial Activity of Curcumin

Critical infections due to multidrug-resistant bacteria can be tormenting and demands innovative scientific solutions to smartly evade this crisis. Every year, nearly 70,000 individuals who get infected by MDR bacteria succumb worldwide and this is higher than demise caused due to measles, tetanus and cholera in total. This condition may further become so complicated that by the year 2050 nearly 10 million lives may depart each year due to raising multidrug resistance thus, surpassing the current 8.2 million lives that die from cancer in a year. This medical crisis may be specifically addressed by naturally produced antibacterial molecule such as curcumin and their nanoformulations that have special and unique mechanism of antibacterial action against various MDR bacterial strains. Literature analysis indicated the broad spectrum and multi-targeting antibacterial action of curcumin that can easily get around the bacterial multi-drug resistance system. Pseudomonas aeruginosa that can establish resilient biofilm is a severe risk to public health care system especially in hospital settings treating immunocompromised patients. P. aeruginosa is the fourth most hazardous nosocomial pathogen and can cause multiple hospital borne infections. Curcumin I (dose = 25 μM-100 μM) was effectively able to retard the growth of *P. aeruginosa* by processes that include bacterial cell membrane disintegration and cell death (Tyagi et al. 2015). In a recent investigation, it was demonstrated that curcumin can bind with peptidoglycan present in bacterial cell wall and drive membrane disruption and lysis of cell (Figure 2) (Duracka et al. 2019). Bacterial when treated with curcumin in combination with light mediated high reactive oxygen species formation resulting in disordering of iron homeostasis, interference of synthesis of iron-sulphur cluster and death of bacteria (Shlar et al. 2017). Curcumin using a principle similar to bacterial apoptosis could kill cells by kill bacterial cells using processes such as influx of calcium inside the cell, bacterial membrane depolarization and DNA fragmentation (Yun and Lee 2016). Quorum sensing (QS) serves as an important communication process for controlling cell adhesion, biofilm establishment and multi-drug resistance and hence is an essential therapeutic target. Abdulrahman et al. reported that a mixed therapy of light and curcumin could retard biofilm formation by blocking the bacterial Quorum Sensing apparatus by processes that involve synthesis of singlet oxygen and reduction of extracellular polysaccharides present in the biofilm (Abdulrahman et al. 2020). Using animal and plant-based pathogenicity model, the biofilm inhibition capacity of curcumin against *P. aeruginosa* by applying mechanisms that include blocking generation of pyocyanin, inhibiting elastase/protease activity, and interfering acyl homoserine lactone (HSL) synthesis (Rudrappa and Bais 2008). Also, curcumin was capable of blocking the biofilm and growth of *P. aeruginosa* by processes that involves inhibiting the quorum sensing apparatus as well as enhancing the sensitivity of *P. aeruginosa* to azithromycin (Packiavathy et al. 2014). Curcumin can also downregulate the bacterial QS apparatus by blocking the protein named acyl-homoserine-lactone synthase coded by LuxI gene (Ding et al. 2017).

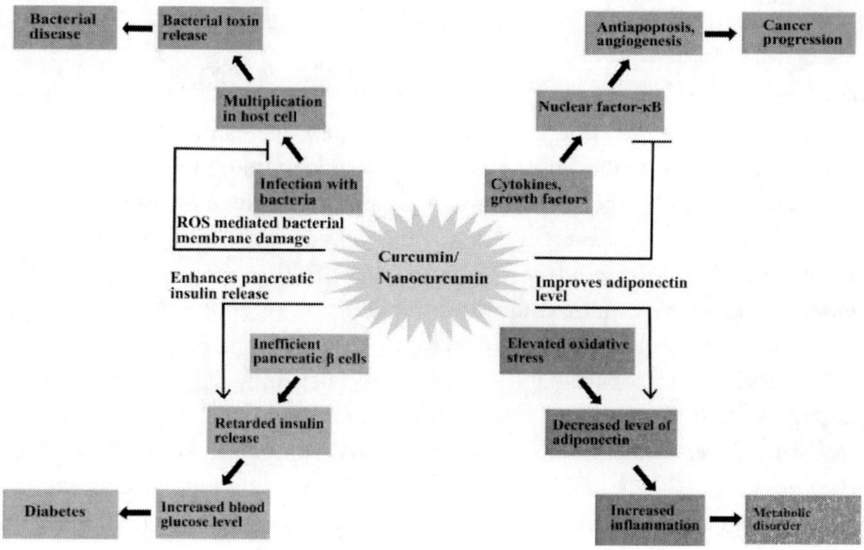

Figure 2. Essential therapeutic targets of curcumin for curing bacterial infection, cancer, diabetes and inflammatory diseases.

Nanocurcumin synthesized using crude curcumin can be defined as the improved form of curcumin that has small size of particle, enhanced dissolution in water, increased bioavailability, decrease hydrodynamic size and increased stability that facilitates easy and efficient entry into the bacterial cell and increased antibacterial/anti-biofilm activity. Moreover, nanocurcumin can also be conjugated to another bioactive nanoparticle that can further improve the aforementioned activity. In context of this, Targhi et al. reported that encapsulated curcumin and metal nanoparticles (silver/copper nanoparticles) prepared by thin film hydration method exhibited very good antibacterial and antibiofilm activity compared to their free form (Targhi et al. 2021). Nanoconjugates of gallium and curcumin showed improved stability of curcumin and superior antibacterial/antibiofilm efficacy against *P. aeruginosa* (MIC= 82.75 μg/ml) by mechanisms that include bacterial cell membrane disintegration and cell organization damage (Ramesh et al. 2022). Curcumin nanoparticles (size=300 nm) micronized and fabricated with solution enhanced dispersion by supercritical CO_2 showed increased level of antibacterial activity against *P. aeruginosa* under both *in-vitro* and *in-vivo* conditions suggesting the enhanced disease healing efficiency of curcumin nanoparticles compared to their crude form (Xue et al. 2020). The primary cause of non-success of dental implant treatments are the subsequent infections that occur after placing implant. To address this issue, nanocurcumin seems very promising since implants treated with nanocurcumin showed remarkable antibacterial activity with more than 99% efficacy when compared to control groups, thus, suggesting the future use of nanocurcumin inside the implant fixture for successful cure of dental ailment (Negahdari et al. 2021). Curcumin nanoparticles green synthesized using supernatant of *Bacillus subtilis* culture showed very good antibacterial activity against *Staphylococcus aureus*, *Bacillus subtilis*, *Pseudomonas aeruginosa*, *Salmonella enterica,* thus, indicating the addition of curcumin nanoparticles as dietary supplements for quails (Reda et al. 2020). Nanocurcumin was ligated to ZnO nanoparticles to synthesize curcumin-ZnO nanocomposites having small hydrodynamic size and improved bioavailability, showed very good anti-*E. coli* and anti-*S. aureus* activity compared to crude curcumin (Shome et al. 2021b, 2021a). Stable and biocompatible silver-curcumin nanoconjugate synthesized using novel and eco-friendly method showed increased antibacterial activity in comparison to pure silver nanoparticle (Abdellah et al. 2018). ZnO-curcumin core shell nanoparticles having size of about 55 to 60 nm exhibited more notable antibacterial efficacy than that of commercially available antibiotic called amoxicillin, thereby suggesting their future use in biomedical industry (Varaprasad et al. 2019). Chitosan-curcumin-C3 nanoparticles prepared using an amalgamation of three types of curcuminoids encapsulated in chitosan showed very good curcumin entrapment and drug release efficiency as well as highly appreciable antioxidant and antibacterial activity against *S. aureus* and *E. coli,* thus, suggesting the use of such nanoparticles for curing inflammatory and bacterial diseases (Reddy et al. 2020).

Anticancer Activity of Curcumin

Cancer is considered as the principal factor of death and is a major hindrance to enhancing life span in many countries around the world (Bray et al. 2021). World Health Organization (WHO) in 2019 estimated that most people before they attain the age of 70 suffer from cancer disease which is the first/second major root of mortality in about 112 countries while third/fourth reason of death in another group of 23 countries (Sung et al. 2021). This rising risks of death due to cancer indicates that deaths occurring due to other factors such as heart disease and stroke is declining when compared to cancer in several countries (Sung et al. 2021). Cancer in the pancreas is considered as one of the most life-threatening cancers globally and surgical resection is the only healing procedure if diagnosed at an early stage (Bimonte et al. 2016). Multiple investigations have demonstrated the anticancer activity of curcumin against pancreatic cancer as curcumin can reduce oxidative stress, inhibit excessive angiogenesis and induce apoptosis (Figure 2) (Bimonte et al. 2016). Hepatocellular cancer is also one of the top risk to public health worldwide and it was demonstrated that curcumin along with resveratrol had the potential to induce intrinsic and extrinsic apoptosis, increase ROS synthesis and down regulate XIAP and survivin in hepatocytes (Du et al. 2013). Nasopharyngeal cancer (NPC) is an important form of head and neck cancer that is majorly treated using radiotherapy, however in some cases the cancer may be radio-resistant and difficult to cure. Multiple reports indicated that curcumin can enhance the sensitivity of nasopharyngeal cancer cells by mechanisms involving regulating genetic expression using non-coding RNAs, altering the dynamics of ROS synthesis thereby suggesting the employability of curcumin along with radiotherapy/chemotherapy for efficient cancer curing (Momtazi-Borojeni et al. 2018). Gastric cancer is considered as a principal reason of death due to cancer globally as this disease suffers from the issue of being poorly diagnosed that result in a high rate of detection of patients with advanced/metastatic stage of gastric cancer during diagnosis. In context of this, a study indicated that combined therapy of curcumin and quercetin significantly inhibited gastric cell proliferation due to modulation of membrane potential of mitochondria, increased cytochrome c release and reduced AKT phosphorylation (Zhang et al. 2015). Breast cancer cases alone contribute to about 30% amongst new instances of cancer and are considered being the most deadly and widespread malignant tumour, killing large number of women worldwide. In context of this, a study indicated that curcumin showed colony forming blocking and anti-proliferation activities in breast cancer cell lines. Curcumin also had the potential to inhibit cancer cell metastasis and its stem-like characteristics, thereby, indicating the use of curcumin as an anti-metastasis drug for breast cancer (Figure 2) (Hu et al. 2019).

Although curcumin has potential and broad anticancer activity, its clinical efficacy is largely retarded due to its reduced solubility in water, retarded bioavailability, quick degradation, poor intestinal absorption and rapid systemic elimination. To solve these issues, a more advanced form of curcumin, namely nanocurcumin and its nanoconjugates/nanocomposites can be developed and its cancer inhibiting efficiency may be tested. In context of this, Yallapu et al. prepared a new CUR-loaded magnetic nanoparticle and tested its anticancer efficacy in pancreas cancer. The results indicated that CUR-loaded magnetic nanoparticle showed improved internalization and efficient anticancer activity in pancreatic cancer cells (HPAF-II and Panc-1 cells) by retarding the proliferation of B-cell lymphoma-extra large (Bcl-xL), proliferating cell nuclear antigen (PCNA) and inducing cell surface–associated Mucin 1 (MUC1) and myeloid leukemia cell differentiation protein (Mcl-1) etc. (Yallapu et al. 2013). Acrylamide (AC) is an artificial environment contaminating carcinogenic compound used largely in industries and can induce cancer in vital organs such as the liver, brain and heart, etc. Recently, it was demonstrated that acrylamide could mediate induction of liver cancer by increasing the expression of P53, cleaved caspase-3, CYP2E1, COL1A1, aspartate aminotransferase and serum alanine aminotransferase. The results confirmed that treatment using nanocurcumin had the potential to block cancer progress by reversing these conditions, thereby suggesting the hepatoprotective and anticancer efficacy of curcumin nanoparticles (Atia et al. 2022). In case of advanced-stage nasopharyngeal cancer, chemotherapy is the most important method of treatment available as no significant progress has been made in its effective curing since a decade. Curcumin, based on its therapeutic efficacy against nasopharyngeal cancer, is considered as an efficient substitute for chemotherapeutics. But due to reduced tumour penetrability and absence of tissue specificity, the efficacy gets retarded to some extent. To address this issue, a therapeutic sub-30 nm lipid nanoparticle loaded with curcumin specific for scavenger receptor class B member 1 (SR-B1) was developed. The results indicated that the synthesized drug was more nasopharyngeal cancer cell specific and inhibited cancer cell proliferation due to increased apoptosis (Luo et al. 2021). Gastric cancer is considered as the 5th most important form of cancer and in case of cancer mediated deaths, gastric cancer occupies third position. Gastric cancer is a deadly disease caused majorly due to *Helicobacter pylori* infection and unhealthy habits/life style (smoking, alcohol consumption, obesity) with surgical resection using chemo/radiation therapy being the potential treatment measures available. Alam et al. demonstrated that curcumin encapsulated into biocompatible co-polymer PLGA nanoparticle could efficiently inhibit *H pylori* (MIC= μg/ml) that resulted in remarkable inhibition of cancer in gastric cells with increasing time for up to 72 hours (IC_{50} = 18.78 μM) as compared to free curcumin (IC_{50} = 24.20 μM) (Alam et al. 2022).

Anti-Inflammatory Activity of Curcumin and Its Important Nanoformulations

Large number of investigations related to anti-inflammatory and antioxidant effect of curcumin and its various nanoformulations on several chronic diseases have been carried out till date. Studies showed that the hydroxyphenyl component of curcumin is very important for mediating anti-inflammatory effect of curcumin since any modification such as acylation and alkylation of this group largely retarded the anti-inflammatory effect of curcumin (Mukhopadhyay et al. 1982). Reports indicated that curcumin can mediate the downregulation of the lipoxygenase and cyclooxygenase pathway by blocking the generation of pro-inflammatory leukotrienes and prostaglandins, respectively (Chainani-Wu 2003). Acute inflammation and high oxidative stress greatly contribute in the process of establishment of metabolic syndrome and a study showed that treatment using nano-micelle curcumin was able to improve the adiponectin level and total antioxidant capacity, thereby, reducing the inflammatory and oxidative stress in the treated groups (Figure 2) (Bateni et al. 2022). Migraine is an important neuroinflammatory disease that consists of repeated strikes of painful sessions. Such inflammation and neurogenic pain are caused largely due to elevated expression of two key factors, namely COX-2 and iNOS. In connection to this, Abdolahi et al. showed that a combined therapy consisting of nanocurcumin and omega-3 fatty acids could down regulate the expression of COX-2 and iNOS mRNA that lowered their levels in the serum, thereby, significantly reducing the repetition, length and intensity of migraine pain (Abdolahi et al. 2019). Curcumin/nanocurcumin exhibits potential anti-inflammatory effects by blocking the action of various inflammation inducing cytokines like interleukin (IL)-1, IL-6, tumour necrosis factor-alpha (TNF-α), IL-12, IL-2, IL-8 and monocyte chemo-attractant protein, thus, decreasing the intensity of inflammatory reaction (Jurenka 2009). In context of this, Valizadeh et al. also reported that treatment of patients suffering from coronavirus disease 2019 using nanocurcumin showed a decrease in both mRNA expression and release in serum of key inflammatory regulators such as IL-6 and IL-8, thus, speeding and improving the recovery process of such patients (Valizadeh et al. 2020). Literature survey indicated that curcumin had the potential to block the transcription factor NF-κB that catalyzes the transcription of several inflammatory factors like COX-2 and iNOS (Shome et al. 2016). Doxorubicin is an important chemotherapeutic drug that is widely utilized for treating several malignant tumours. However, this drug suffers from a very notable disadvantage, as it is highly cardiotoxic. In connection to this, reports indicated that a combined therapy of nanocurcumin along with doxorubicin could ameliorate the cardiotoxicity due to doxorubicin by applying processes such as anti-inflammatory and antioxidant effects, thus, suggesting the potential application of nanocurcumin as a cardio-protective molecule (Moutabian et al. 2022). Osteoarthritis is characterized by gradual degeneration of joints and non-steroidal anti-inflammatory drugs are utilized for curing this ailment. But such non-steroidal anti-inflammatory drugs suffer from a major disadvantage that includes gastrointestinal bleeding. In context of this, nano-micelle curcumin having improved bioavailability was able to cure and heal the chronic symptoms of osteoarthritis (Hashemzadeh et al. 2019). Cystic fibrosis is considered as a serious genetic disorder characterized with production of defective CFTR proteins and increased inflammation (Talebi et al. 2021). Curcumin and its nanoformulations had the potential to find very potential application in curing cystic fibrosis due to its well established anti-inflammatory effects (Talebi et al. 2021). A flavonoid called rotenone that is routinely used in Parkinson's Disease (PD) research also had the potential to cause neurotoxic damage to dopaminergic cells (Bollimpelli et al. 2016). Curcumin loaded lactoferrin nanoparticles of average particle size of 43-60 nm having improved drug loading and release efficiency was able to exhibit notable neuroprotective effect due to its anti-inflammatory and antioxidant properties in dopaminergic neurons treated with rotenone (Bollimpelli et al. 2016). Bovine mastitis is considered as the bacteria induced inflammation of the mammary glands and is a critical financial loss to the dairy industry (Suresh et al. 2018). In context of this, curcumin loaded PLGA nanoparticle synthesized using solid-in-oil-in-water emulsion process had the potential to reduce the severity of *S. aureus* induced mastitis in the mouse model by decreasing the level of pro-inflammatory cytokines (Suresh et al. 2018). Coliform mastitis is another form of critical ailment of the mammary gland worldwide (Lebda et al. 2021). In connection to this, Lebda et al. demonstrated that nanocurcumin having improved solubility and oral bioavailability was able efficiently attenuate lipopolysaccharide induced coliform mastitis in rat model by decreasing the synthesis of pro-inflammatory cytokines and inhibiting lipid peroxidation (Lebda et al. 2021). Copper (Cu) although is an important for several biological processes; but due to elevated redoxreactivity can be possibly toxic. High dosage of copper has been implicated for being cardiotoxic by inducing necrosis and cellular stress in cardiocytes (Sarawi et al. 2021). In connection to this, it was shown that nanocurcumin had the potential to ameliorate copper induced cardiotoxicity by inhibiting the imflammatory response, oxidative injury and cell death (Sarawi et al. 2021).

Antidiabetic Activity of Curcumin

Available testimonials suggested that in the year 2000 the frequency of diabetes was estimated to be about 2.8% and by the year 2030, this occurrence may rise to 4.4%. Series of *in-vitro* and *in-vivo* investigations carried out by research globally have established the capability of curcumin as hypoglycaemic agent (Den Hartogh et al. 2020; Pari and Murugan 2005). Best et al. reported that pancreatic islets isolated from Sprague–Dawley when treated with 10 μM of curcumin for 30 minutes showed elevated insulin release in response to 4 mM of glucose by regulating chloride ion dependent membrane depolarization (Best et al. 2007). Primary pancreatic islets of mouse when pre-treated with curcumin (10 μM) for about 24 hours exhibited enhanced insulin secretion and islet viability under streptozotocin treatment possibly by reduction of oxidative stress by downregulating ROS generation due to enhanced superoxide dismutase level (Figure 2) (Meghana et al. 2007). Pancreatic islet transplantation is a very potential remedy for type 1 diabetes and this process has a key drawback of poor islet cryopreservation and subsequent recovery after thawing. In context of this, Kanitkar et al. treatment of primary mouse islets with curcumin during the process of cryopreservation caused enhanced recovery of healthy islets having normal morphology by mechanisms consisting of reduced ROS generation, increased response to glucose and enhanced insulin secretion and increased heat shock protein 70 (Hsp70) generation (Kanitkar and Bhonde 2008). In a study it was shown that curcumin had the potential to reduce glucose level in blood by mechanisms that includes decreasing the extent of glucose in the liver, increasing the process of glucose uptake by upregulating the expression of glucose transporter-2 (GLUT2), GLUT3 and GLUT4 genes, increasing the action of AMP kinase, activating ligand binding activity of peroxisome proliferator-activated receptor-γ (PPAR-γ), retarding inflammation due to hyperglycaemia, increasing release of insulin from cells of the pancreas and decreasing insulin resistance (Ghorbani et al. 2014). In another study, it was shown that a curcumin derivative having improved aqueous solubility exhibited anti-hyperglycaemic effect in induced type 1 diabetes mellitus model by decreasing ROS generation, blocking lipid peroxidation, up regulating insulin level in plasma and decreasing plasma glucose level (Abdel

Aziz et al. 2013). Curcumin, in combination with pure phytocompound extracted from *Abroma augusta* had the potential to synergistically reduce level of glucose concentration (Ali Hussain 2002).

Metabolic syndrome is a very complicated disease characterized by multiple metabolic disorders having symptoms such as insulin resistance, high level of glucose, low high-density lipoprotein cholesterol, increased blood pressure and high level of triglyceride that collectively contribute to the establishment of type 2 diabetes and cardiovascular disease (Kheiripour et al. 2021; Javandoost et al. 2018). In context of this, Kheiripou et al. showed that treatment of patients suffering from metabolic syndrome with nanocurcumin (dosage = 80 mg/day for two months) caused an enhancement in insulin sensitivity, decrease in fasting plasma glucose and lowered serum afamin level suggesting the applicability of nanocurcumin in managing and treating metabolic syndrome (Kheiripour et al. 2021). Gouda et al. using *in-vivo* system consisting of rats demonstrated that treatment of nanocurcumin in induced diabetic rats had the potential to enhance the expression of genes coding for insulin and receptors of insulin with respect to suitable control (Gouda et al. 2019). Curcumin loaded chitosan nanoparticles was also reported to mediate remarkable enhancement in GLUT-4 translocation to the surface of skeletal muscle and increased phosphorylation of key downstream targets, thus exhibiting appreciable anti-hyperglycemic effects (Chauhan et al. 2018). Irregularities in insulin synthesis and insulin resistance are key characteristics of type 2 diabetes mellitus (T2DM). Moreover, apelin further contributes to the development of insulin resistance (Shamsi-Goushki et al. 2020). In connection to this, one study demonstrated that both nanocurcumin and curcumin were successful in countering insulin resistance and reducing the lipid profile with nanocurcumin was more efficient in reducing insulin resistance, apelin, lipid profile and serum levels of fasting blood sugar (Shamsi-Goushki et al. 2020). In one investigation carried out by Chauhan et al. in which they tried to improve the efficacy and bioavailability of crude curcumin by synthesizing chitosan loaded curcumin-ZnO nanoparticle having an average size of 43 nm and evaluated its antidiabetic and antioxidant effect (Chauhan et al. 2019). The results suggested that induced diabetic rats treated with chitosan loaded curcumin-ZnO nanoparticle for 28 days significantly retarded the blood glucose level and also normalized the lipid profile (Chauhan et al. 2019). A study consisting of comparing the antidiabetic efficacy of nanocurcumin and gliclazide using diabetic albino rats induced with streptozotocin showed that nanocurcumin had the potential to reduce the body weight, fasting blood glucose as well as enhance the expression of insulin, insulin receptor A glucokinase, and glucose transporter 2 (GLUT2) (Afifi et al. 2020). This remarkable therapeutic efficacy exhibited by nanocurcumin treated group was similar to that of gliclazide group, thus suggesting the potential clinical application of nanocurcumin for treating diabetes (Afifi et al. 2020).

Conclusion

Curcumin can thus be considered as a molecule of immense potential having anticancer, antibacterial, antidiabetic and anti-inflammatory effects. However, these pharmacological and therapeutic effects of curcumin are limited due to its large size of particle that decreases its solubility, bioavailability, stability and therapeutic efficacy. Nanocurcumin and its several nanoconjugates having small particle size and enhanced therapeutic efficacy can be defined as the improved form of curcumin that addresses all the aforesaid drawbacks associated with crude curcumin. Nanoconjugates as well as nanocomposites of curcumin/nanocurcumin synthesized using another or multiple bioactive nanomaterials can exhibit unique and multi-targeting therapeutic mechanism against chronic diseases. More future *in-vitro* and *in-silico* studies using nanocurcumin and novel nanoconjugates/nanocomposites synthesized using more improved and optimized methods against severe ailments needs to be demonstrated for better understanding the efficacy and mechanism of action.

References

Abdel Aziz, M. T., El-Asmar, M. F., Rezq, A. M., Mahfouz, S. M., Wassef, M. A., Fouad, H. H., Ahmed, H. H., and Taha, F. M. (2013). The effect of a novel curcumin derivative on pancreatic islet regeneration in experimental type-1 diabetes in rats (long term study). *Diabetology and Metabolic Syndrome* 5 (1):1–14. doi:10.1186/1758-5996-5-75/FIGURES/9.

Abdellah, A. M., Sliem, M. A., Bakr, M., and Amin, R. M. (2018). Green synthesis and biological activity of silver–curcumin nanoconjugates. *Future Medicinal Chemistry* 10 (22):2577–2588. doi:10.4155/FMC-2018-0152.

Abdolahi, M., Jafarieh, A., Sarraf, P., Sedighiyan, M., Yousefi, A., Tafakhori, A., Abdollahi, H., Salehinia, F., and Djalali, M. (2019). The Neuromodulatory Effects of ω-3 Fatty Acids and Nano-Curcumin on the COX-2/ iNOS Network in Migraines: A Clinical Trial Study from Gene Expression to Clinical Symptoms. *Endocrine,*

Metabolic & Immune Disorders - Drug Targets 19 (6):874–884. doi:10.2174/1871530319666190212170140.

Abdulrahman, H., Misba, L., Ahmad, S., and Khan, A. U. (2020). Curcumin induced photodynamic therapy mediated suppression of quorum sensing pathway of Pseudomonas aeruginosa: An approach to inhibit biofilm in vitro. *Photodiagnosis and Photodynamic Therapy* 30:101645. doi:10.1016/j.pdpdt.2019.101645.

Afifi, M., Alkaladi, A., Abomughaid, M. M., and Abdelazim, A. M. (2020). Nanocurcumin improved glucose metabolism in streptozotocin-induced diabetic rats: a comparison study with Gliclazide. *Environmental Science and Pollution Research* 27 (20):25271–25277. doi:10.1007/S11356-020-08941-8.

Alam, J., Dilnawaz, F., Sahoo, S. K., Singh, D. V., Mukhopadhyay, A. K., Hussain, T., and Pati, S. (2022). Curcumin Encapsulated into Biocompatible Co-Polymer PLGA Nanoparticle Enhanced Anti-Gastric Cancer and Anti-Helicobacter Pylori Effect. *Asian Pacific Journal of Cancer Prevention* 23 (1):61–70. doi:10.31557/APJCP.2022.23.1.61.

Ali Hussain, H. E. M. (2002). Hypoglycemic, hypolipidemic and antioxidant properties of combination ofCurcumin from*Curcuma longa*, Linn, and partially purified product fromAbroma augusta, Linn. in streptozotocin induced diabetes. *Indian Journal of Clinical Biochemistry 2002 17:2* 17 (2):33–43. doi:10.1007/BF02867969.

Atia, M. M., Abdel-Tawab, H. S., Mostafa, A. M., and Mobarak, S. A. (2022). Nanocurcumin and curcumin prevent N, N'-methylenebisacrylamide-induced liver damage and promotion of hepatic cancer cell growth. *Scientific Reports* 12 (1):1–17. doi:10.1038/s41598-022-12406-y.

Bateni, Z., Behrouz, V., Rahimi, H. R., Hedayati, M., Afsharian, S., and Sohrab, G. (2022). Effects of nano-curcumin supplementation on oxidative stress, systemic inflammation, adiponectin, and NF-κB in patients with metabolic syndrome: A randomized, double-blind clinical trial. *Journal of Herbal Medicine* 31:100531. doi:10.1016/J.HERMED.2021.100531.

Best, L., Elliott, A. C., and Brown, P. D. (2007). Curcumin induces electrical activity in rat pancreatic beta-cells by activating the volume-regulated anion channel. *Biochemical pharmacology* 73 (11):1768–1775. doi:10.1016/J.BCP.2007.02.006.

Bimonte, S., Barbieri, A., Leongito, M., Piccirillo, M., Giudice, A., Pivonello, C., De Angelis, C., Granata, V., Palaia, R., and Izzo, F. (2016). Curcumin AntiCancer Studies in Pancreatic Cancer. *Nutrients* 8 (7):433. doi:10.3390/NU8070433.

Bollimpelli, V. S., Kumar, P., Kumari, S., and Kondapi, A. K. (2016). Neuroprotective effect of curcumin-loaded lactoferrin nano particles against rotenone induced neurotoxicity. *Neurochemistry International* 95:37–45. doi:10.1016/J.NEUINT.2016.01.006.

Bray, F., Laversanne, M., Weiderpass, E., and Soerjomataram, I. (2021). The ever-increasing importance of cancer as a leading cause of premature death worldwide. *Cancer* 127 (16):3029–3030. doi:10.1002/CNCR.33587.

Chainani-Wu, N. (2003). Safety and anti-inflammatory activity of curcumin: a component of tumeric (*Curcuma longa*). *Journal of alternative and complementary medicine* 9 (1):161–168. doi:10.1089/107555303321223035.

Chauhan, P., Mahajan, S., and Prasad, G. B. K. S. (2019). Preparation and characterization of CS-ZnO-NC nanoparticles for imparting anti-diabetic activities in experimental diabetes. *Journal of Drug Delivery Science and Technology* 52:738–747. doi:10.1016/J.JDDST.2019.05.020.

Chauhan, P., Tamrakar, A. K., Mahajan, S., and Prasad, G. B. K. S. (2018). Chitosan encapsulated nanocurcumin induces GLUT-4 translocation and exhibits enhanced anti-hyperglycemic function. *Life Sciences* 213:226–235. doi:10.1016/J.LFS.2018.10.027.

Den Hartogh, D. J., Gabriel, A., and Tsiani, E. (2020). Antidiabetic Properties of Curcumin I: Evidence from In Vitro Studies. *Nutrients 2020, Vol. 12, Page 118* 12 (1):118. doi:10.3390/NU12010118.

Ding, T., Li, T., Wang, Z., and Li, J. (2017). Curcumin liposomes interfere with quorum sensing system of Aeromonas sobria and in silico analysis. *Scientific Reports* 7 (1):1–16. doi:10.1038/s41598-017-08986-9.

Du, Q., Hu, B., An, H. M., Shen, K. E. P., Xu, L., Deng, S., and Wei, M. M. (2013). Synergistic anticancer effects of curcumin and resveratrol in Hepa1-6 hepatocellular carcinoma cells. *Oncology Reports* 29 (5):1851–1858. doi:10.3892/OR.2013.2310/HTML.

Duracka, M., Lukac, N., Kacaniova, M., Kantor, A., Hleba, L., Ondruska, L., and Tvrda, E. (2019). Antibiotics Versus Natural Biomolecules: The Case of In Vitro Induced Bacteriospermia by Enterococcus Faecalis in Rabbit Semen. *Molecules* 24 (23):1–20. doi:10.3390/MOLECULES24234329.

Furman, D., Campisi, J., Verdin, E., Carrera-Bastos, P., Targ, S., Franceschi, C., Ferrucci, L., Gilroy, D. W., Fasano, A., Miller, G. W., Miller, A. H., Mantovani, A., Weyand, C. M., Barzilai, N., Goronzy, J. J., Rando, T. A., Effros, R. B., Lucia, A., Kleinstreuer, N., and Slavich, G. M. (2019). Chronic inflammation in the etiology of disease across the life span. *Nature Medicine 2019 25:12* 25 (12):1822–1832. doi:10.1038/s41591-019-0675-0.

Ghorbani, Z., Hekmatdoost, A., and Mirmiran, P. (2014). Anti-hyperglycemic and insulin sensitizer effects of turmeric and its principle constituent curcumin. *International journal of endocrinology and metabolism* 12 (4). doi:10.5812/IJEM.18081.

Gouda, W., Hafiz, N. A., Mageed, L., Alazzouni, A. S., Khalil, W. K. B., Afify, M., and Abdelmaksoud, M. D. E. (2019). Effects of nano-curcumin on gene expression of insulin and insulin receptor. *Bulletin of the National Research Centre* 43 (1):1–10. doi:10.1186/S42269-019-0164-0.

Handa, A., Bhullar, K. K., Kaur, S., Kaur, R., and Malhotra, S. (2021). Scope of nanotechnology in dentistry - A review of literature. *Baba Farid University Dental Journal* 11 (1):59–63. doi:10.5958/2230-7273.2021.00010.7.

Hashemzadeh, K., Davoudian, N., Jaafari, M. R., and Mirfeizi, Z. (2019). The Effect of Nanocurcumin in Improvement of Knee Osteoarthritis: A Randomized Clinical Trial. *Current Rheumatology Reviews* 16 (2):158–164. doi:10.2174/1874471013666191223152658.

Hu, C., Li, M., Guo, T., Wang, S., Huang, W., Yang, K., Liao, Z., Wang, J., Zhang, F., and Wang, H. (2019). Anti-metastasis activity of curcumin against breast cancer via the inhibition of stem cell-like properties and EMT. *Phytomedicine* 58:152740. doi:10.1016/J.PHYMED.2018.11.001.

Javandoost, A., Afshari, A., Saberi-Karimian, M., Sahebkar, A., Safarian, H., Moammeri, M., Fathi Dizaji, B., Tavalaei, S., Ferns, G. A., Pasdar, A., Mohammad Reza Parizadeh, S., Ghayour-Mobarhan, M., and Dizaji, F. B. (2018). The effects of curcumin and a modified curcumin formulation on serum Cholesteryl Ester Transfer Protein concentrations in patients with metabolic syndrome: A randomized, placebo-controlled clinical trial. *Avicenna Journal of Phytomedicine* 8 (4):330–337.

Jurenka, J. S. (2009). Anti-inflammatory properties of curcumin, a major constituent of *Curcuma longa*: a review of preclinical and clinical research. *Alternative Medicine Review : a Journal of Clinical Therapeutic* 14 (2):141–153.

Kanitkar, M. and Bhonde, R. R. (2008). Curcumin treatment enhances islet recovery by induction of heat shock response proteins, Hsp70 and heme oxygenase-1, during cryopreservation. *Life Sciences* 82 (3–4):182–189. doi:10.1016/J.LFS.2007.10.026.

Kheiripour, N., Khodamoradi, Z., Ranjbar, A., and Borzouei, S. (2021). The positive effect of short-term nano-curcumin therapy on insulin resistance and serum levels of afamin in patients with metabolic syndrome. *Avicenna Journal of Phytomedicine* 11 (2):146–153. doi:10.22038/AJP.2020.16698.

Lebda, M. A., Elmassry, I. H., Taha, N. M., and Elfeky, M. S. (2021). Nanocurcumin alleviates inflammation and oxidative stress in LPS-induced mastitis via activation of Nrf2 and suppressing TLR4-mediated NF-κB and HMGB1 signaling pathways in rats. *Environmental Science and Pollution Research* 29 (6):8294–8305. doi:10.1007/S11356-021-16309-9.

Luo, H., Lu, L., Liu, N., Li, Q., Yang, X., and Zhang, Z. (2021). Curcumin loaded sub-30 nm targeting therapeutic lipid nanoparticles for synergistically blocking nasopharyngeal cancer growth and metastasis. *Journal of Nanobiotechnology* 19 (1):1–14. doi:10.1186/S12951-021-00966-6/FIGURES/6.

Majumdar, S. and Keller, A. A. (2021). Omics to address the opportunities and challenges of nanotechnology in agriculture. *Critical Reviews in Environmental Science and Technology* 51:2595–2636. doi:10.1080/10643389.2020.1785264.

Meghana, K., Sanjeev, G., and Ramesh, B. (2007). Curcumin prevents streptozotocin-induced islet damage by scavenging free radicals: a prophylactic and protective role. *European journal of pharmacology* 577 (1–3):183–191. doi:10.1016/J.EJPHAR.2007.09.002.

Momtazi-Borojeni, A. A., Ghasemi, F., Hesari, A., Majeed, M., Caraglia, M., and Sahebkar, A. (2018). Anti-Cancer and Radio-Sensitizing Effects of Curcumin in Nasopharyngeal Carcinoma. *Current Pharmaceutical Design* 24 (19):2121–2128. doi:10.2174/1381612824666180522105202.

Moutabian, H., Ghahramani-Asl, R., Mortezazadeh, T., Laripour, R., Narmani, A., Zamani, H., Ataei, G., Bagheri, H., Farhood, B., Sathyapalan, T., and Sahebkar, A. (2022). The cardioprotective effects of nano-curcumin against doxorubicin-induced cardiotoxicity: A systematic review. *BioFactors* 48 (3):597–610. doi:10.1002/BIOF. 1823.

Mukhopadhyay, A., Basu, N., Ghatak, N., and Gujral, P. K. (1982). Anti-inflammatory and irritant activities of curcumin analogues in rats. *Agents and actions* 12 (4):508–515. doi:10.1007/BF01965935.

Nagraik, R., Sharma, A., Kumar, D., Mukherjee, S., Sen, F., and Kumar, A. P. (2021). Amalgamation of biosensors and nanotechnology in disease diagnosis: Mini-review. *Sensors International* 2:100089. doi:10.1016/J.SINTL.2021.100089.

Negahdari, R., Ghavimi, M. A., Barzegar, A., Memar, M. Y., Balazadeh, L., Bohlouli, S., Sharifi, S., and Maleki Dizaj, S. (2021). Antibacterial effect of nanocurcumin inside the implant fixture: An in vitro study. *Clinical and Experimental Dental Research* 7 (2):163–169. doi:10.1002/CRE2.348.

Packiavathy, I. A. S. V., Priya, S., Pandian, S. K., and Ravi, A. V. (2014). Inhibition of biofilm development of uropathogens by curcumin - An anti-quorum sensing agent from *Curcuma longa*. *Food Chemistry* 148:453–460. doi:10.1016/j.foodchem.2012.08.002.

Pari, L. and Murugan, P. (2005). Effect of tetrahydrocurcumin on blood glucose, plasma insulin and hepatic key enzymes in streptozotocin induced diabetic rats. *Journal of basic and clinical physiology and pharmacology* 16 (4):257–274. doi:10.1515/JBCPP.2005.16.4.257.

Raj, S., Jose, S., Sumod, U. S., and Sabitha, M. (2012). Nanotechnology in cosmetics: Opportunities and challenges. *Journal of Pharmacy & Bioallied Sciences* 4 (3):186. doi:10.4103/0975-7406.99016.

Ramesh, G., Kaviyil, J. E., Paul, W., Sasi, R., and Joseph, R. (2022). Gallium–Curcumin Nanoparticle Conjugates as an Antibacterial Agent against Pseudomonas aeruginosa: Synthesis and Characterization. *ACS Omega*. doi:10.1021/ACSOMEGA.1C06398.

Reda, F. M., El-Saadony, M. T., Elnesr, S. S., Alagawany, M., and Tufarelli, V. (2020). Effect of Dietary Supplementation of Biological Curcumin Nanoparticles on Growth and Carcass Traits, Antioxidant Status, Immunity and Caecal Microbiota of Japanese Quails. *Animals* 10 (5):754. doi:10.3390/ANI10050754.

Reddy, D. N. K., Huang, F.-Y., Wang, S.-P., and Kumar, R. (2020). Synergistic Antioxidant and Antibacterial Activity of Curcumin-C3 Encapsulated Chitosan Nanoparticles. *Current Pharmaceutical Design* 26 (39):5021–5029. doi:10.2174/1381612826666200609164830.

Rudrappa, T. and Bais, H. P. (2008). Curcumin, a known phenolic from *Curcuma longa*, attenuates the virulence of Pseudomonas aeruginosa PAO1 in whole plant and animal pathogenicity models. *Journal of Agricultural and Food Chemistry* 56 (6):1955–1962. doi:10.1021/jf072591j.

Sarawi, W. S., Alhusaini, A. M., Fadda, L. M., Alomar, H. A., Albaker, A. B., Aljrboa, A. S., Alotaibi, A. M., Hasan, I. H., and Mahmoud, A. M. (2021). Nano-Curcumin Prevents Cardiac Injury, Oxidative Stress and Inflammation, and Modulates TLR4/NF-κB and MAPK Signaling in Copper Sulfate-Intoxicated Rats. *Antioxidants* 10 (9):1414. doi:10.3390/ANTIOX10091414.

Shamsi-Goushki, A., Mortazavi, Z., Mirshekar, M. A., Mohammadi, M., Moradi-Kor, N., Jafari-Maskouni, S., and Shahraki, M. (2020). Comparative Effects of Curcumin versus Nano-Curcumin on Insulin Resistance, Serum Levels of Apelin and Lipid Profile in Type 2 Diabetic Rats. *Diabetes, Metabolic Syndrome and Obesity: Targets and Therapy* 13:2337. doi:10.2147/DMSO.S247351.

Shlar, I., Droby, S., and Rodov, V. (2017). Modes of antibacterial action of curcumin under dark and light conditions: A toxicoproteomics approach. *Journal of Proteomics* 160:8–20. doi:10.1016/j.jprot.2017.03.008.

Shome, S., Talukdar, A. Das, Choudhury, M. D., Bhattacharya, M. K., and Upadhyaya, H. (2016). Curcumin as potential therapeutic natural product: a nanobiotechnological perspective. *Journal of pharmacy and pharmacology* 68 (12):1481–1500. doi:10.1111/jphp.12611.

Shome, S., Talukdar, A. Das, Tewari, S., Choudhury, S., Bhattacharya, M. K., and Upadhyaya, H. (2021a). Conjugation of micro/nanocurcumin particles to ZnO nanoparticles changes the surface charge and hydrodynamic size thereby enhancing its antibacterial activity against Escherichia coli and Staphylococcus aureus. *Biotechnology and Applied Biochemistry* 68 (3):603–615. doi:10.1002/BAB.1968.

Shome, S., Talukdar, A. Das, and Upadhyaya, H. (2021b). Antibacterial activity of curcumin and its essential nanoformulations against some clinically important bacterial pathogens: A comprehensive review. *Biotechnology and applied biochemistry* 1–30. doi:10.1002/BAB.2289.

Singh, T., Shukla, S., Kumar, P., Wahla, V., and Bajpai, V. K. (2017). Application of nanotechnology in food science: Perception and overview. *Frontiers in Microbiology* 8 (AUG):1–7. doi:10.3389/FMICB.2017.01501/BIBTEX.

Stephen, B. J., Suchanti, S., Mishra, R., and Singh, A. (2020). Cancer Nanotechnology in Medicine: A Promising Approach for Cancer Detection and Diagnosis. *Critical Reviews™ in Therapeutic Drug Carrier Systems* 37 (4):375–405. doi:10.1615/CRITREVTHERDRUGCARRIERSYST.2020032634.

Sung, H., Ferlay, J., Siegel, R. L., Laversanne, M., Soerjomataram, I., Jemal, A., and Bray, F. (2021). Global Cancer Statistics 2020: GLOBOCAN Estimates of Incidence and Mortality Worldwide for 36 Cancers in 185 Countries. *CA: A Cancer Journal for Clinicians* 71 (3):209–249. doi:10.3322/CAAC.21660.

Suresh, S., Sankar, P., Telang, A. G., Kesavan, M., and Sarkar, S. N. (2018). Nanocurcumin ameliorates Staphylococcus aureus-induced mastitis in mouse by suppressing NF-κB signaling and inflammation. *International Immunopharmacology* 65:408–412. doi:10.1016/J.INTIMP.2018.10.034.

Talebi, S., Safarian, M., Jaafari, M. R., Sayedi, S. J., Abbasi, Z., Ranjbar, G., and Kianifar, H. R. (2021). The effects of nano-curcumin as a nutritional strategy on clinical and inflammatory factors in children with cystic fibrosis: the study protocol for a randomized controlled trial. *Trials* 22 (1):1–11. doi:10.1186/S13063-021-05224-6/FIGURES/2.

Targhi, A. A., Moammeri, A., Jamshidifar, E., Abbaspour, K., Sadeghi, S., Lamakani, L., and Akbarzadeh, I. (2021). Synergistic effect of curcumin-Cu and curcumin-Ag nanoparticle loaded niosome: Enhanced antibacterial and anti-biofilm activities. *Bioorganic Chemistry* 115:105116. doi:10.1016/J.BIOORG.2021.105116.

Tyagi, P., Singh, M., Kumari, H., Kumari, A., and Mukhopadhyay, K. (2015). Bactericidal activity of curcumin I is associated with damaging of bacterial membrane. *PLoS ONE* 10 (3):1–15. doi:10.1371/journal.pone.0121313.

US7273630B2 - Process for cleaning and disinfecting food products - Google Patents (n.d.). Available at https://patents.google.com/patent/US7273630B2/en (Accessed 7 July 2020).

Valizadeh, H., Abdolmohammadi-vahid, S., Danshina, S., Ziya Gencer, M., Ammari, A., Sadeghi, A., Roshangar, L., Aslani, S., Esmaeilzadeh, A., Ghaebi, M., Valizadeh, S., and Ahmadi, M. (2020). Nano-curcumin therapy, a promising method in modulating inflammatory cytokines in COVID-19 patients. *International Immunopharmacology* 89:1–12. doi:10.1016/J.INTIMP.2020.107088.

Varaprasad, K., Yallapu, M. M., Núñez, D., Oyarzún, P., López, M., Jayaramudu, T., and Karthikeyan, C. (2019). Generation of engineered core–shell antibiotic nanoparticles. *RSC Advances* 9 (15):8326–8332. doi:10.1039/C9RA00536F.

Varudkar, H. A., Umadevi, G., Nagaraju, P., Dargad, J. S., and Mote, V. D. (2020). Fabrication of Al-doped ZnO nanoparticles and their application as a semiconductor-based gas sensor for the detection of ammonia. *Journal of Materials Science: Materials in Electronics 2020 31:15* 31:12579–12585. doi:10.1007/S10854-020-03808-7.

Wong, K. V., Perilla, N., and Paddon, A. (2014). Nanoscience and Nanotechnology in Solar Cells. *Journal of Energy Resources Technology* 136 (1):1–9. doi:10.1115/1.4024715.

Xue, B., Huang, J., Zhang, H., Li, B., Xu, M., Zhang, Y., Xie, M., and Li, X. (2020). Micronized curcumin fabricated by supercritical CO2 to improve antibacterial activity against Pseudomonas aeruginosa. *Artificial Cells, Nanomedicine, and Biotechnology* 48 (1):1135–1143. doi:10.1080/21691401.2020.1815755.

Yallapu, M. M., Ebeling, M. C., Khan, S., Sundram, V., Chauhan, N., Gupta, B. K., Puumala, S. E., Jaggi, M., and Chauhan, S. C. (2013). Novel curcumin-loaded magnetic nanoparticles for pancreatic cancer treatment. *Molecular Cancer Therapeutics* 12 (8):1471–1480. doi:10.1158/1535-7163.MCT-12-1227/84858/AM/NOVEL-CURCUMIN-LOADED-MAGNETIC-NANOPARTICLES-FOR.

Yetisen, A. K., Qu, H., Manbachi, A., Butt, H., Dokmeci, M. R., Hinestroza, J. P., Skorobogatiy, M., Khademhosseini, A., and Yun, S. H. (2016). Nanotechnology in Textiles. *ACS Nano* 10 (3):3042–3068. doi:10.1021/acsnano.5b08176.

You Must Eat Fresh Turmeric Pickle Daily, Read Its Amazing Benefits (n.d.). Available at https://www.onlymyhealth.com/health-benefits-of-eating-turmeric-pickle-and-recipe-1587616156 (Accessed 7 July 2020).

Yun, D. G. and Lee, D. G. (2016). Antibacterial activity of curcumin via apoptosis-like response in Escherichia coli. *Applied Microbiology and Biotechnology* 100 (12):5505–5514. doi:10.1007/s00253-016-7415-x.

Zhang, J. Y., Lin, M. T., Zhou, M. J., Yi, T., Tang, Y. N., Tang, S. L., Yang, Z. J., Zhao, Z. Z., and Chen, H. B. (2015). Combinational Treatment of Curcumin and Quercetin against Gastric Cancer MGC-803 Cells in Vitro. *Molecules* 20 (6):11524–11534. doi:10.3390/MOLECULES200611524.

Chapter 8

Promises and Challenges of Curcumin

Gulmi Chakraborty[1,2] and Soumen Ghosh[1,*]

[1]Centre for Surface Science, Physical Chemistry Section, Department of Chemistry, Jadavpur University, Kolkata, West Bengal, India
[2]Department of Chemistry, C.V. Raman Global University, Odisha, India

Abstract

Turmeric (*Curcuma longa* L. (Zingiberaceae)) is a popular spice with medicinal properties that has been extensively used in Ayurveda and Chinese traditional medicine for centuries. Curcumin or [(E,E)-1,7-bis(4-hydroxy-3-methoxy-phenyl)-1,6-heptadiene-3,5-ione] is the active component of turmeric and is widely used in the pharmaceutical industry. It is a highly versatile pigment with medicinal properties viz., anticancer, anti-inflammatory, anti-microbial and so on. Curcumin absorbs strongly near 425 nm and, due to its ligand binding properties, it has found extensive use in textile industry as well. It also exhibits strong emission near 570 nm which makes it an excellent choice for cellular imaging and spectroscopic study. However, despite such multifold applications, one of the greatest challenges posed in the application of curcumin is its poor bioavailability. Being a phenolic moiety, curcumin is predominantly hydrophobic which limits its availability in aqueous or biological media. Research is now being focused upon developing media such as microemulsions, mixed micelle systems etc., to increase the solubility of curcumin. This review gives an overview of the application of curcumin in health, the existing challenges in relation to bioavailability of curcumin and current research being done to overcome the same.

---

[*] Corresponding Author's Email: gsoumen70@hotmail.com.

In: Curcumin and Its Role in Health and Disease
Editor: Kathryn Woltjer
ISBN: 979-8-88697-491-1

Introduction

Curcumin is a natural polyphenolic compound derived from the powdered rhizome of turmeric, also known as *Curcuma longa.* For thousands of years, turmeric has been actively studied in Ayurveda and Chinese medicine [1, 2]. That the active component of turmeric is curcumin was discovered only around two centuries ago [3]. Curcumin has the unique ability to modulate important molecular targets such as cytokines [4], cell cycle proteins [5], receptors [6], enzymes [7] etc. As a result, it has far reaching effects in the treatment of arthritis [8], diabetes [9], Crohn's disease [10], autodegerative cardiovascular diseases [11] etc. Apart from these, curcumin is also widely studied due to its remarkable anti-inflammatory and cancer-preventive properties. Curcumin is found to constrain cancerous growth in various cancer models both alone and when combined with other plant-derived phenolic compounds [12]. Anticancerous properties of curcumin includes inhibition of angiogenesis by limiting the blood supply to malignant cancerous cells [13], stimulating Phase I and Phase II detox systems, e.g., inhibition of COX-1 and COX-2 enzymes and glutathione S-transferase [14], inhibition of protein kinases [15], etc. Curcumin neutralizes carcinogenic free radicals such as, the reactive oxygen species (ROS, viz., superoxide, peroxyl and hydroxyl radicals) [16, 17] or nitric oxide, peroxynitrite etc., via H-atom donation form its phenolic sites [18] While phenolic moiety is generally considered chemically responsible for the free radical scavenging, H-atom donation from the β-diketone moiety of curcumin to lipid peroxyl radical or alkyl lipid radical is also considered potential cause for the observed antioxidant activity of curcumin [19].

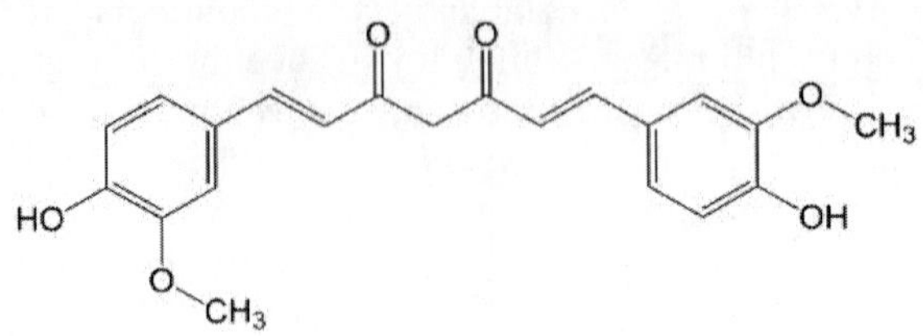

Scheme 1. Chemical structure of curcumin.

The IUPAC name for curcumin is (E,E)-1,7-bis(4-hydroxy-3-methoxy-phenyl)-1,6-heptadiene-3,5-ione]; besides, 1,7-bis(4-hydroxy-3-methoxyphenyl)-1,6-heptadiene-3,5-dione and/or diferuloylmethane are also used to denote the same. It consists of two phenolic rings with an acidic H (Scheme 1). Its taxonomy is as follows:

Class	Liliopsida
Subclass	Commelinids
Order	Zingiberales
Family	Zingiberaceae
Genus	Curcuma

Promises of Curcumin

Curcumin has been extensively employed in the treatment of inflammation [20], oxidative stress [21], eye diseases [22], and diseases concerning the central nervous system, such as, Alzheimer's disease [23], Dejerine-Sottas disease [24], depression [25], anxiety [26], respiratory diseases [27], cardiovascular protection [28, 29] gastrointestinal diseases[30], and as discussed, in the different forms of cancer [31]. Excellent literature is available on clinical trials of curcumin in the treatment of various diseases [32]. Due to the hydrophobic nature of curcumin, bioavailability remains one of the major challenges in harnessing its potential therapeutic effects [33], and great emphasis is now placed on improving curcumin absorption through various modified agencies.

Curcumin: A Potential Antiviral against SARS-CoV-2

Since 'severe acute respiratory syndrome coronavirus' or 2SARS-CoV-2 was first identified in Wuhan, China, in latter part of 2019, its unprecedented spread has led to one of the most serious pandemics in human history. SARS-CoV-2 mainly targets tissues that express high levels of Angiotensin-Converting Enzyme 2 or ACE2 – the human receptor that the virus uses to gain host cell entry. Since the airways express high levels of ACE2, individuals who experience severe disease often develop viral pneumonia or acute respiratory distress syndrome leading to respiratory failure. SARS-CoV-2 is an enveloped β-coronavirus composed of four structural proteins: spike (S), envelope (E), membrane (M), and nucleocapsid (N) proteins [34]. Several recent studies have suggested that natural polyphenolic compounds like catechins (GTCs; Green Tea Catechins) and curcumin (diferuloylmethane; from turmeric) have antiviral activities against a broad spectrum of viruses such as Human Immunodeficiency Virus (HIV), Herpes Simplex Virus, Influenza Virus, Hepatitis B and C Viruses (HBV and HCV respectively) [35], Adenovirus [36] and Chikungunya virus [37].

During the SARS-CoV-2 infection, an enhanced number of Th17 cells and their related inflammatory responses mediated by the production of interleukin (IL)-17, IL-21, IL-22, and granulocyte-macrophage colony-stimulating factor (GM-CSF) cytokines elicit the cytokine storm, which is followed by hyper-inflammation, respiratory system dysfunction, and acute respiratory distress syndrome (ARDS). On the other hand, dysfunction of regulatory T (Treg) cells and disturbance ratio of T helper (Th) 17/Treg cells are considered to be other important causes for disease progression [38] Before and after treatment, Th17 cell-related factors (RAR-related orphan receptor γt, interleukin [IL]-17, IL-21, IL-23, and granulocyte-macrophage colony-stimulating factor), and the serum levels of cytokines were measured in both nanocurcumin and placebo-treated groups. A significant decrease in the number of Th17 cells, down regulation of Th17 cell-related factors, and decreased levels of Th17 cell-related cytokines were found in mild and severe COVID-19 patients treated by nanocurcumin compared to the placebo group. Moreover, the above mentioned parameters were significantly decreased in the nanocurcumin-treated group after treatment versus before treatment. Curcumin could reduce the frequency of Th17 cells and their related inflammatory factors in both mild and severe COVID-19 patients [39].

In another study headed by Valizadeh et al., it was observed that the mRNA expression and cytokine secretion of IL-1β, IL-6, TNF-α, and IL-18 were significantly increased in COVID-19 patients compared with the healthy control group. After treatment with Nano-curcumin, a significant decrease in IL-6 expression and secretion in serum and in supernatant ($P = 0.0003$, 0.0038, and 0.0001, respectively) and IL-1β gene expression and secretion level in serum and supernatant ($P = 0.0017$, 0.0082, and 0.0041, respectively) was observed. However, nano-curcumin had no effect on IL-18 mRNA expression and TNF-α concentration [40]. It was concluded that nano-curcumin, as an anti-inflammatory herbal-based agent, is capable of modulating the increased rate of inflammatory cytokines especially IL-1β and IL-6 mRNA expression and cytokine secretion in COVID-19 patients, which may cause an improvement in clinical manifestation and overall recovery. Assessment of in-vivo examination of curcumin suspension in anionic surfactants and synthesised bi-cells have demonstrated potential cytotoxicity against Vero E6 cells [41].

Curcumin-loaded functionalized carbon quantum dots have been recently reported to have potential antiviral properties [42, 43]. The immunimodulatory and anticytokine potential of hydrazinocurcumin was revealed from a docking study with target proteins ACE2 and PAR-1 [44]. Further molecular docking studies revealed that specific binding of curcumin with ACE2 receptor which has high potential to compete with the spike protein of SARS-CoV-2 inhibiting its membrane fusion and consequent endocytosis [45].

Inflammation

The nuclear factor NF-κB which regulates the expression of Kappa light chain in mature β cells and plasma cells [46] is expressed in almost all tissues and cells [47]. Studies show that NF-κB activation is translated to situation-specific response and is responsible for the expression of pro-inflammatory genes such as cytokines, chemokines, and adhesion molecules [48]. Curcumin is able to decrease the NF-κB pathway along with other vital pathways such as cyclooxygenase (COX) and lipoxygenase pathways reducing cytokine levels and decreasing production of prostaglandin, a lipid compound responsible for inflammation [49, 50]. In a study of Trinitrobenzene sulfonate (TNBS) induced colitis in mice, it was found that treatment with curcumin both prevented and improved the histopathological signs of colon inflammation with suppressed $CD4^+$ T cells infiltration and NF-κB activation in the colonic mucosa [51]. Furthermore, attenuation of epidermal swelling induced by 2,4,6-trinitrochlorobenzene (TNBC) was observed upon treatment with curcumin, which is found to inhibit epigen and amphiregulin [52]. which are peptides responsible for inflammation [53]. The $CD4^+$ T cells play vital role in the regulation of effective immunity against pathogens and a perturbation of its balance is known to cause inflammatory bowel disease [54]. A clinical trial on over 50 patients showed that curcumin combined with mesalamine is a superior treatment of ulcerative colitis (UC) compared to mesalamine and placebo and induced clinical and endoscopic remission in cases with mild-to-moderate UC [55, 56]. Other clinical trials as well as laboratory studies have validated the safe use of curcumin as an anti-inflammatory agent without any adverse side effects [57, 58].

Oxidative Stress

Reactive oxygen species (ROS) such as free radicals such as hydroxyl radical (OH•), oxide anion radicals (O_2^{2-} •) and non-radical species such as hydrogen peroxide (H_2O_2) and singlet oxygen ($^1O_2$) are highly reactive molecules which are produced as by-products during normal cellular metabolism and cause potential damage to living tissues if not scavenged [59, 60]. Oxidative stress is defined as a disruption in the balance of free radicals (reactive oxygen species) and antioxidant defenses [61]. Adverse effects of oxidative stress include lipid peroxidation causing multiple sclerosis [62], neurodegenerative disorders like Alzheimer's disease and Parkinson's disease [63], cardio-vascular diseases like hypertension, congestive heart failures etc. [64], to name a few, along with DNA oxidation and protein oxidation [61].

Curcumin is widely studied for its eminent antioxidant properties viz., free radical scavenging, metal chelation, etc. Curcumin prevents the oxidative degradation of lipids by peroxides via free electron donation [60]. Curcumin actively forms metal chelate with the Fe^{2+} ion and prevents ferrous to ferric oxidation [65] (Scheme 2).

The heptadienone moiety of curcumin exhibits keto-enol tautomerism (Scheme 3) i.e., under neutral and acidic conditions, the keto form is dominant, which is an extremely potential H-atom donor [60, 66]. A laboratory test with hydrogen peroxide scavenging assay has shown that curcumin possesses strong scavenging ability. Curcumin at 15 μg/mL can scavenge 28.4 ± 3.9% H_2O_2, which is greater than the traditional efficient scavenger Trolox (6-hydroxy-2,5,7,8-tetramethylchroman-2-carboxylic acid) i.e., 25.6 ± 3.3% [60].

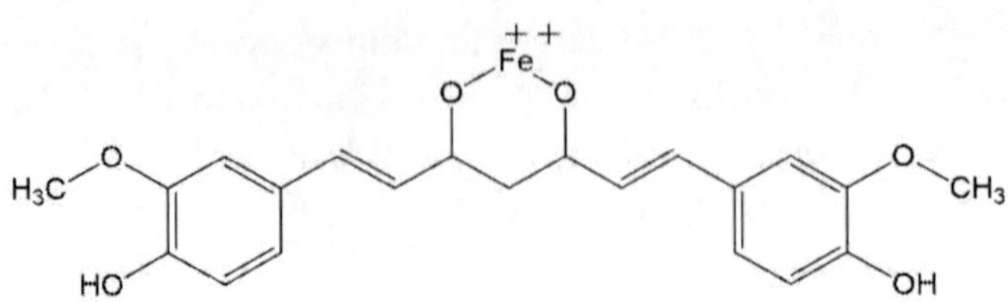

Scheme 2. Curcumin-Fe^{2+} chelate complex.

The antioxidant property of curcumin is used in treatment of knee osteoarthritis (OA) in patients with metabolic syndrome (MetS) [67]. The MetS include central obesity, dyslipidemia or abnormal amount of blood lipid, impaired fasting glucose and hypertension. Treatment with curcumin significantly lowered superoxide dismutase (SOD) activity and enhanced plasma total antioxidant capacity, which reduced oxidative stress [49]. A powerful inhibitory effect of curcumin against damage in human keratinocytes and fibroblasts induced by H_2O_2 has been reported [68].

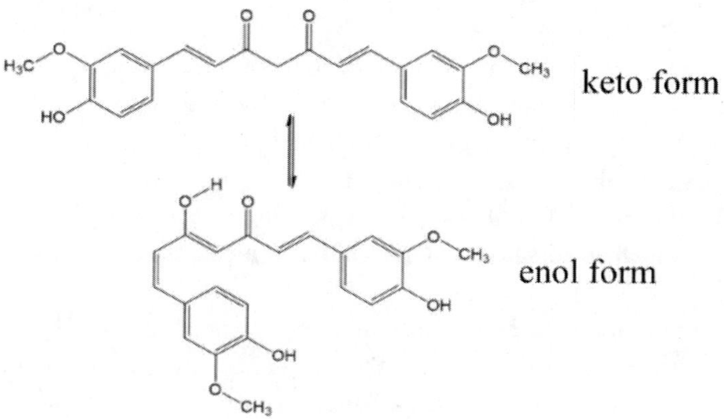

Scheme 3. Keto-enol tautomerism of curcumin.

Curcumin and Cancer

Despite tremendous advancements in research and medical science, cancer remains one of the most important public health problems all over the world. Increasingly, research is being focused on identifying and developing natural sources to combat cancer [69]. Curcumin was found to strongly induce apoptosis on the breast cancer cell line MDA-MB-231 and reduce IκB and p65 phosphorylation, resulting in decreased activation of the NF-κB pathway in an *in vitro* study [70]. Dietary administration of commercial curcumin, i.e., 77% curcumin, 17% demethoxycurcumin, and 3% bisdemethoxycurcumin can reduce the size of carcinogen benzo(a)pyrene-induced forestomach tumors in C57BL/6 mice by up to 67%, N-ethyl-N′-nitro-N-nitrosoguanidine-induced duodenal tumor growth in C57BL/6 mice up to 77% and azoxymethane (AOM) induced colon tumor in CF1 mice by up to 66%, with doses as low as 2% [71]. Another study on AOM-induced carcinoma in male F344 rats showed that oral administration of 2000 ppm of curcumin could significantly inhibit adenocarcinomas and reduce the multiplicity of both invasive and non-invasive adenocarcinomas [72]. Therefore dietary chemoprevention of curcumin is strongly recommended since dissemination of metastatic cells occur long before diagnosis of the primary tumor.

The fibroblast growth factors (FGFs) or signaling proteins are responsible for the formation of new endothelial cells or proliferation of the same [73]. Curcumin and its derivatives (0.5-10 μM) viz., tetrahydrocurcumin, bisdemethoxycurcumin and demethoxycurcumin have shown to inhibit basic fibroblast growth factor (bFGF) induced proliferation in bovine capillary endothelial cell lines and inhibit corneal neovascularization in C57BL6 male mice, which suggests that curcumin and its derivatives act as potent *in vivo* angiogenesis inhibitors [13]. In another study, curcumin (5-20 μmol/L) was found to suppress differentiation in 3T3-L1 adipocyte cell lines and caused inhibition as well as apostasies of adipokine-induced angiogenesis in epithelial cells of human umbilical veins [74].

Excellent literature on successful clinical trials of curcumin as chemo preventive agents are available [75, 76, 77]. A clinical trial on human patients with pre-malignant lesions has established that oral consumption of curcumin up to a dose of 8000 gm/day for up to three months is non-toxic while being chemo preventive [78].

Challenges: Poor Bioavailability and Overcoming Strategy

Curcumin is the most active lipophilic polyphenol compound constituting 2-5% of turmeric which is primarily responsible for the medicinal benefits. Synthetic analogues of curcumin viz., sodium curcuminate, diacetyl curcumin, triethylcurcumin and tetrahydrocurcumin have potent medicinal activity [79]. Due to its rapid metabolism and fast elimination from the body, curcumin is poorly absorbed within the body and its availability is curtailed [80]. Moreover, the route of administration of curcumin plays an important role in dictating its bioavailability [81]. A study has found that oral administration of curcumin leads to >20% intracellular accumulation, resulting in poor availability in serum [82]. In recent years, more emphasis has been made on enhancing the bioavailability of curcumin to meet the potential medicinal benefits. These include encapsulation of curcumin in molecular aggregates viz., liposome [83], micelles [84], vesicles [85] etc., of surface active agents etc.

Nanoparticle Suspension

The homogeneous small size (208-246 nm) nanosuspension (NS) of curcumin in the presence of d-α-Tocopherol polyethylene glycol 1000 succinate (TPGS) stabilizer has been shown to have enhanced the solubility of curcumin from 0.6 μg/mL in pure water to 260 μg/mL in the NS (curcumin:TPGS 1:10) [86]. Solid dispersion systems of curcumin with Polyvinylpyrrolidone (PVP) (1:9) are reported to highly improve the solubility of and bio-absorption of curcumin [87, 88]. The PVP bound curcumin shows promising antibacterial efficiency via photodynamic inactivation [89]. A 50 μM concentration of PVP - curcumin with an incubation period of 15-20 min is found to completely eradicate the Gram (+) bacteria *Staphylococcus aureus,* while in the case of Gram (-) bacteria *Escherichia coli*, a significant drop in the bacterial count was obtained in the presence of $CaCl_2$ as sensitizer [89].

Piperine loaded cubosome nanoparticles (mean size 153 nm) have been found to significantly improve oral bioavailability and tissue distribution of curcumin compared to suspension of curcumin and piperine and bioabsorption especially in the spleen [90].

Micellar Composition

The micellar conjugate of poly lactic acid (PLA) via a hydrophobic Tris(hydroxymethyl) aminomethane (Tris) block that binds with the drug and a hydrophilic block (methoxy-poly(ethylene glycol) (mPEG), has been shown to be a highly efficient curcumin carrier with improved intracellular delivery and chemo preventive activity on human hepatocellular carcinoma (HepG2) [84].

Another micellar composition of methoxypoly(ethylene glycol)-b-poly(ε-caprolactone-co-p-dioxanone) [MPEG-P(CL-co-PDO)] copolymers have been found to demonstrate high encapsulation efficiency (>95%) for curcumin and effectively inhibit the cancerous growth in PC-3 human prostate cancer cells in a dose-dependent manner [91]. A 900-fold increase in solubility of curcumin compared to that in aqueous medium was observed when conjugated to the highly water soluble polysaccharide, gum arabic, while the curcumin-gum arabic conjugate showed profound anticancer activity against human hepatocellular carcinoma cells (HepG2) [92].

Vesicles and Liposomes

An important molecular aggregates studied in delivery of curcumin are vesicles. Curcumin decorated phosphaditidyl choline based nanoliposomes have been reported to have high affinity towards the amyloid-β-42 peptide and be used effectively in the treatment of Alzheimer's disease [93].

Biocompatible mixed cationic vesicles of quarternary ammonium ion with long alkyl chain (n = 12 - 18) have been shown to improve the loading capacity, stability, and antioxidant properties of curcumin [94].

Curcumin bioavailability enhancement to meet medicinal benefits is still being researched extensively [95].

Coating liposomal curcumin comprising soybean phosphotidylcholine, cholesterol, and D-α-tocopheryl polyethylene glycol 1000 succinate with trimethyl chitosan has resulted in a marked improvement in curcumin dissolution with entrapment efficiency (86.67%) and effective drug loading of 2.33%. The coated liposomal curcumin showed a maximum plasma concentration of 46.13 μg/L compared to 32.12 μg/L for uncoated liposomes, however, with an increased elimination of half-life of $t_{1/2}$ = 12.05 hours compared to 9.79 hrs for uncoated liposomes [96]. Another strategy to enhance liposomal bioavailability is the co-encapsulation of curcumin with other target drug molecules. The co-encapsulation of curcumin with resveratrol in a 5:1 ratio resulted in an overall entrapment efficiency of 80.4% [97]. Liposomes with curcumin co-loaded with paclitaxel showed enhanced cytotoxicity against cancer cell and induced significantly higher earlier and late apostasies compared to singly loaded curcumin liposomes [98]. Curcumin encapsulated in phosphatidylcholine measuring up to 200 nm showed a significantly higher anti-inflammatory response compared to non-liposomal curcuminoids [99]. Cyclodextrin encapsulated curcumin has been found to induce apoptotic cell death in tissue cancer cells and has been effectively used as a drug carrier in the treatment of osteosarcoma [100].

Conclusion

Curcumin has been used as a therapeutic agent in traditional medicine for many decades. In the recent years, it has been extensively used in the treatment of a number of physiological conditions as well as in treatment of cancer. The biggest hurdle in the applicative aspect of curcumin is the bioavailability which is highly restricted due to its hydrophobic nature. The present chapter provides an overview of the health benefits of curcumin and an understanding of current approaches for increasing the bioavailability of curcumin for its use in the pharmaceutical industry.

Acknowledgment

GC thanks DST-SERB for the NPDF fellowship (File no. PDF/2018/001014).

Conflict of Interest

There are no conflicts of interest to declare.

References

[1] Ammon, H. P. T., Wahl, M. A., Pharmacology of *Curcuma longa*. *Planta Med* 1991, 57 (01), 1-7.

[2] Shishodia, S., Sethi, G., Aggarwal, B. B., Curcumin: Getting Back to the Roots. *Annals of the New York Academy of Sciences* 2005, 1056 (1), 206-217.

[3] Gupta, S. C., Patchva, S., Koh, W., Aggarwal, B. B., Discovery of curcumin, a component of golden spice, and its miraculous biological activities. *Clinical and Experimental Pharmacology and Physiology* 2012, 39 (3), 283-299.

[4] Jobin, C., Bradham, C. A., Russo, M. P., Juma, B., Narula, A. S., Brenner, D. A., Sartor, R. B., Curcumin Blocks Cytokine-Mediated NF-κB Activation and Proinflammatory Gene Expression by Inhibiting Inhibitory Factor I-κB Kinase Activity. *The Journal of Immunology* 1999, 163 (6), 3474.

[5] Moragoda, L., Jaszewski, R., Majumdar, A. P., Curcumin induced modulation of cell cycle and apoptosis in gastric and colon cancer cells. *Anticancer Res* 2001, 21 (2A), 873-878.

[6] Wang, R., Xu, Y., Wu, H. L., Li, Y. B., Li, Y. H., Guo, J. B., Li, X. J., The antidepressant effects of curcumin in the forced swimming test involve 5-HT1 and 5-HT2 receptors. *European Journal of Pharmacology* 2008, 578 (1), 43-50.

[7] Mitra, S. P., Binding and stability of curcumin in presence of bovine serum albumin. *Journal of Surface Science and Technology* 2007, 23(3-4), 91-110.

[8] Jackson, J. K., Higo, T., Hunter, W. L., Burt, H. M., The antioxidants curcumin and quercetin inhibit inflammatory processes associated with arthritis. *Inflammation Research* 2006, 55 (4), 168-175.

[9] Chiu, J., Khan, Z. A., Farhangkhoee, H., Chakrabarti, S., Curcumin prevents diabetes-associated abnormalities in the kidneys by inhibiting p300 and nuclear factor-κB. *Nutrition* 2009, 25 (9), 964-972.

[10] Aggarwal, B. B., Sung, B., Pharmacological basis for the role of curcumin in chronic diseases: an age-old spice with modern targets. *Trends in Pharmacological Sciences* 2009, 30 (2), 85-94.

[11] Aggarwal, B. B., Harikumar, K. B., Potential therapeutic effects of curcumin, the anti-inflammatory agent, against neurodegenerative, cardiovascular, pulmonary,

metabolic, autoimmune and neoplastic diseases. *The International Journal of Biochemistry & Cell Biology* 2009, 41 (1), 40-59.

[12] Jovanovic, S. V., Boone, C. W., Steenken, S., Trinoga, M., Kaskey, R. B., How Curcumin Works Preferentially with Water Soluble Antioxidants. *Journal of the American Chemical Society* 2001, 123 (13), 3064-3068.

[13] Arbiser, J. L., Klauber, N., Rohan, R., van Leeuwen, R., Huang, M. T., Fisher, C., Flynn, E., Byers, H. R., Curcumin Is an *In Vivo* Inhibitor of Angiogenesis. *Molecular Medicine* 1998, 4 (6), 376-383.

[14] Venkatesan, N., Curcumin attenuation of acute adriamycin myocardial toxicity in rats. *British Journal of Pharmacology* 1998, 124 (3), 425-427.

[15] Hasmeda, M., Polya, G. M., Inhibition of cyclic AMP-dependent protein kinase by curcumin. *Phytochemistry* 1996, 42 (3), 599-605.

[16] Masuda, T., Hidaka, K., Shinohara, A., Maekawa, T., Takeda, Y., Yamaguchi, H., Chemical Studies on Antioxidant Mechanism of Curcuminoid: Analysis of Radical Reaction Products from Curcumin. *Journal of Agricultural and Food Chemistry* 1999, 47 (1), 71-77.

[17] Ghosh, S., Mondal, S., Spectroscopic study on the interaction of medicinal pigment curcumin with various surfactants: an overview. *Journal of Surface Science and Technology* 2012, 28, 179-195.

[18] Barzegar, A., Moosavi-Movahedi, A. A., Intracellular ROS Protection Efficiency and Free Radical-Scavenging Activity of Curcumin. *Plos One* 2011, 6 (10), e26012.

[19] Jovanovic, S. V., Steenken, S., Boone, C. W., Simic, M. G., H-Atom Transfer Is A Preferred Antioxidant Mechanism of Curcumin. *Journal of the American Chemical Society* 1999, 121 (41), 9677-9681.

[20] Ghosh, S., Banerjee, S., Sil, P. C., The beneficial role of curcumin on inflammation, diabetes and neurodegenerative disease: A recent update. *Food and Chemical Toxicology* 2015, 83, 111-124.

[21] Soetikno, V., Sari, F. R., Lakshmanan, A. P., Arumugam, S., Harima, M., Suzuki, K., Kawachi, H., Watanabe, K., Curcumin alleviates oxidative stress, inflammation, and renal fibrosis in remnant kidney through the Nrf2–keap1 pathway. *Molecular Nutrition & Food Research* 2013, 57 (9), 1649-1659.

[22] Radomska-Leśniewska, D. M., Osiecka-Iwan, A., Hyc, A., Góźdź, A., Dąbrowska, A. M., Skopiński, P., Therapeutic potential of curcumin in eye diseases. *Central European Journal of Immunology* 2019, 44 (2), 181-189.

[23] Mishra, S., Palanivelu, K., The effect of curcumin (turmeric) on <i>Alzheimer's disease</i>: An overview. *Annals of Indian Academy of Neurology* 2008, 11 (1), 13-19.

[24] Burns, J., Joseph, P. D., Rose, K. J., Ryan, M. M., Ouvrier, R. A., Effect of Oral Curcumin on Déjérine-Sottas Disease. *Pediatric Neurology* 2009, 41 (4), 305-308.

[25] Ng, Q. X., Koh, S. S. H., Chan, H. W., Ho, C. Y. X., Clinical Use of Curcumin in Depression: A Meta-Analysis. *Journal of the American Medical Directors Association* 2017, 18 (6), 503-508.

[26] Haider, S., Naqvi, F., Batool, Z., Tabassum, S., Sadir, S., Liaquat, L., Naqvi, F., Zuberi, N. A., Shakeel, H., Perveen, T., Pretreatment with curcumin attenuates

anxiety while strengthens memory performance after one short stress experience in male rats. *Brain Research Bulletin* 2015, 115, 1-8.

[27] Lelli, D., Sahebkar, A., Johnston, T. P., Pedone, C., Curcumin use in pulmonary diseases: State of the art and future perspectives. *Pharmacological Research* 2017, 115, 133-148.

[28] Venkatesan, N., Punithavathi, D., Babu, M., Protection From Acute And Chronic Lung Diseases By Curcumin. In *The Molecular Targets and Therapeutic Uses of Curcumin in Health and Disease*, Aggarwal, B. B., Surh, Y. J., Shishodia, S., Eds. Springer US: Boston, MA, 2007; pp 379-405.

[29] Wongcharoen, W., Phrommintikul, A., The protective role of curcumin in cardiovascular diseases. *International Journal of Cardiology* 2009, 133 (2), 145-151.

[30] Irving, G. R. B., Karmokar, A., Berry, D. P., Brown, K., Steward, W. P., Curcumin: The potential for efficacy in gastrointestinal diseases. *Best Practice & Research Clinical Gastroenterology* 2011, 25 (4), 519-534.

[31] Anand, P., Sundaram, C., Jhurani, S., Kunnumakkara, A. B., Aggarwal, B. B., Curcumin and cancer: An "old-age" disease with an "age-old" solution. *Cancer Letters* 2008, 267 (1), 133-164.

[32] Salehi, B., Stojanović-Radić, Z., Matejić, J., Sharifi-Rad, M., Anil Kumar, N. V., Martins, N., Sharifi-Rad, J., The therapeutic potential of curcumin: A review of clinical trials. *European Journal of Medicinal Chemistry* 2019, 163, 527-545.

[33] Prasad, S., Tyagi, A. K., Aggarwal, B. B., Recent Developments in Delivery, Bioavailability, Absorption and Metabolism of Curcumin: the Golden Pigment from Golden Spice. *Cancer Res Treat* 2014, 46 (1), 2-18.

[34] Chen, Y., Liu, Q., Guo, D., Emerging coronaviruses: Genome structure, replication, and pathogenesis. *Journal of Medical Virology* 2020, 92 (4), 418-423.

[35] Song, J. M., Anti-infective potential of catechins and their derivatives against viral hepatitis. *Clin Exp Vaccine Res* 2018, 7 (1), 37-42.

[36] Steinmann, J., Buer, J., Pietschmann, T., Steinmann, E., Anti-infective properties of epigallocatechin-3-gallate (EGCG), a component of green tea. *British Journal of Pharmacology* 2013, 168 (5), 1059-1073.

[37] Weber, C., Sliva, K., von Rhein, C., Kümmerer, B. M., Schnierle, B. S., The green tea catechin, epigallocatechin gallate inhibits chikungunya virus infection. *Antiviral Research* 2015, 113, 1-3.

[38] Tan, M., Liu, Y., Zhou, R., Deng, X., Li, F., Liang, K., Shi, Y., Immunopathological characteristics of coronavirus disease 2019 cases in Guangzhou, China. *Immunology* 2020, 160 (3), 261-268.

[39] Tahmasebi, S., El-Esawi, M. A., Mahmoud, Z. H., Timoshin, A., Valizadeh, H., Roshangar, L., Varshoch, M., Vaez, A., Aslani, S., Navashenaq, J. G., Aghebati-Maleki, L., Ahmadi, M., Immunomodulatory effects of nanocurcumin on Th17 cell responses in mild and severe COVID-19 patients. *Journal of Cellular Physiology* 2021, 236 (7), 5325-5338.

[40] Valizadeh, H., Abdolmohammadi-vahid, S., Danshina, S., Ziya Gencer, M., Ammari, A., Sadeghi, A., Roshangar, L., Aslani, S., Esmaeilzadeh, A., Ghaebi, M., Valizadeh, S., Ahmadi, M., Nano-curcumin therapy, a promising method in

modulating inflammatory cytokines in COVID-19 patients. *International Immunopharmacology* 2020, 89, 107088.

[41] Mahmoud, D. B., Bakr, M. M., Al-karmalawy, A. A., Moatasim, Y., El Taweel, A., Mostafa, A., Scrutinizing the Feasibility of Nonionic Surfactants to Form Isotropic Bicelles of Curcumin: a Potential Antiviral Candidate Against COVID-19. *AAPS Pharm Sci Tech* 2021, 23 (1), 44.

[42] Lin, C. J., Chang, L., Chu, H. W., Lin, H. J., Chang, P. C., Wang, R. Y. L., Unnikrishnan, B., Mao, J. Y., Chen, S. Y., Huang, C. C., High Amplification of the Antiviral Activity of Curcumin through Transformation into Carbon Quantum Dots. *Small* 2019, 15 (41), 1902641.

[43] Łoczechin, A., Séron, K., Barras, A., Giovanelli, E., Belouzard, S., Chen, Y. T., Metzler-Nolte, N., Boukherroub, R., Dubuisson, J., Szunerits, S., Functional Carbon Quantum Dots as Medical Countermeasures to Human Coronavirus. *ACS Applied Materials & Interfaces* 2019, 11 (46), 42964-42974.

[44] Noor, H., Ikram, A., Rathinavel, T., Kumarasamy, S., Nasir Iqbal, M., Bashir, Z., Immunomodulatory and anti-cytokine therapeutic potential of curcumin and its derivatives for treating COVID-19 – a computational modeling. *Journal of Biomolecular Structure and Dynamics* 2021, 1-16.

[45] Utomo, R. Y. I., M., Meiyanto, E., *Revealing the Potency of Citrus and Galangal Constituents to Halt SARS-CoV-2 Infection*.

[46] Sen, R., Baltimore, D., Multiple nuclear factors interact with the immunoglobulin enhancer sequences. *Cell* 1986, 46 (5), 705-716.

[47] Oeckinghaus, A., Ghosh, S., The NF-κB Family of Transcription Factors and Its Regulation. *Cold Spring Harbor Perspectives in Biology* 2009, 1 (4).

[48] Lawrence, T., The Nuclear Factor NF-κB Pathway in Inflammation. *Cold Spring Harbor Perspectives in Biology* 2009, 1 (6).

[49] Sanidad, K. Z., Sukamtoh, E., Xiao, H., McClements, D. J., Zhang, G., Curcumin: Recent Advances in the Development of Strategies to Improve Oral Bioavailability. *Annual Review of Food Science and Technology* 2019, 10 (1), 597-617.

[50] Singh, S., Aggarwal, B. B., Activation of Transcription Factor NF-κB Is Suppressed by Curcumin (Diferuloylmethane). *Journal of Biological Chemistry* 1995, 270 (42), 24995-25000.

[51] Sugimoto, K., Hanai, H., Tozawa, K., Aoshi, T., Uchijima, M., Nagata, T., Koide, Y., Curcumin prevents and ameliorates trinitrobenzene sulfonic acid–induced colitis in mice. *Gastroenterology* 2002, 123 (6), 1912-1922.

[52] Sakai, H., Sato, K., Sato, F., Kai, Y., Mandokoro, K., Matsumoto, K., Kato, S., Yumoto, T., Narita, M., Chiba, Y., Curcumin inhibits epigen and amphiregulin upregulated by 2,4,6-trinitrochlorobenzene associated with attenuation of skin swelling. *Inflammation Research* 2017, 66 (8), 663-678.

[53] Kuemmerle, J. F., Barnard, J. A., McHugh, K. M., Chapter 8 - Growth Factors in the Gastrointestinal Tract. In *Physiology of the Gastrointestinal Tract (Fifth Edition)*, Johnson, L. R., Ghishan, F. K., Kaunitz, J. D., Merchant, J. L., Said, H. M., Wood, J. D., Eds. Academic Press: Boston, 2012; pp 199-277.

[54] Imam, T., Park, S., Kaplan, M. H., Olson, M. R., Effector T Helper Cell Subsets in Inflammatory Bowel Diseases. *Frontiers in Immunology* 2018, 9, 1212.

[55] Lang, A., Salomon, N., Wu, J. C. Y., Kopylov, U., Lahat, A., Har-Noy, O., Ching, J. Y. L., Cheong, P. K., Avidan, B., Gamus, D., Kaimakliotis, I., Eliakim, R., Ng, S. C., Ben-Horin, S., Curcumin in Combination With Mesalamine Induces Remission in Patients With Mild-to-Moderate Ulcerative Colitis in a Randomized Controlled Trial. *Clinical Gastroenterology and Hepatology* 2015, 13 (8), 1444-1449.e1.

[56] Hanai, H., Iida, T., Takeuchi, K., Watanabe, F., Maruyama, Y., Andoh, A., Tsujikawa, T., Fujiyama, Y., Mitsuyama, K., Sata, M., Yamada, M., Iwaoka, Y., Kanke, K., Hiraishi, H., Hirayama, K., Arai, H., Yoshii, S., Uchijima, M., Nagata, T., Koide, Y., Curcumin Maintenance Therapy for Ulcerative Colitis: Randomized, Multicenter, Double-Blind, Placebo-Controlled Trial. *Clinical Gastroenterology and Hepatology* 2006, 4 (12), 1502-1506.

[57] Kohli, K., Ali, J., Ansari, M., Raheman, Z., Curcumin: A natural antiinflammatory agent. *Indian Journal of Pharmacology* 2005, 37 (3), 141-147.

[58] Holt, P. R., Katz, S., Kirshoff, R., Curcumin Therapy in Inflammatory Bowel Disease: A Pilot Study. *Digestive Diseases and Sciences* 2005, 50 (11), 2191-2193.

[59] Birben, E., Sahiner, U. M., Sackesen, C., Erzurum, S., Kalayci, O., Oxidative Stress and Antioxidant Defense. *World Allergy Organization Journal* 2012, 5 (1), 9-19.

[60] Ak, T., Gülçin, İ., Antioxidant and radical scavenging properties of curcumin. *Chemico-Biological Interactions* 2008, 174 (1), 27-37.

[61] Betteridge, D. J., What is oxidative stress? *Metabolism* 2000, 49 (2, Supplement 1), 3-8.

[62] Toshniwal, P. K., Zarling, E. J., Evidence for increased lipid peroxidation in multiple sclerosis. *Neurochemical Research* 1992, 17 (2), 205-207.

[63] Sayre, L. M., Smith, M. A., Perry, G., Chemistry and Biochemistry of Oxidative Stress in Neurodegenerative Disease. *Current Medicinal Chemistry* 2001, 8 (7), 721-738.

[64] Dhalla, N. S., Temsah, R. M., Netticadan, T., Role of oxidative stress in cardiovascular diseases. *Journal of Hypertension* 2000, 18 (6).

[65] Jiao, Y., Wilkinson, J., Christine Pietsch, E., Buss, J. L., Wang, W., Planalp, R., Torti, F. M., Torti, S. V., Iron chelation in the biological activity of curcumin. *Free Radical Biology and Medicine* 2006, 40 (7), 1152-1160.

[66] Kawano, S. I., Inohana, Y., Hashi, Y., Lin, J. M., Analysis of keto-enol tautomers of curcumin by liquid chromatography/mass spectrometry. *Chinese Chemical Letters* 2013, 24 (8), 685-687.

[67] Hejazi, J., Rastmanesh, R., Taleban, F. A., Molana, S. H., Hejazi, E., Ehtejab, G., Hara, N., Effect of Curcumin Supplementation During Radiotherapy on Oxidative Status of Patients with Prostate Cancer: A Double Blinded, Randomized, Placebo-Controlled Study. *Nutrition and Cancer* 2016, 68 (1), 77-85.

[68] Phan, T. T., See, P., Lee, S. T., Chan, S. Y., Protective Effects of Curcumin against Oxidative Damage on Skin Cells *In Vitro:* Its Implication for Wound Healing. *Journal of Trauma and Acute Care Surgery* 2001, 51 (5).

[69] Cutler, S. E., Cutler, H. (Ed.), *Biologically Active Natural Products*. Boca Raton: CRC Press: 2000.

[70] Bachmeier, B. E., Nerlich, A. G., Iancu, C. M., Cilli, M., Vene, R., Dell; Eva, R., Jochum, M., Albini, A., Pfeffer, U., The chemopreventive polyphenol curcumin prevents hematogenous breast cancer metastases in immunodeficient mice. *Cancer Epidemiology Biomarkers & Prevention* 2006, 15 (12 Supplement), A67.

[71] Huang, M. T., Lou, Y. R., Ma, W., Newmark, H. L., Reuhl, K. R., Conney, A. H., Inhibitory Effects of Dietary Curcumin on Forestomach, Duodenal, and Colon Carcinogenesis in Mice. *Cancer Research* 1994, 54 (22), 5841.

[72] Rao, C. V., Rivenson, A., Simi, B., Reddy, B. S., Chemoprevention of Colon Carcinogenesis by Dietary Curcumin, a Naturally Occurring Plant Phenolic Compound. *Cancer Research* 1995, 55 (2), 259.

[73] Coleman, Stacey J., Bruce, C., Chioni, A. M., Kocher, Hemant M., Grose, Richard P., The ins and outs of fibroblast growth factor receptor signalling. *Clinical Science* 2014, 127 (4), 217-231.

[74] Ejaz, A., Wu, D., Kwan, P., Meydani, M., Curcumin Inhibits Adipogenesis in 3T3-L1 Adipocytes and Angiogenesis and Obesity in C57/BL Mice. *The Journal of Nutrition* 2009, 139 (5), 919-925.

[75] Shehzad, A., Wahid, F., Lee, Y. S., Curcumin in Cancer Chemoprevention: Molecular Targets, Pharmacokinetics, Bioavailability, and Clinical Trials. *Archiv der Pharmazie* 2010, 343 (9), 489-499.

[76] Hatcher, H., Planalp, R., Cho, J., Torti, F. M., Torti, S. V., Curcumin: From ancient medicine to current clinical trials. *Cellular and Molecular Life Sciences* 2008, 65 (11), 1631-1652.

[77] Hsu, C. H., Cheng, A. L., Clinical Studies With Curcumin. In *The Molecular Targets and Therapeutic Uses of Curcumin in Health and Disease*, Aggarwal, B. B., Surh, Y. J., Shishodia, S., Eds. Springer US: Boston, MA, 2007; pp 471-480.

[78] Hsieh, C. Y., Phase I clinical trial of curcumin, a chemopreventive agent, in patients with high-risk or pre-malignant lesions. *Anticancer Res* 2001, 21, 2895-2900.

[79] Mukhopadhyay, A., Basu, N., Ghatak, N., Gujral, P. K., Anti-inflammatory and irritant activities of curcumin analogues in rats. *Agents and Actions* 1982, 12 (4), 508-515.

[80] Anand, P., Kunnumakkara, A. B., Newman, R. A., Aggarwal, B. B., Bioavailability of Curcumin: Problems and Promises. *Molecular Pharmaceutics* 2007, 4 (6), 807-818.

[81] Prasad, S., Tyagi, A. K., Aggarwal, B. B., Recent developments in delivery, bioavailability, absorption and metabolism of curcumin: the golden pigment from golden spice. *Cancer research and treatment* 2014, 46 (1), 2-18.

[82] Wahlang, B., Pawar, Y. B., Bansal, A. K., Identification of permeability-related hurdles in oral delivery of curcumin using the Caco-2 cell model. *European Journal of Pharmaceutics and Biopharmaceutics* 2011, 77 (2), 275-282.

[83] Patra, D., El Khoury, E., Ahmadieh, D., Darwish, S., Tafech, R. M., Effect of Curcumin on Liposome: Curcumin as a Molecular Probe for Monitoring Interaction of Ionic Liquids with 1,2-Dipalmitoyl-sn-Glycero-3-Phosphocholine Liposome. *Photochemistry and Photobiology* 2012, 88 (2), 317-327.

[84] Yang, R., Zhang, S., Kong, D., Gao, X., Zhao, Y., Wang, Z., Biodegradable Polymer-Curcumin Conjugate Micelles Enhance the Loading and Delivery of Low-Potency Curcumin. *Pharmaceutical Research* 2012, 29 (12), 3512-3525.

[85] Zhao, Y. Z., Lu, C. T., Zhang, Y., Xiao, J., Zhao, Y. P., Tian, J. L., Xu, Y. Y., Feng, Z. G., Xu, C. Y., Selection of high efficient transdermal lipid vesicle for curcumin skin delivery. *International Journal of Pharmaceutics* 2013, 454 (1), 302-309.

[86] Shin, G. H., Li, J., Cho, J. H., Kim, J. T., Park, H. J., Enhancement of Curcumin Solubility by Phase Change from Crystalline to Amorphous in Cur-TPGS Nanosuspension. *Journal of food science* 2016, 81 (2), N494-501.

[87] Xu, D. H., Wang, S., Mei, X. T., Luo, X. T., Xu, S. B., [Studies on solubility enhancement of curcumin by Polyvinylpyrrolidione K30]. *Zhong Yao Cai* 2008, 31 (3), 438-442.

[88] Hernandez-Patlan, D., Solis-Cruz, B., Pontin, K. P., Latorre, J. D., Baxter, M. F. A., Hernandez-Velasco, X., Merino-Guzman, R., Méndez-Albores, A., Hargis, B. M., Lopez-Arellano, R., Tellez, G., Evaluation of a Solid Dispersion of Curcumin With Polyvinylpyrrolidone and Boric Acid Against Salmonella Enteritidis Infection and Intestinal Permeability in Broiler Chickens: A Pilot Study. *Frontiers in Microbiology* 2018, 9, 1289.

[89] Winter, S., Tortik, N., Kubin, A., Krammer, B., Plaetzer, K., Back to the roots: photodynamic inactivation of bacteria based on water-soluble curcumin bound to polyvinylpyrrolidone as a photosensitizer. *Photochemical & Photobiological Sciences* 2013, 12 (10), 1795-1802.

[90] Tu, Y. S., Fu, J. W., Sun, D. M., Zhang, J. J., Yao, N., Huang, D. E., Shi, Z. Q., Preparation, characterisation and evaluation of curcumin with piperine-loaded cubosome nanoparticles. *J Microencapsul* 2014, 31 (6), 551-559.

[91] Song, L., Shen, Y., Hou, J., Lei, L., Guo, S., Qian, C., Polymeric micelles for parenteral delivery of curcumin: Preparation, characterization and *in vitro* evaluation. *Colloids and Surfaces A: Physicochemical and Engineering Aspects* 2011, 390 (1), 25-32.

[92] Sarika, P. R., James, N. R., Kumar, P. R. A., Raj, D. K., Kumary, T. V., Gum arabic-curcumin conjugate micelles with enhanced loading for curcumin delivery to hepatocarcinoma cells. *Carbohydrate Polymers* 2015, 134, 167-174.

[93] Mourtas, S., Canovi, M., Zona, C., Aurilia, D., Niarakis, A., La Ferla, B., Salmona, M., Nicotra, F., Gobbi, M., Antimisiaris, S. G., Curcumin-decorated nanoliposomes with very high affinity for amyloid-β1-42 peptide. *Biomaterials* 2011, 32 (6), 1635-1645.

[94] Kumar, A., Kaur, G., Kansal, S. K., Chaudhary, G. R., Mehta, S. K., Enhanced solubilization of curcumin in mixed surfactant vesicles. *Food Chemistry* 2016, 199, 660-666.

[95] Her, C., M. C. V. J. A. E. R., Improvement of Curcumin Bioavailability for Medical Applications. *Medicinal & Aromatic Plants* 2018, 7 (6).

[96] Chen, H., Wu, J., Sun, M., Guo, C., Yu, A., Cao, F., Zhao, L., Tan, Q., Zhai, G., N-trimethyl chitosan chloride-coated liposomes for the oral delivery of curcumin. *Journal of Liposome Research* 2012, 22 (2), 100-109.

[97] Huang, M., Liang, C., Tan, C., Huang, S., Ying, R., Wang, Y., Wang, Z., Zhang, Y., Liposome co-encapsulation as a strategy for the delivery of curcumin and resveratrol. *Food & Function* 2019, 10 (10), 6447-6458.

[98] Ruttala, H. B., Ko, Y. T., Liposomal co-delivery of curcumin and albumin/ paclitaxel nanoparticle for enhanced synergistic antitumor efficacy. *Colloids and Surfaces B: Biointerfaces* 2015, 128, 419-426.

[99] Basnet, P., Hussain, H., Tho, I., Skalko-Basnet, N., Liposomal Delivery System Enhances Anti-Inflammatory Properties of Curcumin. *Journal of Pharmaceutical Sciences* 2012, 101 (2), 598-609.

[100] Dhule, S. S., Penfornis, P., Frazier, T., Walker, R., Feldman, J., Tan, G., He, J., Alb, A., John, V., Pochampally, R., Curcumin-loaded γ-cyclodextrin liposomal nanoparticles as delivery vehicles for osteosarcoma. *Nanomedicine: Nanotechnology, Biology and Medicine* 2012, 8 (4), 440-451.

Biographical Sketches

Gulmi Chakraborty

Affiliation: C. V. Raman Global University, Odisha

Education: PhD (Chemistry)

Business Address: Bidyanagar, Mahura, District- Khordha, Bhubaneshwar 752054

Research and Professional Experience:
6 years doctoral research, 3 years post-doctoral research, 1 year experience as Assistant Professor.

Professional Appointments:
Convener of Departmental research committee, undergraduate students' mentor, Post graduate course design and conduction of Environmental Chemistry, Examiner of semester examination.

Honors:

1. 2020, Indian Chemical Society Research Excellence Award for oral presentation entitled "Relevance of pi stacking in tuning the neighboring structural pattern of soft nanoaggregates" in International Webinar on

'Recent Advances in Chemistry and Material Sciences' held from 2nd-21st August 2020.

2. 2019, DST-SERB National Post-Doctoral Fellowship (N-PDF) by Science and Engineering Research Board, Government of India, (Award numberPDF/2018/001014), 2019.
3. 2015, Award for best scientific oral presentation in 22nd West Bengal Science and Technology Congress 2015, held at University of North Bengal during February 28-March 01, 2015.
4. 2014, Award for best scientific oral presentation in International Conference on "Emerging trends in Science and Technology" held at Biratnagar, Nepal during March 22-23, 2014.
5. 2013, UGC-Basic Science Research Awarded Fellowship for Meritorious students by University Grants Commission (UGC), New Delhi, India, 2013. (Award number: F.4-1/2006(BSR)/7-133/2007(BSR)), 2013.

Publications from the Last 3 Years:

1. Dipanjan Mukherjee, Gulmi Chakraborty, Md. Nur Hasan, Uttam Pal, Priya Singh, Tatini Rakshit, Reem I. Alsantali, Tanusri Saha Dasgupta, Saleh. A. Ahmed, Ranjan Das* and Samir Kumar Pal*, Reversible photoswitching of spiropyran in biomolecular interfaces: Acombined spectroscopy and computational study, *Journal of Photochemistry & Photobiology, A,* 2022, 430, 113958.
2. Gulmi Chakraborty, Ajaya Bhattarai,* and Ranjit De*. Polyelectrolyte–Dye Interactions: An Overview, *Polymers,* 2022, 14, 598.
3. Gulmi Chakraborty, Soumik Bardhan and Swapan K. Saha. Unfolding of tryptophanoctyl ester and elastic deformation of host micelles via RR′3N+…π interaction: Conceivable relevance to wrapping process of receptor mediated endocytosis, *Chem Phys Chem*, 2021, 22, 2535-2549.
4. Gulmi Chakraborty, Soumik Bardhan, Soumen Ghosh and Swapan K.Saha, Relevance of π-stacking in tuning the neighboring structural pattern of soft nano-aggregates. *J. Molecular Liquids.,* 2020, 317, 114013.
5. Bidyut Debnath, Gulmi Chakraborty, Solution properties and rheological behaviour of polyacrylamide in 1,4-dioxane + water mixed solvent media, *J. Macromolecular Sciences Part A*, 2020, 57, 628-635.

Soumen Ghosh

Affiliation: Jadavpur University

Education: PhD (Chemistry)

Business Address: Department of Chemistry, Physical Chemistry Section, Chemical Engineering Building, 1st Floor, Jadavpur University, Kolkata - 700032

Research and Professional Experience:

Prof. Ghosh was awarded his PhD in Colloidal Chemistry in 1999, from Jadavpur University. He has been associated with teaching in the same institute since 2001 till date.

He has guided 14 PhD scholars, 3 Postdoctoral scholars and 21 Postgraduate students. Till now, he published more than 100 papers, one book Chapter and two Proceedings in reputed national and international journals.

He teaches Thermodynamics, Electrochemistry, Chemical Kinetics, Photochemistry, Kinetic theory of Gas, Liquid, Solid, Adsorption and Colloid Chemistry to the undergraduate and postgraduate curriculum.

His broad area of research is surface and biophysical chemistry.

Professional Appointments:

2016 to Continuing Professor, Jadavpur University

Honors:

Awarded By	*Award name*	*Year*
Scientists by Stanford University, USA	Selected as top 2% World Ranking Scientist	2020
Chemical Research Society of India	Bronze Medal	2020
Indian Society for Surface Science and Technology	Editor of Journal of Surface Science and Technology	2015
American Chemical Society	American Chemical Society Membership Award	2015
StFX University, Canada	Chair Professor	2015
Research Excellence Program, USC - India (PEIN)	Selected for a short-term visit at University of Santiago de Compostela, Spain	2014
Indian Science Congress Association, Kolkata	Dr. B. C. Deb Memorial Award for Soil/Physical Chemistry of ISCA for the year 2013-2014	2014

Indian Chemical Society, Kolkata	Professor B. N. Ghosh 80th Birthday Commemoration Award for the year 2012	2013
American Scientific Publishers	Editorial Board Member of Journal of Nanofluids	2012
FCT, Portugal	Postdoctoral Fellowship (University of Porto, Portugal)	2008
Fast Track, Dept. of Science and Technology, Govt. of India	Young Scientist	2006
Dept. of Science and Technology, Govt. of India	BOYSCAST Fellowship (University of Hull, UK, 2004-2005)	2003
Dept. of Biotechnology, Govt. of India	Postdoctoral Fellowship (Bose Institute, Calcutta, 1999-2001)	1999

Publications from the Last 3 Years:

1. Arpan Mal, Ankita Saha, Gargi Dinda and Soumen Ghosh, Effect of carbohydrate based polymers on worm-like micelles of cetyltrimethylammonium p-toluenesulfonate in aqueous media: Detail physicochemical and antimicrobial properties survey, *J. Molecular Liquids* 299 (2020) 112153-112164.
2. Manas Barai, Manas Kumar Mandal, Habiba Sultana, Emili Manna, Sourav Das, Kaushik Nag, Soumen Ghosh, Anuttam Patra, and Amiya Kumar Panda, Theoretical approaches on the synergistic interaction between double-headed anionic amino acid-based surfactants and hexadecyltrimethylammonium bromide, *J. Surfactants and Detergents* 23 (2020) 891-902.
3. Ankita Saha, Arpan Mal and Soumen Ghosh, An elaborate investigation on the transition of rod-like micelle of cetyltrimethylammonium p-toluenesulfonate in presence of different additives, *J. Molecular Liquids* 309 (2020) 113084-113094.
4. Gulmi Chakraborty, Soumik Bardhan, Soumen Ghosh and Swapan K. Saha, Relevance of π -stacking in tuning the neighboring structural pattern of soft nano-aggregates, *J. Molecular Liquids* 317 (2020) 114013-114021.
5. Sourav Das, Nitai Patra, Arnab Banerjee, Bijan Das and Soumen Ghosh, Studies on the self-aggregation, interfacial and thermodynamic properties of a surface active imidazolium-based ionic liquid in aqueous solution: Effects of salt and temperature, *J. Molecular Liquids* 320 (2020) 114497-114512.
6. Satyajit Mondal and Soumen Ghosh, Spectroscopic study on the interaction of curcumin with single chain and gemini surfactants, *Chemical Physics Letters* 762 (2021) 138144-138150.

7. Arpan Mal, Soumen Ghosh, and Satya Priya Moulik, Time dependent physicochemical changes of SDS-CTAB interacted self-assembled vesicles: Ostwald ripening effect, *Colloids and Surfaces A: Physicochemical and Engineering Aspects* 617 (2021) 126328-126337.
8. Apensu Dey, Rajesh Banik and Soumen Ghosh, Temperature comparative studies on self-assembly of sodium dodecyl sulphate and didodecyl dimethyl ammonium bromide in aqueous, brine and trifluoroethanol media, *J. Surfactants and Detergents* 24 (2021) 459-472.
9. Sandip Paul, Pritam Roy, Sourav Das, Soumen Ghosh, Pinki Saha Sardar and Anjoy Majhi, Addressing the exigent role of a coumarin fluorophore toward finding the suitable microenvironment of biomimicking and biomolecular systems: steering to project the drug designing and drug delivery study, *ACS Omega* 6 (2021) 11878-11896.
10. Sonali Mondal, Partha Pyne, Animesh Patra, Rajib Kumar Mitra and Soumen Ghosh, "Effect of surfactant tail length on the hydroxypropyl cellulose-mediated premicellar aggregation of sodium *n*-alkyl sulfate surfactants, *Langmuir* 37 (2021) 6168-6177.
11. Nitai Patra, Arpan Mal, Sourav Das and Soumen Ghosh, Detailed physicochemical interaction of inulin with some conventional surfactants and surface active ionic liquid, *J. Molecular Liquids* 340 (2021) 116849-116857.
12. Sourav Das and Soumen Ghosh, A detailed assessment on the interaction of sodium alginate with a surface-active ionic liquid and a conventional surfactant: a multitechnique approach, *Physical Chemistry Chemical Physics* 24 (2022) 13738-13762.

Book Chapter

1. Chapter entitled "Advancement in Biosensors Based on Emerging Polymers" in the e-book series on materials entitled "Advances in Material Research and Technology" in the *Volume Advanced Polymers* edited by Shadia Jamil Ikhmayies, Springer Publisher (Accepted, 2022).

Index

D

E

F